Moodeen Sheriff

A Catalogue of Indian Synonymes of the Medicinal Plants, Products, Inorganic Substances

Salzwasser

Moodeen Sheriff

A Catalogue of Indian Synonymes of the Medicinal Plants, Products, Inorganic Substances

1. Auflage | ISBN: 978-3-84604-952-5

Erscheinungsort: Frankfurt, Deutschland

Erscheinungsjahr: 2020

Salzwasser Verlag GmbH

Reprint of the original, first published in 1869.

A
CATALOGUE OF INDIAN
SYNONYMES

OF THE MEDICINAL PLANTS, PRODUCTS, INORGANIC SUBSTANCES, &c., PROPOSED TO BE INCLUDED IN THE PHARMACOPŒIA OF INDIA

By

MOODEEN SHERIFF

CONTENTS.

PREFACE.

A few years since, I had an occasion to pay attention to the vernacular synonymes in some works on Materia Medica and Botany. While I was much impressed with the importance and usefulness of the subject, I found it blended with a great inaccuracy and confusion. I was about rectifying these defects in a work, when it was my privilege to be called upon officially to contribute to the Pharmacopœia of India, *vide* Circular Memorandum No. 2824, dated 7th August 1865, from the Secretary to the Principal Inspector General of the Medical Department, which was accompanied with the 'Proceedings of the Madras Government, Financial Department, 28th July 1865,' and Dr. E. J. Waring's lists of medicinal plants, &c.

On the receipt of these documents, I immediately thought of the subject I was previously meditating upon, and with a wish to see the Pharmacopœia as free as possible from the defects just alluded to, I prepared a Table of Vernacular Synonymes of the medicinal plants, drugs, &c., proposed to be included in that work. The Table was composed of 12 languages, besides the Latin and English ; viz., Arabic, Persian, Hindustani, Dukhni, Tamil, Telugu, Malyalim, Canarese, Bengali, Mahratti, Guzratti, and Burmese, and the synonymes in all these languages were expressed in their native characters as well as in English.

In preparing this Table, although I consulted a few works, yet, for the reason already mentioned, I thought it advisable .to depend chiefly upon the names found out by myself. With this view, I had personally examined with several native practitioners, druggists, &c., all the plants known as medicinal in many localities of Madras, eluding the Agri-horticultural Society's and other gardens, and ascertained their names without any reference to books. The drugs in the bazaar, together with several other plants which were sent for from distant places, were next examined, and their names found out in the same manner.

The Table was then forwarded, as a part of my contribution, to the Committee of the Pharmacopœia of India, on the 7th February 1866, and returned to me on the 9th July of the same year, with a copy of the following Despatches and Orders :—

' *Proceedings of the Madras Government, Financial Department,* *6th July* 1866.

No. 7. Read the following Despatch from the Right Honorable the Secretary of State for India, to His Excellency the Right Honorable the Governor in Council, Fort Saint George ; dated India Office, London, 31st May 1866, No. 43.

I forward herewith copies of correspondence with Surgeon E. J. Waring, M.D., with enclosures in original, and I have to request that the necessary measures may be taken by you for meeting, if practicable, the wishes of the Pharmacopœia of India Committee, in regard to the printing at Madras of Mr. Moodeen Sheriff's Table of Medicinal Plants, under that Officer's supervision.

Letters from Dr. Waring, dated the 26th April and 15th May 1866, with enclosures in originals.
Letter to Dr. Waring, dated the 4th May 1866.

From Surgeon E. J. Waring, M.D., Editor of the Pharmacopœia of India, to the Under Secretary of State for India, &c., &c., &c. ; dated 3A, Talbot Road, Bayswater, 26th April 1866.

By desire of the " Pharmacopœia of India" Committee, I have the honor herewith to transmit a Table compiled by Native Surgeon Moodeen Sheriff of Triplicane Dispensary, Madras, containing the names of upwards of four hundred Medicinal plants of India, in twelve Eastern languages, in Vernacular and English characters

A
CATALOGUE OF INDIAN SYNONYMES
OF THE MEDICINAL PLANTS, PRODUCTS,
INORGANIC SUBSTANCES, &c., PROPOSED TO BE
INCLUDED IN THE PHARMACOPŒIA
OF INDIA.

Affixes and Prefixes required in each language to designate plants or their parts and products, &c.

I. TREE, SHRUB, OR HERBACEOUS PLANT.—
Shajar شجر , *plur.* Ashjár اشجار ; Nabát نبات , *plur.*
Nabátát نباتات . *(Arab.)* Darakht درخت , *plur.*
Darakhtahá درختها or Darakhtán درختان . *(Pers.)* Pér
پیڑ , *plur.* Péréṅ پیڑین ; Búṭi بوٹی , *plur.* Buṭiyáṅ بوٹیان
(Hind.) Jhár جهاڑ , *plur.* Jháráṅ جهاڑان . *(Duk.)*
Maram மரம், *plur.* Marangal மரங்கள் ; Chedi செடி, *plur.*
Chedigal செடிகள். *(Tam.)* Mánu మాను, *plur.* Mánulu
మానులు ; Cheṭṭu చెట్టు, *plur.* Cheṭlu చెట్లు. *(Tel.)*
Maram മരം, *plur.* Marannal മരങ്ങള്‍; Cheṭi ചെടി, *plur.*
Cheṭikal ചെടികള്‍. *(Malyal.)* Mará ಮರ, *plur.* Maragalu
ಮರಗಳು; Giḍá ಗಿಡ, *plur.* Giḍa-galu ಗಿಡಗಳು. *(Can.)*
Gáchh ; Brikhya. *(Beng.)* Vrikshaha, *plur.* Vriksháha.
(Sans.) Jháḍa, *plur.* Jháḍi. *(Mah.)* Jháḍa, *plur.* Jháḍá.
(Guz.) Gahá, *plur.* Gas. *(Cing.)* Ṣippiṇ, *plur.* Ṣippiṇ-
miyáá ; Apiṇ, *plur.* Apiṇ-miyáá——or in combination,
Piṇ, *plur.* Piṇ-miyáá ; Biṇ, *plur.* Biṇ-miyáá. *(Bur.)*

II. CREEPER, TWINING OR CLIMBING PLANT.

Yaqṭin يقطين, *plur.* Yaqáṭín يقاطين. (*Arab.*) Biyárah
بيار, *plur.* Biyárahá بيارها. (*Pers.*) Bél بيل, *plur.* Béléṅ
بيلين; Latá لتا. (*Hind.*) Bél بيل, *plur.* Béláṅ بيلان
(*Duk.*) Koḍi கொடி, *plur.* Koḍigaḷ கொடிகள். (*Tam.*)
Tíge తీగ, *plur.* Tígelu తీగెలు. (*Tel.*) Valḷi വള്ളി, *plur.*
Vaḷḷikaḷ വള്ളികൾ. (*Malyal.*) Baḷḷi ಬಳ್ಳಿ, *plur.* Baḷḷigaḷu
ಬಳ್ಳಿಗಳ; Hambu ಹಂಬು, *plur.* Hambugaḷu ಹಂಬುಗಳ.
(*Can.*) Latá. (*Beng.*) Latú, *plur.* Latáha. (*Sans.*) Véla,
plur. Vélá. (*Mah.*) Vél, *plur.* Vélo. (*Guz.*) Vel. (*Cing.*)
Anóye, *plur.* Anóye-miyáú—or *in* combination, Nóye,
plur. Nóye-miyáú. (*Bur.*).

III. GRASS.—Tibn تبن, *plur.* Atbán اتبان; Hashísh

حشيش, *plur.* Hasháyash حشايش. (*Arab.*) Káh كاہ,
plur. Káhá كاها; Giyáh گياہ, *plur.* Giyáhá گياها. (*Pers.*)
Ghás گھاس, *plur.* Ghásén گھاسين. (*Hind.*) Ghans
گھنس, *plur.* Ghánsáṅ گھانسان. (*Duk.*) Pullu புல்லு,
plur. Pullugaḷ புல்லுகள். (*Tam.*) Gaḍḍi గడ్డి, *plur.* Gaḍḍilu
గడ్డిలు; Kasuvu కసువు, *plur.* Kasuvulu కసువులు. (*Tel.*)
Pullu പുല്ല്, *plur.* Pullukaḷ പുല്ലുകൾ. (*Malyal.*) Hullu
ಹುಲ್ಲು, *plur.* Hullugaḷu ಹುಲ್ಲುಗಳ. (*Can.*) Gháns; Khér.
(*Beng.*) Triṇam, *plur.* Triṇáni. (*Sans.*) Gavat. (*Mah.*)
Gháns. (*Guz.*) Tana or Tanakol. (*Cing.*) Miye, *plur.*
Miye-miyáú. (*Bur.*).

IV. FRUIT (*not including Pod or Legume*).—

Ṣamar ثمر, *plur.* Aṣmár اثمار. (*Arab.*) Bar بر, *plur.* Barhá
برها. (*Pers.*) Phal پھل. (*Hind.*) Panḍu پنڈو, *plur.*
Panḍuváṅ پنڈوان. (*Duk.*) Pazham பழம், *plur.* Pazhaṅgaḷ
பழங்கள். (*Tam.*) Panḍu పండు, *plur.* Pandlu పండ్లు. (*Tel.*)
Pazham പഴം, *plur.* Pazhaṅṅaḷ പഴങ്ങൾ; Káya കായ,

plur. Káyakal കായകൾ. (*Malyal.*) Haṇṇu ಹಣ್ಣು, *plur.*
Haṇṇugaḷu ಹಣ್ಣುಗಳು. (*Can.*) Phal. • (*Beng.*) *Phalam,*
plur. *Phálání* (*Sans.*) Panḍú ; *Phal, plur. Phalá.*
(*Mah.*) *Phal, plur. Phalá.* (*Guz.*) Gaḍi ; Ká or Káya.
(*Cing.*) Aṣi, *plur.* Aṣi-miyáá ; ati, *plur.* ati-miyáá.——*or in*
combination, Ṣi, *plur.* Ṣi-miyáá ; Ti, *plur.* Ti-miyáá. (*Bur.*).

V. POD OR LEGUME.—*Gẖiláful-quṭnít* غلاف القطنيت
Gẖiláfuṣṣamar غلا ف الثمر. (*Arab.*) Séngrí سٿينگري, *plur.*
Séngríyáň سٿينگريان ; Séngi سٿينگی, *plur.* Séngiyáň سٿينگريان.
(*Hind.*) Phallí پهلی, *plur.* Phalliyáň پهليان. (*Duk.*)
Káy காய், *plur.* Káygaḷ காய்கள். (*Tam.*) Káya కాయ
plur. Káyalu కాయలు. (*Tel.*) Káya കായ, *plur.* Káyakaḷ
കായകൾ. (*Malyal.*) Káyi ಕಾಯಿ, *plur.* Káyigaḷu ಕಾಯಿಗಳು.
(*Can.*) Sim ; Ṣhim ; Simbi. (*Beng.*) Sing, *plur.* Singo ;
Kái, *plur.* Káilá. (*Guz.*) Péḍoṇ, *plur.* Péḍoṇ-miyáá ; Aṣi,
plur. Aṣi-miyáá ;——*or in combination,* Ṣi, *plur.* Ṣi-
miyáá. (*Bur.*).

VI. SEEDS.—Bazr بزر or Baẕr بذر , *plur.* Buzúr
بزور or Buẕúr بذور ; Ḥab حب , *plur.* Ḥubúb حبوب .
(*Arab.*) Tukhm تخم, *plur.* Tukhmhá تخمها ; Dánah دانه,
plur. Dánahá دانها. (*Pers.*) Bíj بيج ; Bínj بينج ; Dánah دانه,
plur. Dáné دانے. (*Hind.*) Binj بينج, *plur.* Binjáň
بينجان. (*Duk.*) Virai விளை, *plur.* Viraigaḷ விளைகள்.
(*Tam.*) Vittu విత్తు, *plur.* Vittanamulu విత్తనములు or Vittulu
విత్తులు ; Ginja గింజ, *plur.* Ginjalu గింజలు. (*Tel.*) Vitta
വിത്ത, *plur.* Vittukaḷ വിത്തുകൾ ; Bijam ബീജം,
plur. Bijaṇṇaḷ ബീജങ്ങൾ. (*Malyal.*) Bijá ಬೀಜ, *plur.*
Bijagaḷu ಬೀಜಗಳು ; Káḷu ಕಾಳು, *plur.* Káḷugaḷu ಕಾಳುಗಳು.

(*Can.*) Bíj ; Bíchi. (*Beng.*) Bíjam, *plur.* Bíjáni. (*Sans.*) Bí, *plur.* Byá ; Bíj, *plur.* Bíjá. (*Mah.*) Bíj ; Bí. (*Guz.*) Aṭṭa ; Bíja. (*Cing.*) Asi, *plur.* Asi-miyáá——*or in combination,* Zi, *plur.* Zi-miyáá ; Si, *plur.* Si-miyáá. (*Bur.*)

VII. NUT.—Ḥab حب, *plur.* Ḥubúb حبوب. (*Arab.*) Khastah خسته, *plur.* Khastahá خستها ; Ustakhán استخوان, *plur.* Ustakhánhá استخوانها. (*Pers.*) Guṭhli كنّهلي *plur.* Guṭhliyán كنّهليان. (*Hind.*) Guṭlí كنّلي, *plur.* Guṭliyán كنّليان. (*Duk.*) Koṭṭai கொட்டை, *plur.* Koṭṭaigaḷ கொட்டைகள். (*Tam.*) Kuru கரு, *plur.* Kurukkaḷ கருக்கள்; Anṭi அண்டி, *plur.* Anṭikaḷ அண்டிகள். (*Malyal.*) Goṭṭi ಗೊಟ್ಟಿ, *plur.* Goṭṭigalu ಗೊಟ್ಟಿಗಳು; Váṭe ವಾಟೆ, *plur.* Váṭegalu ವಾಟೆಗಳು. (*Can.*) Anthóli, *plur.* Anthólá. (*Mah.*) Góṭli, *plur.* Gúṭliyo. (*Guz.*) Aṭṭa ; Koṭṭa. (*Cing.*) Asi, *plur.* Asi-miyáá—*or in combination,* Zi, *plur.* Zi-miyáá. (*Bur.*).

VIII. FLOWERS.—Vard ورد, *plur.* Varúd ورود. (*Arab.*) Gul گل, *plur.* Gulhá گلها. (*Pers.*) Phál پهول (*Hind.*) Phúl پهول, *plur.* Phúlán پهولان. (*Duk.*) Pú பூ, *plur.* Púkkaḷ பூக்கள். (*Tam.*) Puvvu పువ్వు or Pú పూ, *plur.* Puvvulu పువ్వులు or Púvulu పూవులు. (*Tel.*) Pushpam പുഷ്പം, *plur.* Pushpaṇṇaḷ പുഷ്പണ്ണള്; Pú പൂ, *plur.* Púkkaḷ പൂക്കള്. (*Malyal.*) Huvvu ಹುವ್ವು, *plur.* Huvvagaḷu ಹುವ್ವಗಳು. (*Can.*) Phúl. (*Beng.*) Pushpam, *plur.* Pushpáṇi. (*Sans.*) Phúla, *plur.* Phúlá. (*Mah.*) Phúl, *plur.* Phúlá. (*Guz.*) Mal. (*Cing.*) Pán, *plur.* Pán-miyáá ; Apóén, *plur.* Apóén-miyáá——*or in combination,* Póén, *plur.* Póén-miyáá. (*Bur.*).

IX. BUDS.—Zahr زهر, *plur.* Azhár ازهار. (*Arab.*) Ghunchah غنجه, *plur.* Ghunchahá غنجها. (*Pers.*) Kali كلي,

plur. Kaliyán كليان. (*Hind.*) Kalli كلي, *plur.* Kalliyán كليان.
(*Duk.*) Moggu மொக்கு, *plur.* Moggugaḷ மொக்குகள். (*Tam.*)
Mogga ముగ్గ, *plur.* Moggalu ముగ్గలు. (*Tel.*) Moṭṭa മൊട്ട,
plur. Moṭṭukaḷ മൊട്ടുകൾ. (*Malyal.*) Moggú ಮುಗ್ಗ, *plur.*
Moggugaḷu ಮುಗ್ಗಗಳ; Magge ಮಗ್ಗ; *plur.* Maggégaḷu ಮಗ್ಗೆಗ
ಳ. (*Can.*) Kali (*Beng.*) Mukulam, *plur.* Mukaláni. (*Sans.*)
Kali, *plur.* Kaḷé (*Mah.*) Kali, *plur.* Káḷiyo. (*Guz.*)
Moṭṭa. (*Cing.*) Áṇoun or Ang-oun, *plur.* Áṇoun-miyáá or
Ang-oun-miyáá. (*Bur.*).

X. LEAVES —Varaq ورق, *plur.* Ouráq اوراق. ا
(*Arab.*) Barg برگ, *plur.* Bargahá برگها. (*Pers.*) Pát پات;
Patti پتي, *plur.* Pattiyán پتيان. (*Hind.*) Pattá پتا,
plur. Patté پتے. (*Duk.*) Ilai இலை *plur.* Ilaigaḷ இலைகள்!
(*Tam.*) Áku ఆకు, *plur.* Ákulu ఆకులు. (*Tel.*) Ela, എല,
plur. Elakaḷ എലകൾ. (*Malyal.*) Yalé ಯಲೆ, *plur.*
Yalegaḷu ಯಲೆಗಳ. (*Can.*) Pátá. (*Beng.*) Patram, *plur.*
Patráni. (*Sans.*). Pána, *plur.* Páná. (*Mah.*) Pánḍru, *plur.*
Pánḍrá. (*Guz.*) Kola. (*Cing.*) Ayo-e, *plur.* Ayo-e-miyáá
——or in combination, Yo-e, *plur.* Yo-e-miyáá. (*Bur.*).

XI. BARK.—Qishr قشر, *plur.* Qushúr قشور. (*Arab.*)
Póst-e-draḵht پوست درخت, *plur.* Pósthúé-draḵht
پوستهائے درخت (*Pers.*) Chhál چھال, *plur.* Chháléñ.
چھالين (*Hind.*) Chhilká چھلكا, *plur.* Chhilké چھلكے
(*Duk.*) Paṭṭai பட்டை, *plur.* Paṭṭaigaḷ பட்டைகள். (*Tam.*)
Paṭṭa పట్ట, *plur.* Paṭṭalu పట్టలు. (*Tel.*) Tóla തോല, *plur.*
Tólukaḷ തോലുകൾ; Toli തോലി; *plur.* Tolikal തോലി
കൾ. (*Malyal.*) Paṭṭe ಪಟ್ಟೆ, *plur.* Paṭṭegaḷu ಪಟ್ಟೆಗಳ.
(*Can.*) Sál or Chhál; Bákal. (*Beng.*) Valkalam, *plur.* Val-
kaláni; Tvakam, *plur.* Tvakáni. (*Sans.*) Paṭṭa, *plur.* Paṭṭe.
(*Mah.*) Chál, *plur.* Chálo; Chilṭu, *plur.* Chilṭá. (*Guz.*)

Pottà. *(Cing.)* Akhàv *or* Khàv, *plur.* Akhàv-miyáá *or* Kkàv-miyáá; Ṣikhàv *or* Ṭikhàv, *plur.* Ṣikhàv-miyáá *or* Ṭikhàv-miyáá. *(Bur.).*

XII. ROOT OR RHIZOME—Aṣl اصل , *plur.* Uṣúl اصول۰ *(Arab.)* Bikh بيخ , *plur.* Bíkhhá بيخها. *(Pers.)* Jar جر, *plur.* Jaréň جڑين *(Hind.)* Jar جڑ, *plur.* Jaṛáň جڑان. *(Duk.)* Vér வேர், *plur.* Vérgaḷ வேர்கள். *(Tam.)* Véru, వేరు, *plur.* Vérulu వేరులు. *(Tel.)* Véra വേര, *plur.* Vérukaḷ, വേരുകൾ; Múlam മൂലം, *plur.* Múlaṇṇaḷ മൂലങ്ങൾ. *(Malyal.)* Béru ಬೇರು, *plur.* Bérugalu ಬೇರುಗಳು. *(Can.)* Ṣhikar; Jar; Múl; Hiṅar. *(Beng.)* Múlam, *plur.* Múláni. *(Sans.)* Muḷï, *plur.* Muḷé. *(Mah.)* Jaḍ, *plur.* Jaḍo. *(Guz.)* Múl. *(Cing.)* Amie, *plur.* Amie-miyáá; Anú, *plur.* Anú miyáá,—*or in combination,* Mi, *plur.* Mi miyáá. *(Bur.).*

XIII. BULB OR TUBER.—Aṣlussiṭabr اصل السطبر, *plur.* Uṣúlussiṭabr اصول السطبر; Aṣlul-mudavvar اصل المدور, *plur.* Uṣúlul-mudavvar اصول المدور. *(Arab.)* Bikhe-mudavvar بيخ مدور, *plur.* Bíkhháé-muddavar بيخهاے مدور. *(Pers.)* Kand كند. *(Hind.)* Gaḍḍah گڈه, *plur.* Gaḍḍé گڈے. *(Duk.)* Kizhaṇgu கிழங்கு, *plur.* Kizhaṇgugaḷ கிழங்குகள். *(Tam.)* Gaḍḍa గడ్డ, *plur.* Gaḍḍalu గడ్డలు. *(Tel.)* Kizhaṇṇa കിഴങ്ങ, *plur.* Kizhaṇṇukaḷ കിഴങ്ങുകൾ. *(Malyal.)* Gaḍḍe ಗಡ್ಡೆ, *plur.* Gaḍḍegaḷu ಗಡ್ಡೆಗಳು. *(Can.)* Gól-múl *(Beng.)* Kandaha, *plur.* Kandáha *(Sans.)* Gaḍḍá, *plur.* Gaḍḍé *(Mah.)* Kan; Gaḍḍá, *plur.* Gaḍḍo. *(Guz.)* Ala. *(Cing.)* Aú. *or* U, *plur.* Aúmiyáá *or* U-miyáá. *(Bur.).*

XIV. WOOD.—Khashab خشب. *(Arab.)* Chób چوب, *plur.* Chóbhá چوبها. *(Pers.)* Lakṛi لكڑى, *plur.* Lakṛiyáň لكڑيان. *(Hind. and Duk.)* Kaṭṭai கட்டை, *plur.* Kaṭṭaigaḷ

கட்டைகள்; *Chakkai* சக்கை, *plur. Chakkaigal* சக்கைகள். *(Tam.)* Katta கட்ட, *plur.* Kattalu கட்டலு; Chekka சెக்க, *plur.* Chekkalu செக்கலு. *(Tel.)* Mutti ஓடி, *plur.* Muttikal ஓடிகள்; Tati தடி, *plur.* Tatikal தடிகள். *(Malyal.)* Kattige கட்டிಗೆ, *plur.* Kattigegalu கட்டிಗೆಗಳು. *(Can.)* Káth: Káshtha. *(Beng.)* Káshtam, *plur.* Káshtáni. *(Sans.)* Lákada, *plur.* Lákadé. *(Mah.)* Lákdu, *plur.* Lákdá *(Guz.)* Thén, *plur.* Thén-miyáá; Sissa. *plur.* Sissa-miyáá. *(Bur.).*

XV. GUM OR RESIN.—Samagh صمغ, *plur.* Sumúgh صموغ; Aalak علك, *plur.* Aulúk علوك. *(Arab.)* Kouj كوج, *plur.* Koujhá كوجها; Samagh صمغ, *plur.* Samaghhá صمغها. *(Pers.)* Gónd گوند, *plur.* Góndén گوندين. *(Hind.)* Gónd گوند, *plur.* Góndán گوندان. *(Duk.)* Pishin பிசின், *plur.* Pishingal பிசின்கள். *(Tam.)* Pisunu పిసును; Banka బంక. *(Tel.)* Pasha പശ, *plur.* Pashakal പശകൾ. *(Malyal.)* Góndu ಗೊಂದು, *plur.* Góndagalu ಗೊಂದಗಳು; Antu ಅಂಟು, *plur.* Antagalu ಅಂಟಗಳು. *(Can.)* Gun; Lásá. *(Beng.)* Niryásam, *plur.* Niryásáni. *(Sans.)* Gónda, *plur.* Góndá; Dink. *(Mah.)* Gún; Gúndar. *(Guz.)* Melliyam. *(Cing.)* Así, *plur.* Así-miyáá; —— *or in combination,* Sí, *plur.* Sí-miyáá. *(Bur.).*

XVI. OIL.—Dohan دهن, *plur.* Adhán ادهان—— *Essential oil,* Aitr عطر. *(Arab.)* Róghan روغن, *plur* Róghanhá روغنها——*Essential oil,* Aitr عطر. *(Pers.)* Tél تيل, —— *Essential oil,* Aitr عطر *or* Atar عطر. *(Hind. and Duk.)* Enney எண்ணெய், *plur.* Enneygal எண்ணெய்கள் —— *Essential oil,* Tailam தைலம். *(Tam.)* Núne నూనె, —— *Essential oil,* Tailamu తైలము. *(Tel.)* Enna എണ്ണ, *plur.* Ennakal എണ്ണകൾ —— *Essential oil,* Tailam തൈലം, *plur.* Tailangal തൈലങ്ങൾ. *(Malyal.)* Yanne

ಯಣ್ಣೆ, *plur.* Yaṇṇegalu ಯಣ್ಣೆಗಳು; *Dhrati* ಧೃತಿ, *plur.* Dhrati-galu ಧೃತಿಗಳು. *(Can.)* Tail; Tél. *(Beng.)* Tailam, *plur.* Tailáni. *(Sans.)* Téla. *(Mah.)* Tél. *(Guz.)* Tel. *(Cing.)* Ṣi, *plur.* Ṣi-miyáá. *(Bur.)*.

XVII. SPIRIT.—Ḳhamar خمر, *plur.* Ḳhumúr خمور; Sharáb شراب, *plur.* Sharábát شرابات. *(Arab.)* Mai مي, *plur.* Maihá ميها; Sharáb شراب, *plur.* Sharábhá شرابها. *(Pers.)* Sharáb شراب, *plur.* Sharábéṅ شرابين. *(Hind.)* Dárú دارو, *plur.* Dárúváṅ داروان. *(Duk.)* Ṣháṛáyam சாரூயம், *plur.* Ṣháṛáyangal சாரூயங்கள். *(Tam.)* Sáráyi సారాయి. *(Tel.)* Cháráyam ചാരായം, *plur.* Cháráyannal ചാരായങ്ങൾ; Tákaram താകരം, *plur.* Tákarannal താക രങ്ങൾ. *(Malyal.)* Sáráyi ಸಾರಾಯಿ *plur.* Sáráyigalu ಸಾರಾಯಿಗಳು. *(Can.)* Mad; Suráp. *(Beng.)* Madyam. *(Sans.)* Dáru. *(Mah.)* Dáru. *(Guz.)* Arak *or* Araku. *(Cing.)* Aye, *plur.* Aye-miyáái. *(Bur.)*.

XVIII. MILKY JUICE.—Laban لبن, *plur.* Albán البان. *(Arab.)* Shír شير, *plur.* Shírhá شيرها. *(Pers.)* Dúdh دوده. *(Hind. and Duk.)* Pál பால், *plur.* Pálgal பால்கள். *(Tam.)* Pálu పాలు. *(Tel.)* Pál പാൽ, *plur.* Pálkal പാലകൾ; Kshíram ക്ഷീരം, *plur.* Kshírannal. ക്ഷീരങ്ങൾ. *(Mal-yal.)* Hálú ಹಾಲು, *plur.* Hálugalu ಹಾಲುಗಳು. *(Can.)* Khír; Dúdh. *(Beng.)* Kshíram, *plur.* Kshíráni. *(Sans.)* Dúda. *(Mah.)* Dúdh. *(Guz.)* Kiri. *(Cing.)*· No. *(Bur.)*.

XIX. WHITE.—Abyaẓ ابيض. *(Arab.)* Supéd سپيد. *(Pers.)* Suféd سفيد. *(Hind.)* Ujlá اجلا, *or* Ujlí اجلي. *(Duk.)* Vellai வெள்ளை; Venmai வெண்மை. *(Tam.)* Tella తెల్ల. *(Tel.)* Ven വെൺ; Vel വെൾ; Vella വെള്ള. *(Malyal.)* Bili ಬಿಳಿ. *(Can.)* Dhóp; Sádá. *(Beng.)* Shvéta;

Dh-oulam. *(Sans.)* Pándhara. *(Mah.)* Ujlo; *Dhólo;*
Saphéd. *(Guz.)* Sudu. *(Cing.)* Aphiyu *or Phiú. (Bur.).*

XX. BLACK.—Asvad اسود. *(Arab.)* Siyáh سياه.
(Pers.) Kálá كالا *or* Káli كالى. *(Hind. and Duk.)* Karuppu
கருப்பு; Karu கரு. *(Tam.)* Nalla నల్ల. *(Tel.)* Kaṛa కఠ;
Kaṛuppa കറുപ്പ. *(Malyal.)* Kappu ಕಪ್ಪು; Kari ಕರಿ. *(Can.)*
Kálá; Kál. *(Beng.)* Krishṭṇa; Kála. *(Sans.)* Kála.
(Mah.) Kálo. *(Guz.)* Kalu. *(Cing.)* Amé, Ané, *or*
Né. *(Bur.).*

XXI. RED.—Aḥmar احمر. *(Arab.)* Surkh سرخ. *(Pers.)*
Lál لال. *(Hind. and Duk.)* Ṣhivappu சிவப்பு. *(Tam.)*
Erra ఎఱ. *(Tel.)* Chem ചെം; Chovanna ചൊവന്ന.
(Malyal.) Kempu ಕೆಂಪು. *(Can.)* Rakto; Lál. *(Beng.)*
Lóhita; Rakta. *(Sans.)* Támbaḍa. *(Mah.)* Lál. *(Guz.)*
Rat *or* Rata. *(Cing.)* Ani *or* Ni. *(Bur.).*

XXII. YELLOW.—Aṣfar اصفر. *(Arab.)* Zard زرد. *(Pers.)*
Pílá پيلا *or* Píli پيلي. *(Hind. and Duk.)* Maṇjá மஞ்சா.
(Tam.) Pasupu పసుపు. *(Tel.)* Maṇṇa മഞ്ഞ. *(Malyal.)*
Haḷadi ಹಳದಿ. *(Can.)* Haldiá; Jard. *(Beng.)* Píta.
(Sans.) Pívaḷa. *(Mah.)* Píḷu. *(Guz.)* Kahá *or* Kahápáṭa.
(Cing.) Avá *or* Vá. *(Bur.).*

XXIII. GREEN.—Akhẓar اخضر. *(Arab.)* Sabz سبز.
(Pers.) Hará هرا *or* Harí هري. *(Hind. and Duk.)* Pach-ch-ai
பச்சை. *(Tam.)* Pach-cha పచ్చ. *(Tel.)* Pach-cha പച്ച.
(Malyal.) Hasaru ಹಸರು. *(Can.)* Hará; Sabujh. *(Beng.)*
Harita. *(Sans.)* Hirva. *(Mah.)* Sabaz; Haru. *(Guz.)*
Pach-cha; Kola-páṭa. *(Cing.)* Asaiṅ, Saiṅsi *or* Sénzi.
(Bur.)

XXIV. BLUE OR PURPLE.—Azraq ازرق; **Arzaq** ارزق. *(Arab.)* **Nilgún** نیلگون; **Kabúdi** کبودي. *(Pers.)* **Nilá** نیلا *or* **Nili** نیلي; **Udá** اودا *or* **Udi** اودي. *(Hind. and Duk.)* **Nila** நீல. *(Tam.)* **Nila** నీల. *(Tel.)* **Nila** നീല. *(Malyal.)* **Nili** ನೀಲಿ. *(Can.)* **Nilá.** *(Beng.)* **Nila; Shámalá.** *(Sans.)* **Nila; Vúdá** *(Mah.)* **Udu.** *(Guz.)* **Nil** *or* **Nilpáta.** *(Cing.)* **Piyá** *or* **Biya.** *(Bur.).*

XXV. SWEET.—Haló حلو. *(Arab.)* **Shírin** شیرین. *(Pers.)* **Mithá** میٹھا *or* **Mithí** میٹھي. *(Hind.)* **Mitthá** مٹھا *or* **Mitthí** مٹھي. *(Duk.)* **Tittippu** தித்திப்பு; **Inippu** இனிப்பு. *(Tam.)* **Tiyyani** తియ్యని. *(Tel.)* **Madhura** മധുര. *(Malyal.)* **Shiyáda** ಶಿಯಾದ. *(Can.)* **Mishtá; Míthá.** *(Beng.)* **Madhuryá.** *(Sans.)* **Gulachita.** *(Mah.)* **Mithu; Galu.** *(Guz.)* **Peni.** *(Cing.)* **Akhiyu** *or* **Khiyu.** *(Bur.).*

XXVI. SOUR—Hámiz حامض. *(Arab.)* **Tursh** ترش. *(Pers.)* **Khattá** کھٹا *or* **Khatti** کھٹي. *(Hind. and Duk.)* **Pulippu** புளிப்பு. *(Tam.)* **Pulla** పుల్ల. *(Tel.)* **Puli** പുളി. *(Malyal.)* **Huli** ಹುಳಿ. *(Can.)* **Amlá; Khatá.** *(Beng.)* **Ámlá.** *(Sans.)* **Ambata.** *(Mah.)* **Khátu.** *(Guz.)* **Ambul.** *(Cing.)* **Akhin** *or* **Akhing** *(Bur.).*

XXVII. BITTER.—Murr مُر. *(Arab.)* **Talkh** تلخ. *(Pers.)* **Karvá** کروا *or* **Karvi** کروي. *(Hind. and Duk.)* **Kashappu** கசப்பு. *(Tam.)* **Chédu** చేదు. *(Tel.)* **Kaipa** കൈപ. *(Malyal.)* **Tikta** ತಿಕ್ತ. *(Can.)* **Tito; Títá.** *(Beng.)* **Tikta.** *(Sans.)* **Kadú.** *(Mah.)* **Kadavu; Kadu.** *(Guz.)* **Titta.** *(Cing.)* **Khága** *or* **Akhá.** *(Bur.).*

XXVIII. GREATER OR LARGER.—Kabír کبیر; **Kubár** کبار. *(Arab.)* **Kalán** کلان; **Buzarg** بزرگ. *(Pers.)* **Bará** بڑا *or* **Bari** بڑي. *(Hind. and Duk.)* **Periya** பெரிய;

Peru பெரு; Perin பெரின். *(Tam.)* Pedda పెద్ద. *(Tel.)* Valiya
വലിയ. *(Malyal.)* Doḍḍá ದೊಡ್ಡ. *(Can.)* Baṛa; Mahá.
(Beng) Mahá; Brahata. *(Sans.)* Thóra. *(Mah.)* Móṭu.
(Guz.) Lokka; Mahá. *(Cing.)* Kiġi, Aki, Agi *or* Gi.
(Bur.):

XXIX. LESSER OR SMALLER.—Ṣigḥár صغار; Ṣagḥir
صغير. *(Arab.)* Ḳhurd خرد; Kóchak كوچك. *(Pers.)* Chhóṭá
چهوٹا *or* Chhóṭi چهوٹي. *(Hind. and Duk.)* Ṣhiṛiya சிறிய;
Ṣhiṛu சிறு. *(Tam.)* Sanna సన్న; Chinna చిన్న. *(Tel.)*
Cheṛiya ചെറിയ. *(Malyal.)* Chikka ಚಿಕ್ಕ; Saṇṇa ಸಣ್ಣ;
Puṭṭá ಪುಟ್ಟ. *(Can.)* Chhóṭa. *(Beng.)* Lahana. *(Mah.)*
Nánu. *(Guz.)* Punji *or* Punchi. *(Cing.)* Aṇéṇ *or*
Angéṅ. *(Bur.)*.

XXX. GREEN OR FRESH.—Raṭb رطب *or* Raṭab
رطب. *(Arab.)* Tar تر. *(Pers.)* Kach-chá كچا *or* Kach-chi
كچي. *(Hind. and Duk.)* Pach-ch-ai பச்சை. *(Tam.)*
Paçh-çhani పచ్చని *or* Pach-chi పచ్చి. *(Tel.)* Pach-cha പച്ച.
(Malyal.) Hasaru ಹಸರು; Haṣhi ಹಸಿ. *(Can.)* Káchá.
(Beng.) Karitá *(Savs.)* Hirva. *(Mah.)* Káchu. *(Guz.)*
Pach-chá; Amu *or* Ammu. *(Cing.)* Asiṅ, Siṅ *or* Ziṅ.
(Bur.).

XXXI. DRY OR DRIED.—Yábis ياس. *(Arab.)*
Ḳhushk خشك. *(Pers.)* Súkhá سوكها *or* Súkhi سوكهي.
(Hind.) Súká سوكا *or* Súki سوكي; Sukká سكا *or* Sukkí
سكي. *(Duk.)* Ularnda உலர்ந்த. *(Tam.)* Enḍu ఎండు.
(Tel.) Uṇaṇṇiya ഉണങ്ങിയ. *(Malyal.)* Vaṇa ವಣ.
(Can.) Suká. *(Beng.)* Ṣhushkám, Plur. Ṣhushkáni. *(Sans.)*
Válaṭṭe. *(Mah.)* Sùku. *(Guz.)* Veḷicha *or* Vellich-cha.
(Cing.) Akhiyáv, Ḳháyáv *or* Khiáv. *(Bur.)*.

XXXII. WILD.—Barrí بري ; Ṣaḥrái صحرائي. *(Arab.)* Dashtí دشتي. *(Pers.)* Janglí. جنگلي. *(Hind. and Duk.)* Káṭṭu சாட்டு. *(Tam.)* Adavi అడవి. *(Tel.)* Káṭṭa കാട്ട *(Malyal.)* Káḍu ಕಾಡು; Aḍavi ಅಡವಿ. *(Can.)* Ban; Banér; Janglér; Jangli. *(Beng.)* Aṭaví. *(Sans.)* Rána. *(Mah.)* Jangli. *(Guz.)* Val. *(Cing.)* To. *(Bur.)*.

XXXIII. HILL OR MOUNTAIN. *(Adjective)*.— Jablí جبلي. *(Arab.)* Kohí کوهی. *(Pers.)* Pahári پهاڑی. *(Hind. and Duk.)* Malai மலை. *(Tam.)* Konḍa కొండ. *(Tel.)* Malan മലൻ; Malam മലം. *(Malyal.)* Parvatadá ಪರ್ವತ್ತ.ದಾ; Beṭṭadá ಬೆಟ್ಟದಾ. *(Can.)* Pahárér; Parbbatér. *(Beng.)* Parvatá. *(Sans.)* Ḍóngarácha. *(Mah.)* Pahaḍni. *(Guz.)* Konḍa; Kandu. *(Cing.)* Távún. *(Bur.)*.

XXXIV. EUROPE OR FOREIGN.—Viláyati ولايتي. *(Hind. and Duk.)* Ṣhímai சீமை. *(Tam.)* Ṣhíma శీమ or Síma సీమ. *(Tel.)* Ṣhíma ശീമ. *(Malyal.)* Ṣhíme ಶೀಮೆ or Síme ಸೀಮೆ. *(Can.)* Biláti. *(Beng.)* Viláyati. *(Mah.)* Viláti. *(Guz.)* Raṭa. *(Cing.)* Ṣimbo *or* Ṭimbo. *(Bur.)*.

XXXV. INDIAN OR COUNTRY.—Hindí هندي. *(Arab. Pers. and Hind.)* Náṭ ناٹ. *(Duk.)* Náṭṭu சாட்டு. *(Tam.)* Náṭṭu నాట్టు. *(Tel.)* Náṭṭu നാട്ടു. *(Malyal.)* Náṭ ನಾಟ್. *(Can.)* Banglá. *(Beng.)* Déṣha. *(Sans.)* Mul-kácha. *(Mah.)* Gámni. *(Guz.)* Kala. *(Bur.)*.

A.

1. ABELMOSCHUS ESCULENTUS, *W. et A. (Capsules of)*.

Bámiyá باميا . *(Arab.)* Bámiyah باميه . *(Pers.)* Bhindí ; بهندّ ي Rám-turí رام ترئى *or* Rám-turái رام ترائي . *(Hind.)* Bhéndí بهيندّ ى . *(Duk.)* Veṇḍaik-káy வெண்டைக்காய். *(Tam.)* Benḍa-káya బెండకాయ. *(Tel.)* Veṇṭak-káya വെണ്ടക്കായ. *(Malyal.)* Bendé-káyi ಬೆಂಡೇಕಾಯಿ. *(Can.)* Dhéras *or* Dhéṅras; Rám-torai. *(Beng.)* Dárviká. *(Sans.)* Bhéṇḍá. *(Mah.)* Bhindu. *(Guz.)* Banḍa-ká. *(Cing.)* Youṅ-padi-ṣi *or* Youṅ-padi-ti. *(Bur.)*

The Hindustani and Bengali synonymes *Rám-turí* and *Rám-torai* are also occasionally applied to the fruit of *Luffa acutangula* and *L. pentandra*, but they are correctly applicable only to the capsule of *A. esculentus*. The names of the two former are as follows :—

L. acutangula, *Roxb.* Turí or *Turái*. *(Hind.)* Torai and Jhiṅgá. *(Beng.)*.

L. pentandra, *Roxb.* Ghí-turí or Ghí-turái. *(Hind.)* Ghirta-torai, Ghirta-jhiṅgá, Porul, and Dhundul. *(Beng.)*

2. ABELMOSCHUS MOSCHATUS, *Mœn. (Seeds of)*.

Habbul-mishk حب المشك *or* Habbul-mushk حب المشك . *(Arab.)* Mushk-dánah مشك دانه . *(Pers. and Hind.)* Mushk-bhéndí-ké-binj مشك بهيندّ ي كے بيذج . *(Duk.)* Kastúri-veṇḍaik-káy-virui கஸ்தூரி வெண்டைக்காய்விரை

விளா ; Káṭṭuk-kaśtúri காட்டுக்கஸ்தூரி. (*Tam.*) Kastúri-benda-vittulu కట్టుంబెండ విత్తులు. (*Tel.*) Káṭṭu-kastúri കാട്ടു കസ്തൂരി ; Kastúri-venṭa-vitta കസ്തൂരി വെണ്ട വിത്ത. (*Malyal.*) Mushak-dána. (*Beng.*) Mushak-dáná. (*Guz.*).

Though this plant is occasionally met with in the gardens and fields, and can be very easily cultivated, its seeds are not sold in the bozsars of Santhern India. But what is some times known as *Mushk-dánah* in the bazaars of Madras are the seeds of *Psorglia corylifolia*, which are deceitfully sold under that name by some native druggists who take advantage of their knowledge of both being of the same size, having an aromatic smell, and bearing some resemblance to each other in their appearance. Although the seeds of the variety of *A. moschatus* found in Madras, &c., are of the same size and color as the seeds of *P. corylifolia*, they can be readily distinguished as follows :—

Seeds of A. moschatus.	*Seeds of P. corylifolia.*
1. Kidney shaped, slightly compressed, striated or marked with minute parallel elevated lines of the same color, and present a small but very distinct *hilum* in the concave border.	1. Oval or oblong, and flat.
2. Brown in color, and about two lines in length.	2. Brown or dark brown in color, and about two or two and a half lines in length.
3. Smell like that of the *pure* musk, though very faint, not being distinctly perceptible unless the seeds are put in the mouth and chewed or rubbed between the fingers.	3. Smell aromatic, but musty or unctuous.
4. Taste not bitter.	4. Taste slightly bitterish.

The *Mushk-dánah* of Calcutta; which is one of the few medicines I have not as yet obtained, is said to be much larger (the size of a hemp seed) with a very distinct smell of musk, and will not therefore be easily confounded with the seeds of *P. cory-lifolio* or any other seed.* The seeds of *P. corylifolia* are commonly sold in almost all the large bazaars of India, and their native names will be found in the Catalogue under their proper head.

The names in the text are those that are generally known to the native practitioners, druggists, and others who are acquainted with the nature of the seeds of *A. moschatus;* but the plant is often recognised at Madras by the Tamil names 'Shi-mai-veṇḍaikkáy' (*Europe or Foreign Abelmoschus*) and 'Káṭṭu-veṇḍaikkáy' (*Wild Abelmoschus*), by those that are not acquainted with them. The former name is applied to the plant when it is found in the gardens, and the latter when it is m. t with in the fields.

In many works, including the Materia Indica and Hortus Suburbanus Calcuttensis, &c., 'Kala-kustooree' or 'Kalee-kustoorie' and 'Kal-kusturee' are given as the Hindustani, Bengali, and Dukhni synonyms of the plant; but they are neither correct nor recognisable. Their meaning is *black musk*, but as the musk is black itself, it is not probable that such a name is applied to any plant or seed for the sake of distinction.

The Tamil names found in Rottler and Winslow's Dictionaries, are very incorrect. They are *Poṭṭagat-tutti, Iraṭṭagat-tutti, Vayaṭ-rutti,* and *Vaṭṭat-tutti,* and are applied to *A. moschatus,* under the name of '*Hibiscus abelmoschus, L,*' which is one of its synonyms. From the word '*tutti*' they are likely the names of some species of *Sida* or *Abutilon.*

The Telugu name '*Karpúra-benḍu*' is appiied to the plant in Flora Andhrica, which means *the camphor Abelmoschus.* Whether this name is in use in any place or not, it is not correctly applicable to the plant, since it has no smell of camphor whatever.

Like almost all the plants in Rheed's Hortus Malabaricus, there is also a name assigned to *A. moschatus,* under the head of 'Arab.' (Vol. II. Tab. 38) which will induce the reader to

* I received a specimen of *Mushk-dánah* from Hyderabad just as this part of the Catalogue was passing through the press. There is no difference whatever between these seeds and the seeds of *A. moschatus* at Madras.

think that it is an Arabic name.   In reality there is not a single
Arabic, Persian, or Hindustani name in the whole work, and
what is found under the above head is an attempt to express the
Malyalim names in Arabic or Persian character, which is
generally either very imperfect or incorrect.

The literal meaning of 'ba-lu-wa', the Burmese name found
in Mason's Natural Productions of Burmah, is *a demon's bamboo,*
and therefore it appears to be more applicable to a species of
Bamboo than to the *A. moschatus.*   The same name with a slight
alteration is found in Judson's Burmese Dictionary, page 238,
viz., *ba-lu-leva,* and is applied to the '*musk plant.*'   Whether
this *musk plant* is the *musk-mallow* (*A. moschatus*) or some other
plant, is very doubtful; because the name is generally considered
to be applicable to a plant whose leaves are very *thick* and *broad*;
hence its meaning, *the demon's palm.*

3. ABRUS PRECATORIUS,   *Linn. (Country Liq-uorice bush—Seed of.)*

Aainuddék   عين الديك.   (*Arab.*)   Chashme-ḳhurós
چشم خروس; Surḵh سرخ. (*Pers.*) Ghungchí گهنگچی; Gunj
گنج. (*Hind.*) Gumchí گمچی.(*Duk.*) Gundu-maṇi குண்டுமணி;
Kunṛi-maṇi குன்றிமணி} (*Tam.*)Guri-ginja గురిగింజ;Guru-venda
గురువెంద. (*Tel.*) Kunni-kuru കുന്നിക്കുരു. (*Malyal.*)Gul-ganji
గుల్గంజి. (*Can.*) Kúṅch; Kúṅch-gúlà; Gunj. (*Beng.*)
Káka-chínchi-bíjam; Gunja.   (*Sans.*)   Gunza.   (*Mah.*)
Gumchi; Chano-kaḍi.   (*Guz.*)   Olinda *or* Olinda-aṭṭa.
(*Cing.*)   Yove-si *or* Yu-e-si. (*Bur.*).

Five varieties of this plant are found in the vicinity of
Madras, and I believe this to be the case all over India.   They
are named in all the languages included in the Catalogue according to the color of their seeds. viz.. *red. white, black, yellow,* and
blue or *purple.* The red is the most common variety, and is
generally known by the names inserted in the text without the
distinction of color.

The seeds are named *Aainuddék* and Chashme-ḳhurós in
Arabic and Persian in allusion to their resemblance to a cock's

eye, and the names are restricted to them all over India, except in Bombay and a few other places, where they are also applied to the seeds of *Adenanthera pavonina*, for a similar reason.

In many works (Flora Andhrica, Brown's Telugu Dictionary, Bailey's Malyalim Dictionary, Garret's Canarese Dictionary, Reeves' 'Carnatica' Dictionary, &c.,) the names *Yashṭimadhukam* and *Atimadhuram* are applied either to both the root of *A. precatorius* and of *Glycyrrhiza glabra*, or to the former alone. This is incorrect as well as a source of confusion. The names belong only to the true *Liquorice root* (*G. glabra*), and they cannot be correctly applied to the root of *A. precatorius*, unless the word *Indian* or *Country* is added to them as follows :—

Náṭṭu-yashṭi madhukam, Náṭṭu-atimadhuram. (*Tel.*) *Náṭ-yashṭi-madhukam, Náṭ-atimadhuram, Náṭ-iraṭṭimadhukam.* (*Malyal.*) *Náṭ-yashṭimadhuká, Náṭ-atimadhurá.* (*Can.*).

I have repeatedly examined this root both in the fresh and dry conditions, and found it to be far from 'abounding in sugar' as is generally considered. It does not possess any sweetness at all until it attains a certain size or becomes pretty old, and even then it is not always distinctly perceptible to taste, nor the *saccharine matter* of any kind easily detectable by *chemical tests*. Nevertheless, the root of *A. precatorius* is not only used in some bazaars for adulteration with the root of *G. glabra*, but is also sold indiscriminately under the same names. It is quite possible, therefore, that these roots are sometimes confounded with each other, and this accounts for the misconception as to the amount of sugar in the root of *A. precatorius*. The following distinctions are sufficient to distinguish this root from the true Liquorice :—

Glycyrrhiza glabra.	Abrus precatorius.
1. Generally about the size of a large goose quill or of the little finger, and sometimes as large as a thumb	1. Generally much smaller and seldom acquires the size of a finger.
2. Color greyish or reddish-brown externally, and slightly yellow or yellow internally.	2. Brown externally, and white internally.

3. Taste sweet and muci-laginous.	3. Taste generally not distinctly sweet.

The root of *A. precatorius*, however, still deserves the name of '*Indian or Country Liquorice*,' because it yields an Extract which is nearly similar in medicinal properties to the *Extract of Glycyrrhiza*, though somewhat bitterish in taste. I have succeeded in preparing an Extract not only from the root, but also from the leaves of all the varieties of *A. precatorius*. The leaves being distinctly sweet, the Extract they yield is much superior both in taste and as a medicine. The following is the best way of preparing the Extract from them.

Pour the boiling distilled water on dry leaves till they are sufficiently covered, keep the vessel on a slow fire for six hours, and then strain the liquor while hot through flannel and evaporate on a water bath to a proper consistence.

The Extract prepared from the juice of the fresh leaves is also sweet, but very inferior for medicinal purposes. The Extract of the root is prepared in the same way as recommended in the British Pharmacopœi for the preparation of *Extractum Glycyrrhizæ*.

4. ABUTILON INDICUM, *G. DON.*

Mashtul-*gh-oul* مشط الغول. (*Arab.*) Darakhte-shánah درخت شانه.. (*Pers.*) Kangai كنگنى; Kanghi كنگهي—— leaf of, Kanghi-ká-pát كنگهى كاپات. (*Hind.*) Kangói كنگوئى; Kangói-ká-*jhár* كنگوئى كاجهاڙ; Dabbé-ká-*jhár* كنگوئى كاپتا دبه كا جهاڙ—— leaf of, Kangoi-ká-pattá. (*Duk.*) Tutti தத்தி; Perun-tutti பெருந்தத்தி. (*Tam.*) Tutti తుత్తి; Tutturu-benda తుత్తురుబెండ; Núgu-benda నూగుబెండ: Tuttiri-chettu తుత్తిరిచెట్టు. (*Tel.*) Peṭṭaka-puṭṭi വെട്ടകപുട്ടി; Tutta ഇത്ത; Úram ഊരം. (*Malyal.*) Shrimudrigiḍá ಶ್ರೀಮುದ್ರಿಗಿಡ. (*Can.*) Jhumká-gáchh; Gunji-gáchh; Piṭári-gáchh. (*Beng.*) Kangóyi-nu-*jhádá*. (*Guz.*) Anoda-gahá. (*Cing.*) Bou-khoye or Bou-kho-e (*Bur.*).

Whether the *Abutilon Asiaticum* and *A. populifolium* (*G. Don*) are mere varieties of the above plant or different species, their native names are generally the same; and they are in India, with reference to their medicinal purposes, what the *mallow* and *marsh-mallow* are in Europe. There is one variety, however, which is always known by different names. It is distinguished by a blue or purple color of its stem, branches, petioles, &c., and is generally found growing in the hedges at Madras. It is named according to its color *Údi* or *Káli-kangói-ká-jhár* (*Duk.*), *Karu* or *Karan-tutti* (*Tam.*), Nalla-*tutti* or *Nalla-núgu-benḍa* (*Tel.*).

The names in the text are those that correctly and only belong to *A. Indicum* and its varieties, including *A. Asiaticum* and *A. populifolium;* but some of them are occasionally misapplied in some works (Materia Indica, &c.,) to *Malva* (*Sida*) *Mauritiana.* If the latter is often found in India (?) it should be distinguished by a prefix *Viláyatí* (*Europe or Foreign*); as, *Viláyati-kangói-ká*-jhár, &c. The word *Kanghí* or *Kangói* is not only used incorrectly in some books as synonymous with the Arabic and Persian words Ḳhabbázi خبازي , Khiṭmí خطمي and *Tódari* تودري (*the names of three different drugs*), but is also confounded with the word *Kangóni* كنگوني or 'Coongoonie' as it is generally written. The latter is one of the Dukhni synonyms of the seeds of *Panicum Italicum.*

The Malyalim name *Veḷḷarén* or 'Belluren' which is found in the Hortus Malabaricus (Vol. VI, Tab. 45) is véry incorrect, not being generally recognised as a name of any plant.

The Burmese name applied to this plant in Mason's Natural Productions of Burmah, '*tha-ma-khyoke*,' is the name of a different plant.

5. ACACIA ARABICA, *Willd.* (*Babool tree.*)

Ammugẖilán امغيلان; Mugẖilán مغيلان. (*Arab.*) Ḳháre-mugẖilán خارمغيلان. (*Pers.*) Babúl ببول; Kikar كيكر. (*Hind.*) Káli-kikar كالي كيكر. (*Duk.*) Kuru-vélam கருேவலம்; Karu-vél கருேவல். (*Tam.*) Nalla-tumma నల్లతుమ్మ; Barbúramu బర్బూరము; Tumma-cheṭṭu తుమ్మచెట్టు. (*Tel.*) Karu-vélakam

കൃഷ്ണവേലകം. *(Malyal.)* Karé-jáli-mará ಕರ್ಜಾಲಿಮರಾ; Karé-góbbaḷi-mará ಕರ್ಗೊಬ್ಬಳಿಮರಾ; *(Can.)* Bábúl *or* Bábulér-gáchh. *(Beng.)* Kála-barbúra-vrikshaha. *(Sans.)* Bábli-*ch'a-jh*áḍa. *(Mah.)* Kálobável. *(Guz.)*.

Sh-ou*kul-makkah*, Sh-ou*kul-egrúbiyah*, Sh-ou*kul-miṣríyah*, *qarṣ*, and *Aqáqiyá* are the Arabic names applied to *A. Arabica* in some Persian and other works. The first three are more properly the names of *A. vera* and a few other species which are commonly found in Egypt and Arabia, and the last two, the names of their pod and the juice of the pod respectively.

6.   ACACIA CATECHU, *Willd. (Catechu tree.)*

Kh-air-babúl كهيربهول; *Kh-air-ká-pé*ṛ كهيركاپيڑ —— *wood of, Kh-air* كهير *and* Ka*th-kh-air* كتهكهير. *(Hind.)* Katt*hé*-ki-ki-kar كتهي كي كڈكر. *(Duk.)* Vodalai ஓடலை; Vódaḷam ஓடளம். *(Tam.)* Poḍali-mánu పాడలిమాను; *Khadi*ramu ఖదిరము. *(Tel.)* Kadaram കദരം. *(Malyal.) Kh-air*-gáchh——*wood of, Kh-air. (Beng.) Kh*adira-vrikshaha. *(Sans.)* Khadira——*wood of, Kh-airi. (Mah.) Kh*a-dira——*wood of*, Kihiri. *(Cing.)* Shúzi-biṇ. *(Bur.)*.

This plant is considered by some not to have any Tamil name or not to be a 'Tamil tree,' which means apparently that it does not exist in the Central and Southern Carnatic, where the Tamil is the prevailing language. At present, however, it is found in the Agri-horticultural Society's and other gardens at Madras, and is included in Dr. Cleghorn's Hortus Madras, patensis. I believe also that it is not very rare in the jungles near Veuore, Vouumbody and many other places, but it is not generally noticed by the inhabitants who are not aware of its yielding a *Catechu*. It is more easly recognised in this country by its Tamil names than any other.* See the remarks on *Kadaram* or *Kadara* under *Alangium hexapetalum.*

---

* After I made the above remarks, I have found some more plants in Madras, and they all correspond with the characters of *A. catechu.* This species is much more common in S. India than I thought before.

7. ACACIA CONCINNA, D. C. *(Pods of.)*

Sikí-kái سیکي کائي *or* Siké-kái سیکي کائی. *(Duk.)* Shiká சீகா. *(Tam.)* Shikáya சீகாయ; Chikáya சికாయ. *(Tel.)* Chinik-káya ചിനിക്കായ. *(Malyal.)* Shige-káyi ಶಿಗೆಕಾಯಿ. *(Can.)* Kóch-ái. *(Beng.)* Shiká; Telaséngá. *(Mah.)* Kènbhon-si; Kénbhon-pédon; Kenbon-ti. *(Bur.).*

"Reeta" is the Bengali name assigned to this plant under the head "Acacia rugata" in the Hortus Suburbanus Calcuttensis and some other works, but it is undoubtedly the Hindustani and Bengali name of the *Soapnut (Sapindus emarginatus).* The correct Bengali synonym of the pod of *A. concinna* is the one inserted in the text.

8. ACACIA FARNESIANA, *Willa.*

Gúh-babúl گوہ ببول. *(Hind.)* Gú-kikar گو کیکر. *(Duk.)* Piy-vélam பிய்வேலம், Piy-vél பிய்வேல். *(Tam.)* Piyi-tumma పియితుమ్మ; Kampu-tumma కంపుతుమ్మ; Nága-tumma నాగతుమ్మ. *(Tel.)* Pivélam പിവേലം. *(Malyal.)* Gú-bábúl. *(Beng.)* Gu-bával. *(Guz.)* Nanluñ-maiñ. *(Bur.).*

The smell of the fresh bark and wood of this plant is not quite unlike that of the human ordure; hence the meaning of all its native synonyms. The Telugu name *Kastúri-tumma* which is found in some books and means *a musk Acacia,* cannot be applicable to it, for obvious reasons. Two names are applied to this plant in Mason's Natural Productions of Burmah, one of which (*nánlún-kh-ain*) means *a good smell,* and the other, *a bad smell;* the former is objectionable for the same reason given against the Telugu name *Kastúri-tumma,* and is therefore not included in the text.

The Dukhni name *Gú-kikar* is sometimes applied also to *Parkinsonia aculeata,* but the name by which the latter is more commonly recognised is *Jangli-kikar* جنگلی کیکر.

9. ACACIA FERRUGINEA, *D. C.*

Shimai-veḷvél ஷிமைவெள்வேல். *(Tam.)* Vuni ఒని;
Anasandra అనసంద్ర; Ana-chandra అనచంద్ర. *(Tel.)*.

The Telugu name *Vuni* is often confounded with the *Vanni*
of Tamil, which is the name of *Prosopis spicigera*.

10. ACACIA LEUCOPHLÆA, *Willd.*

Suféd-kikar سفيدكيكر. *(Hind.)* Ujli-kikar اجلي كيكر;
Paṭṭé-ki-kikar پٹے كي كيكر; Sharáb-ki-kikar شراب كي كيكر.
(Duk.) Veḷ-vél வெள்வேல்; Veḷ-vélam வெள்வேலம். *(Tam.)*
Tella-tumma తెల్లతుమ్మ. *(Tel.)* Veḷ-vélam വെൾവേലം.
(Malyal.) Biḷijáli-mará ಬಿಳಿಜಾಲಿಮರಾ. *(Can.)* Saphéd-
bábúl. *(Beng.)* Shvéta-barbára-vrikshaha. *(Sans.)* Pándha-
ra-báblicha-jháda. *(Mah.)* Saphéd-bával. *(Guz.)* Nanloun-
kiyiṇ-aphiju. *(Bur.)*.

11. ACACIA SPECIOSA. *Willd.*

Siris-ká-péṛ سرس كاپيز. *(Hind.)* Sirish-ká-jháṛ
سرش كاجهاڑ; Sirij-ká-jhá سرج كاجهاڑ. *(Duk.)* Káṭṭu-vágai
காட்டுவாகை. *(Tam.)* Dirisana-cheṭṭu దిరిసనచెట్టు; Tella-
dirisana-cheṭṭu తెల్లదిరిసనచెట్టు. *(Tel.)* Veḷu-váke വെളുവാകെ.
(Malyal.) Siris-gáchh. *(Beng.)* Saras-nu-jháda. *(Guz.)*.

From the similarity of its sound, the Dukhni name *Sirij-
ká*-jháṛ is frequently confounded with *Súrij-ká*-jháṛ. The latter
is the name of *Helianthus annuus*, and is synonymous with *Surij-
makkhí*.

In some Persian works, the Arabic names *Leḥaiyetuttis* and
aznábul-khíl are incorrectly applied to *A. speciosa*.

12. ACETUM. *(Vinegar.)*

Khal خل. *(Arab.)* Sirkah سركه. *(Pers.)* Sirká سركا.
(Hind. and Duk.) Kádi காடி. *(Tam.)* Kádi-níḷḷu కాడినిళ్ళు.

(Tel.) Káṭi கஅஸி. *(Malyal.)* Kùdi ಕಡಿ; Huḷirasa ಹುಳಿರಸ.
(Can.) **Sirka.** *(Beng.)* <u>Sirko.</u> *(Guz.)* Venà-kiri ; Kùḍi.
(Cing.) Póṅ-ye. *(Bur.)*.

There are many kinds of *Vinegar* in India ; indeed, almost all the sweet and delicious fruits, in addition to *rice, sugar, honey, &c.,* are made to undergo the acetous fermentation, and the vinegar thus produced is made use of in medicine by native practitioners, particularly the Hakeems. Each kind of vinegar is named after the substance from which it is produced; as, *Tári-kd-sirkah* is *the vinegar of Toddy, &c.* The following are the native synonyms of some of the vinegars generally found in the bazaar.

a. Vinegar of Grapes or Wine-vinegar——Ḳhallul-ḳhamar خل الخمر; Ḳhallul-ganab خل العنب. *(Arab.)* Sirkahe-angúrí سرکهٔانگوري. *(Pers.)* Angúri-sirkah انگوري سرکه. *(Hind. and Duk.)* Diráksha-káḍi திராக்ஷகாடி. *(Tam.)* Dráksha-pulla-niḷḷu ద్రాక్షపుల్లనీళ్ళు. *(Tel.)* Muntirinna-káṭi മുന്തിരിങ്ങകാടി. *(Malyal.)* Drákshi-kàḍi ದ್ರಾಕ್ಷಿಕಡಿ. *(Can.)* Angurér-sirká. *(Beng.)* Drákhnu-sirko. *(Guz.)*.

b. Vinegar of the Palm-wine or the Toddy of Phœnix Sylvestris.——Séndhí-kd-sirkah سيندهي كاسرکه. *(Hind.)* Séndí-kd-sirkah سيندي كاسرکه. *(Duk.)* Íshan-kaḷḷu-káḍi சசங்கள்ளுகாடி; Íshan-káḍi சசங்காடி. *(Tam.)* Íta-káḍi ఈతకాడి; Íta-kaḷḷu-káḍi ఈతకళ్ళుకాడి. *(Tel.)* Ínte-káṭi ഇന്തെകാടി. *(Malyal.)*.

c. Vinegar of Toddy or Palmyra-vinegar——Sirkahe-tárí سرکهٔ تاري. *(Pers.)* Tári-kd-sirkah تاري كاسرکه. *(Hind. and Duk.)* Panan-káḍi பனங்காடி; Panan-kaḷḷu-káḍi பனங்கள்ளு-காடி. *(Tam.)* Táṭi-káḍi తాటికాడి; Taṭi-kaḷḷu-kádi తాటికళ్ళుకాడి. *(Tel.)* Pand-káṭi പനാകാടി. *(Malyal.)* Pané-káḍi ಪನೇಕಡಿ. *(Can.)* Tàl-sirká. *(Beng.)* Tár-nu-sirko. *(Guz.)* Tàl-vend. *(Cing.)* Thán-póṅ-ye. *(Bur.)*.

Of all the liquids known as vinegars, none enjoys a greater reputation in India as a useful medicine than the *Búf-ká-sirkah*

کاسرکه بوت‎ (*Vinegar of the Bengal-gram plant*); but it is not properly a vinegar, with reference to which see the remarks on *Cicer arietinum*.

13. ACHYRANTHES ASPERA. *Linn.*

Atkumah اتکمه. (*Arab.*) Ḵháre-vázhún خاروازون; Ḵháre-vázhgúnah خاروازگونه. (*Pers.*) Chirchirá چرچرا; Chichrá چچرا. (*Hind.*) Agárá اگارا or Aghárá اگهارا (*Duk.*) Ná-yurivi நாயுரிவி. (*Tam*) Utta-réṇi உத்தரேணி; Antisha అంటిష; Apá-márgamu అపామార్గము; Pratyuk-pushpi ప్రత్యుక్పుష్పి. (*Tel.*) Kaṭaláṭi കടലാടി. (*Malyal.*) Utrúṇi-giḍá ಉತ್ರಣಿಗಿಡ. (*Can.*) Chirchiri ; Opang. (*Beng.*) Apámárgaha. (*Sans.*) Utráṇicha-jháḍa (*Mah.*) Jhinjarvaṭṭo. (*Guz.*) Gaskaral-hebbo. (*Cing.*) Kiva-lá-mou *or* Kune-lá-mou. (*Bur.*).

The remarks I have made under *Abelmoschus moschatus* with regard to the Arabic synonyms in the Hortus Malabaricus, are also in some degree applicable to the Mahratti synonyms in the same work. These synonyms are found under the head of 'Bram.' or 'Bra.' written in the Sanscrit (Deva-nagari or Bála-band) character, and are of such nature that more than two-thirds of them are either wrong or not in use at present. The name assigned to the plant under consideration, Káṭe-magaró, is one of the examples of the former. It is the name of a species of *Jasmine*, and this corresponds with the meaning given to it in some Mahratti works (Molesworth's Dictionary, &c.,) except the word *Magaró* which is spelt there as *Mogorí*.

14. ACIDUM BENZOICUM. (*Benzoic Acid.*)

Lóbán-ká-sat لوبان کاست ; Lóbán-ká-phúl لوبان کاپهول. (*Hind.*) Aúd-ká-sat عودکاست. (*Duk.*) Shámbiráṇip-pú சாம்பிராணிப்பூ. (*Tam.*) Sámbráṇi-puvvu సాంబ్రాణిపువ్వు. (*Tel.*).

15. ACIDUM HYDROCHLORICUM. (*Hydrochloric or Muriatic Acid*).

Mául-milḥ ما'الملح. (*Arab.*) Tézábe-namak تیزاب نمک, Aarqe-namak عرق نمک. (*Pers.*) Namak-ká-tézáb. نمک کا تیزاب. (*Hind. and Duk.*) Uppu-dirávakam உப்பு ஜிராவகம்; Lavaṇa-dirávakam லவண ஜிராவகம். (*Tam.*) Lavaṇa-drávakam లవణ ద్రావకం. (*Tel.*) Uppa-drávakam ഉപ്പ ദ്രാവകം. (*Malyal.*) Núnér-téjáb. (*Beng.*) Míḷhá-nu-tézáb. (*Guz.*) Ṣáye-biyán. (*Bur.*).

16. ACIDUM NITRICUM. (*Nitric Acid*).

Mául-abqar ما'الابقر. (*Arab.*) Tézábe-shórah تیزاب شوره; Aarqe-shórah عرق شوره. (*Pers.*) Shóré-ká-tézáb شوریکاتیزاب. (*Hind. and Duk*) Poṭluppu-dirávakam பொற்றுப்பு ஜிராவகம். (*Tam.*) Poṭluppu-drávakam పొట్లుప్పు ద్రావకం; Súrákára-drávakam సూరాకార ద్రావకం. (*Tel.*) V(ṭiyuppa-drávakam വെടിയുപ്പ ദ്രാവകം. (*Malyal.*) Shórár-téjáb. (*Beng.*) Surákhár-nu-tézáb. (*Guz.*) Yánzain-yebiján. (*Bur.*).

17. ACIDUM SULPHURICUM. (*Sulphuric Acid*).

Mául-kibrít ما'الکبریت. (*Arab.*) Tézábe-gogird تیزاب گوگرد; Aarqe-gogird عرق گوگرد. (*Pers.*) Gandhak-ká-tézáb گندهک کا تیزاب; Gandhak-ká-aiṭr گند هک کا عطر. (*Hind.*) Gandak-ká-tézáb گندک کا تیزاب. (*Duk.*) Gendaka-dirávakam கெந்தக ஜிராவகம். (*Tam.*) Gendhaka-drávakam గెంధక ద్రావకం. (*Tel.*) Gandhaka-drávakam ഗന്ധക ദ്രാവകം. (*Malyal.*) Gandrokér-téjáb. (*Beng.*) Gandak-nu-tézáb. (*Guz.*) Kán-gí. (*Bur.*).

18. ACONITUM FEROX, *Wall.* (*Root of*).

Bísh بیش. (*Arab.*) Bishnág بیشناگ. (*Pers.*) Bis بس; Singyá سنگیا; Singyá-bis سنگیابس; Míḷhá-zahar میٹھا زهر; Téliyá-bis تیلیا بس; Bachhnág بچهناگ. (*Hind.*) Bach-nág بجِّنا گ . (*Duk.*) Vaşha-návi வசநாவி; Návi நாவி. (*Tam.*) Vasanábhi వసనాథ; Nábhi నాథ. (*Tel.*) Valsa-nábhi വത്സനാഭി. (*Malyal.*) Vasa-nábhi ವಸನಾಥ. (*Can.*) Bish. (*Beng.*) Vachhnág (*Guz.*) Vachanábhi. (*Cing.*).

The root of this very poisonous plant is found in every large bazaar of India. There are four or more varieties of it, two of which are named as *black* and *white* according to the color of their substance internally. The black variety, which is generally of a reddish brown color, is considered by native practitioners and druggists to be more virulent than the other, and is well known by its Hindustani name *Kálá-bachhnág* كالابجِّنا گ. But, by some mistake, this name is applied in many works, including the Materia Indica, to *Hymenodictyon Excelsum* or *Cinchona Excelsa!*

Although the Hindustani names *Míṭhá-zahar* (*sweet poison* or *A. ferox*) and *Singyá* or *Singyá-bis* (*horny A. ferox*), are often applied to any variety of the root of *A. ferox* without much discretion, yet they are correctly applicable only to two varieties which differ in some particular points from all others. The root called *Míṭhá-zahar* is generally an inch or an inch and a half in length, and its circumference at the base is about the same; it is tapering, slightly compressed, and very rough from wrinkles; brown externally, and pale-brown internally; slightly but distinctly *sweet* in taste, and produces a kind of tingling or peculiar sensation on the tongue when chewed. The *Singyá-bis*, which is also known as *Télíyá-bis*, as its names imply, looks like a small *horn* of a deer or goat, being very hard, smooth, and tapering; and of *dark brown* color. It is generally longer than the sweet variety, but seldom more in thickness; and the color of its substance is dark brown with shining when recently broken. On chewing a very small bit of it, there is a feeling of great acridity on the tongue and lips, which is followed by a kind of numbness or altered sensation. After examining the four varieties I have mentioned, I believe the *Singyá-bis* to be the strongest of all, and the *Míṭházahar* the weakest. Moreover, I have some doubt whether these two varieties are really the produce of *A. ferox,* as is generally considered, or of some other species closely allied to it.

The Telugu name *Ati-rasa* will be found applied in some books to *A. ferox*, whereas it is very familiarly known in all the bazaars of Southern India to be the name of a variety of the root of *A. heterophyllum*, which will be described under the head of that plant. *Ati-vasa* is derived from the word *ati*, excess or great, and *vasa*, sweet-flag or the root of *Acorus calamus*; it means accordingly *the greater or larger sweet-flag*, and is applied to this root on account of some supposed resemblance of its actions to those of the former. The above derivation is according to the usage of the language among the Vaiddiyars, druggists, and other educated persons; but according to some books, the word appears to have been derived from ' *atis*,' because the latter is given as its meaning. *Ati-vasa* is, however, confounded in some books (Flora Andhrica, &c.) with the Sanscrit name *Ati-visha*,* which means *a great poison*, and is derived from *ati*, much or great, and *visha*,* a poison. The word *ati* is the same in both names, but *vasa* and *visha** are two different words. *Vasa* in Flora Andhrica itself is applied to *Acorus calamus*, which is correct.

The above is a serious confusion and should be carefully avoided, because the *Ati-vasa* is sold in the same bazaars together with the root of *A. ferox*, and is frequently used internally in pretty large doses in persons of all ages, including children.

The Cingalese name *Niri-visha* or ' Nerree-weesa' is often applied to the root of *A. ferox*, but it is not restricted to that drug. It is occasionally applied to another root according to its original meaning as explained elsewhere, and thus becomes a source of confusion. I have therefore omitted it from the text. See the remarks on this, as well as other names derived from the Sanscrit name *Nir-visha*,* under the head '*Aconitum. sp. of. (Root of——Jadvar.)*'. See also the remarks under *Gloriosa-superba*.

19. ACONITUM HETEROPHYLLUM, *Wall. (Root of)*.

Vajje-turkí ترکي وج . *(Pers.)*   Atís تيس ا . *(Hind.)*   Atviká ا قو يکا ; Vajje-turkí ترکي وج . *(Duk.)*   Ati-vaḍayam அதிவடயம். *(Tam.)*   Ati-vasa అతివస. *(Tel.)*.

Except *Atís* and *Atviká* all other synonymes in the text are applied in the bazaars of Southern India to a root which I have

---

no doubt is a variety of the root of *A. heterophyllum.* It is a
small tuberous root; from 1 to 2 inches in length and circumference; conical, or ovoid with a tapering point towards one end;
grey externally and white internally with more or less white
scars of rootlets on the surface; inodorous; and bitter in
taste without any acridity or astringency. I have compared
this root with the specimens of *Atis* obtained from Calcutta and
other places, and found it to correspond with them exactly in the
appearance of their substance internally and in taste, but
it differed from some of them in shape and external color.

In one of the specimens, the epidermis was of a brown color,
the roots were smaller and almost oblong, and in some of these
the tendency to be divided into two tubers, as described in some
books, was more distinctly marked than in the roots of any other
specimen. In another specimen, most of the roots were thin and
cylindrical with longitudinal wrinkles and with little or no
point at either end. All these specimens agreed in 3 characters
which were invariable, viz., the whiteness of the substance
internally, the pure bitter taste, and the farinaceous nature.

Atvíká is the name in use in some Bombay districts and a
few other places for this root, as is *Atis* in Calcutta and other
places of Upper India. The meaning of the Persian name *Vajje-
turki* is, *the Turkey-sweet-flag,* and it is accordingly applied to a
variety of the root of *Acorus calamus* all over India, except
in Southern India, where it is confined to the root under
consideration. There is another root in the bazaars of South
India, which is erroneously considered to be a variety of the
above root, and is named accordingly as *Nát-kí-vajje-turki*
ناتُّ کی وج ترکی (*Duk.*), *Náṭṭu-ati-vaḷayam* நாட்டு அதிவளயம்
(*Tam.*), *Náṭṭu-ati-vasa* నాటి అతివస (*Tel.*), &c., which
mean *the root of the country A. heterophyllum.* This is a very
small root and bears more resemblance externally to the
root of *Ipecacuanha* than any other I have seen. It is generally
about the thickness of a small quill; from $\frac{1}{4}$ to $1\frac{1}{2}$ inches long;
annulated; of grey or dark-grey color externally and white
internally; inodorous; and *acrid* in taste. It is clear from
this description that it is not a variety of *A. heterophyllum,*
but probably another species of *Aconitum.* The Hindustani name

Atís is some times incorrectly applied to this root in Hyderabad. See the remarks on the word *Ati-rasa* under *A. ferox.*

20. ACONITUM. *Sp. of. (Root of——Jadvàr.)*

Jadvàr جدوار . (*Arab.*) *Zh*advàr زدوار; or Zadvàr زدوار ; Màfarfiñ مافرفین ; Màh-parviñ مادپروین . (*Pers.*) Nir-bisì نربسي . (*Hind.*).

In many Dictionaries and other works, the Arabic, Persian, and Hindustani names *Jadvár, Máhparvin,* and *Nir-bisi* are applied to the root of *Curcuma zedoaria* of Roxburgh (*Zedoary or Round Zedoary),* but in almost all the bazaars of India they are used for different medicines. I have obtained these medicines from many parts, and found none of them to correspond with the characters of the *Round Zedoary,* which is correctly the *Añbé-haldì* of the bazaar, and the names, therefore, are not applicable to it.

The roots sold under the name of *Jadvár* in most of the Indian bazaars are nearly the same, and the little difference which exists between them, constitutes its varieties. Four or five varieties of it àre spoken of in some Persian and other medical works, but only three are generally used in medicine at present. I believe these to be the roots of some species of *Aconite* like *A. .heterophyllum,* which is not poisonous; but, whether they are really the produce of one species, or of two or more, is not as yet ascertained. Until this is done, I shall describe them as mere varieties.

a. The variety of *Jadvár* which is comparatively cheap and easily procurable at Calcutta, is a very small tuberous root, varying in length from half to one inch; tapering to a sharp point; not round, but very irregularly compressed or shrunken, which together with the deep wrinkles renders its surface very rough and uneven; brown or dark-brown internally and externally; hard and cannot be cut easily with a knife; *slightly bitter in taste without the least acridity or tingling sensation when a bit of it is chewed;* and there is a more or less projection of woody substance in the centre of its base, the remains of the root-stalk.

b. The second variety of *Jadvár* is about the same in size, but round, nearly smooth, and conical dark brown externally and brown internally with occasional spots of grey color; and its taste is slightly but purely bitter like that of the *Atis*, to which it also bears a slight resemblance in its form. From the latter circumstances it may appear to be a variety of *Atis*, but, in addition to the color, it differs from it in not responding to the Iodine-test. It is recognised by the Hakeems as one of the varieties of *Jadvár.*

c. The third variety of *Jadvár* is a larger root, being generally about one or one and a quarter inches in length, and one, one and a half, or two inches in circumference at the base. It is slightly round, conical, and rough with wrinkles and scars of the rootlets; brown in color both externally and internally; slightly but distinctly *sweet* in taste; and somewhat soft so as to be cut easily and smoothly with a knife. When very old, this root often becomes much harder in texture; loses the sweetness, and even acquires a bitterish taste, as if the latter were covered by the former in the fresh or recent condition; and is also attacked by insects some times. The other two varieties of *Jadvár* undergo no material change in course of time.

The first and third varieties I have described, are the *Jad-váre-hindi* جدواردهندي (*Indian*) and *Jadváre-Khatái* جدوارخطاني (*of Northern China*), respectively. The latter is said to be brought from some parts of Northern China, or rather from some parts beyond the Himalayah mountains; and the former is imported into the plains of India from the mountains themselves. According to some Arabic and Persian medical works, the plant of *Jadvár* is always found growing together with *A. ferox*, to which and all other poisons, including the snake poison, &c., it is considered to be the best *antidote;* hence its Hindustani synonym *Nir-bisi* (*nir*, free or without, *bisi*, belonging to *bis* or *A. ferox*).

Jadvár is one of the best, active, and most valuable Indian medicines, and though very dear and scarce in Southern India, it is pretty cheap and easily procurable in several districts of Hindustan Proper and Northern Hindustan. At Madras, it is not sold, if genuine, below four or five Rupees a tolah, and I have known the same quantity to fetch more than ten, at one time. It is generally kept here by the druggists in oil in stopper or other bottles, to prevent, as they allege, its decay or destruction by insects. This precaution, however, is not only injurious to the root, but is also fraudulent, because some other roots, and even the pieces of some blackwood cut out in the shape of *Jadvár*, are kept soaking in oil for a long time, which alters their natural appearance and taste so much that they cannot be easily distinguished from the real drug under the same circumstances. No particular care is necessary in preserving the root, it being sufficient to keep it in a bottle in the ordinary way. *Jadvár* is very seldom attacked by insects on account of its containing a bitter principle, and when it is so, the circumstance may be looked upon as the best criterion to distinguish it from all poisonous roots of similar appearance.

As explained above, *Nir-bisí* and *Mahparvín* are correctly the Hindustani and Persian synonyms of *Jadvár*, and they should not be applied to any other drug but the root or its varieties I have just described. *Nir-bisí*, however, is often confounded with the Sanscrit name *Nir-visha*, and this is partly from the partial analogy that exists between their pronunciation, and partly from their literal and general meaning being nearly the same. *Free from* or *without poison* is the literal meaning of *Nir-visham* or *Nir-visha*, and the meaning generally attached to it in books is *an antidote*. The only difference between the above meaning and the meaning of *Nir-bisí* is, that the Sanscrit word *Visham* or *Visha* is the common name for any poison, whatever it may be, while *bis* in Hindustani is the name of a particular vegetable poison, viz., the root of *A. ferox*. *Nir-visham* is adopted with a slight alteration in some other languages; such as, *Niri-visham* in Tamil, *Niri-visha* or '*Nerree-weesa*' in Cingalese, &c., and although these names appear to have been originally applied to a root which was considered to be *an antidote*, yet, at present, they are given to different drugs in different bazaars of India. For example, the *Niri-visha* I have received from Ceylon is the root of *A. ferox;* and the *Niri-visham* of Madras resembles the root of *Curcuma aromatica* and will be described under that head.

It is to the latter root *(Niri-visham)* the Hindustani name *Nir-bisí* is frequently misapplied at Madras, but its correct name is that which is in use in Hyderabad, Bombay, and many other parts of India, viz., *Madan-mast* مدن مست . In his 'Illustrations of the Botany of the Himalayan mountains,' the late Professor Royle remarks that he found the name *Nirbisí* applied to

Delphinium pauciflorum in the mountains of Sirmoor and Gurwal. The same name, again, is incorrectly applied in the bazaars of Calcutta to a root which bears some resemblance to one of the varieties of *A. ferox;* but, a careful examination will reveal that it is not only different from the roots of all the varieties of that plant, but also from those of other species of *Aconite* included in the Catalogue.

From the above remarks, it is apparent that some precaution is necessary in selecting for medicinal purposes the drug named at the heading of this article. First, it should be obtained under the Arabic name, *Jadvár*, and all its other synonyms avoided as much as possible, being greatly involved in confusion. Secondly, as there are several species of *Aconite*, whose roots resemble each other, *Jadvár* is liable to be confounded with some of them which might be poisonous in nature. To avoid this, no medicine is to be considered as a *genuine Jadvár*, unless it corresponds with the characters of any of its varieties I have described, particularly in *taste* and *color*, which are the best criterions. The former ought to be either *bitter* or *sweet* without the least *acridity, irritation, tingling* or any other *unnatural sensation;* and the latter, more or less *brown* both *externally* and *internally*.

21. ACORUS CALAMUS, *Linn.* (*Root of—Sweet flag.*)

Vajj وج or Vai وج · (*Arab.*) Agre-turki اگوترکي (*Pers.*) Bach بَچ · (*Hind.*) Gand-ki-lakri گند کي لکڑي or Gan-ki-larri گن، کي لکڑي; Vach وج · (*Duk.*) Vaṣhambu வசம்பு. (*Tam.*) Vasa వస; Vadaja వడజ. (*Tel.*) Vaṣhanpa വശമ്പ. (*Malyal.*) Bajé ಬಜೆ. (*Can.*) Bach; Saphéd-bach. (*Benq.*) Ugra-gan*dhaha.* (*Sans.*) Vé*khn*da. (*Mah.*) Vaj; Vach. (*Guz.*) Leiihe, Lene *or* Linhe. (*Bur.*).

In almost all the Vernacular Dictionaries with English, the *sweet-flag* is confounded with the *Orris root.* Besides this, the Arabic name *Vaj* or *Vaji* is erroneously applied to ‘ *Gallangal*’ in Richardson, Shakespear, and Forbes’ Dictionaries, &c. See the remarks on the Persian name *Vajje-turki* وج قرکي under *Aconitum heterophyllum.*

22. ADANSONIA DIGITATA. *Linn.*

Hujéd حجبيد . (*Arab.*) Gorak-amlí گورک املي
(*Hind.*) Háthí-*kh*atyán هاتهي ختيان ; Bará-*kh*at-yán
بڑا ختيان . (*Duk.*) Ánai-puḷiya-maram ஆனைபுளியமரம் ;
Papparap-puḷi பப்பரப்புளி ; Púri-maram புரிமரம். (*Tam.*)
Góraka-ámalí. (*Mah.*) Gorak-amlí. (*Guz.*) Bíla-magi-
ṣí. (*Bur.*).

23. ADENEMA (CICENDIA) HYSSOPIFOLIA,
W. et A.

Chhóṭá-charáyetah چهوٹا چرايته . (*Hind.*) Nái-
ká-pattá نائي کا پتا . (*Duk.*) Veḷḷarugu வெள்ளறுகு.
(*Tam.*) Chevukurti-cheṭṭu చెవుకుతిచెట్టు ; Golimiḍi గొలిమిడి.
(*Tel.*) Chóṭa-kiróṭá. (*Beng.*) Nái-cha-pálá. (*Mah.*)
Nànu-kiryáta; Karo-kiryáta; Nàyi. (*Guz.*).

24. ADHATODA VASICA, *Nees.*

Aḍalsá اڈلسا ; Adalsá ادلسا ; Arúsá ارو سا ; Aḍarsá
اڈرسا . (*Hind. and Duk.*) Áḍáṭoḍai அடாடொடை. (*Tam.*)
Aḍḍasaram అడ్డసరం. (*Tel.*) Áṭa-lóṭakam ആടലോടകം.
(*Malyal.*) Áḍasóge-sappu ಆಡಸೋಗೆಸಪ್ಪು. (*Can.*) Bákas;
Árusá. (*Beng.*) Vaídyamátru-vrikshaha. (*Sans.*) Áḍaṭoḍa;
Pàvaṭṭa. (*Cing.*) Meṣan-biṇ. (*Bur.*).

The above plant is also named *Búṅsá* or *Búṅsah* in some
Persian works; but as that name is commonly in use for the *Bamboo* in many parts of India, I have omitted it from the text.

25. ÆGLE MARMELOS. *Corr. (Fruit of——Bengal*
Quince.)

Safarjale-hindi سفرجل هندي ; Shul شل . (*Arab. and*
Pers.) Bél بيل ; Si-*phal* سيبهل ; Siri-*phal* سرى پهل

(*Hind.*) ·Bél-*phal* بيل پهل . (*Duk.*) Vilva-pazham விலவ-பழம். (*Tam.*) Marédu-pandu మారేదుపండు ; Bilva-pandu బిల్వపండు; (*Tel.*) Kúvalap-pazham കുവളപ്പഴം. (*Malyal.*) Bilapatri-hannu ಬಿಲಪತ್ರಿಹಣ್ಣು. (*Can.*) Bél, Shri-*phal*. (*Beng.*) Bilva-*phalam*. (*Sans.*) Béla ; Bélácha-phalá. (*Mah.*) Bél-*phal* ; Bilinu-*phal*. (*Guz.*) Bélli ; Bélli-ká. (*Cing.*) Oushi-si, Úshi-si *or* Úshi-ti. (*Bur.*).

The cultivated *Ægle marmelos* differs in some respects from the common variety. It is generally free from spines; the leaflets are broadly and abruptly acuminate instead .of oblong or broadly lanceolate, and when bruised have *an agreeable aromatic smell* somewhat like that of the camphor; and the fruit is much larger, globular, and edible. The plant is therefore ·often recognised by different names in Southern India.

This variety is apparently the *Cratæra religiosa* spoken of in the Materia Indica and some other books. In the first named work, again, the *Cratæra marmelos* of Linnæus is mentioned under a separate head as if a different plant from *Ægle marmelos*, but the vernacular names applied to the former are some of those properly belong to the latter. According to all authorities, however, both plants are one and the same species. See the remarks on *C. religiosa.**

26. AGAVE AMERICANA, *Linn.*

Rákas-pattah راكس پته ; Háthi-séngár هاتهي سينگار ; Bará-kanvár بڑا كنوار ; Janglí-kanvár جنگلي كنوار . (*Hind.*) Rakkas-pattah ركس پته . (*Duk.*) Anaik-katrázh-ai ஆனைக கற்றாழை. (*Tam.*) Rákáshi-mattalu రాకాశిమట్టలు. (*Tel.*) Panam-katrázha പനംകറ്റാഴ. (*Malyal*) Bhuttále ಭುತ್ತಾಳೆ.

(*Can.*) Jangli-ananá*sh* *or* Jangli-ánanás ; Bilátipát. (*Beng.*) Jangli-komári. (*Guz.*).

Kétgi كينگي is the name used in some Hyderabad districts for *Agave Americana*, whereas the same name is employed in all other parts of India to designate a variety of *Pandanus odoratissimus*.

In some works, ' Kóyángi' or ' Kóyánji' is assigned as the Burmese synonym of this plant, but it is the name of *Crinum Asiaticum*.

27. AILANTHUS MALABARICUS, *D. C. (Bark of.)*

Peru-marattup-paṭṭai பெருமரத்தப்பட்டை. (*Tam.*) **Pedda-mánu-paṭṭa** పెద్దమానుపట్ట. (*Tel.*) Peru-marat-toli பெരുമரத்தொலி. (*Malyal.*) Kumbalu-potta. (*Cing.*).

Poṇṇalyam பொங்ஙல்யം is the Malyalim name found in the Hortus Malabaricus for the above plant, (Vol. VI, Tab. 15,) which is, at least, not recognisable. The dry bark of the tree which is sold in the bazaar is generally known under the name of *Peru-marat-toli* in the districts of Malabar.

28. AILANTHUS MALABARICUS, *D. C. (Resinous juice of.)*

Maḍḍi-pál மட்டிபால். (*Tam.*) Maḍḍí-pálu మడ్డిపాలు. (*Tel.*) Maṭṭip-pál മട്ടിപ്പാൽ. (*Malyal.*).

29. ALANGIUM DECAPETALUM, *Lam.*

Akólá اكولا *or* Akólah اكولہ. (*Hind. and Duk.*) Azhiṇji-maram அழிஞ்சிமரம். (*Tam.*) Úḍuga-cheṭṭu ఉడుగచెట్టు ; *Amkólam-cheṭṭu* అంకోలంచెట్టు. (*Tel.*) Ayangólam അങ്കോലം;*Azhiṇṇa-maram* അഴിഞ്ഞമരം.(*Malyal.*) *Amkóle* ಅಂಕೋಲೆ (*Can.*) Bágh-ankará. (*Beng.*) Aṇgola (*Cing.*) To-sh-ou-biṇ or Tou-sh-ou-biṇ. (*Bur.*).

30. ALANGIUM HEXAPETALUM, *Lam.*

Akól اكول ; Kálá-akólá كالاكولا or Kálá-akolah
كالاكول. (*Hind. and Duk.*) Karuppu-azhiŋŋi-maram
கருப்பு அழிஞ்சிமரம். (*Tam.*) Nalla-úḍuga-chettu நల்ல ఊడుగ
చెట్టు; Nalla-amkólam-chettu నల్ల అంకోలంచెట్టు. (*Tel.*)
Karutta-ayangólam കറുത്തഅയ്യോലം. (*Malyal*) Kare-
amkóle-giḍá ಕರೆಅಂಕೋಲೆಗಿಡಾ. (*Can.*) Kalu-aṇgola. (*Cing.*).

Kadaru 'കഭ' or rather *Kadaram* കഭരം is the Malyalim
name of *Acacia catechu*; but it is applied to *Alangium hexapetalum* in the Hortus Malabaricus (Vol. IV, Tab. 26).   The correct
name for the latter is *Karutta-ayangólum* കറുത്തഅയ യാലം
(*black Ayangólom*) in contradistinction to *Ayangólam*, which is
the name of *Alangium decapetalum*.

31 ALEURITIS TRILOBA, *Forst.* (*Fruit of——
Bengal Walnut.*)

Ḳhasifc-hindi خسف هندى ; Jouze barri جوز بري .
(*Arab.*) Girdagáne-hindi گردگان هندي ; Chahár-maghze-
hindí چهارمغزهندي (*Pers.*) Hindi-akrót هندي اكروت
Jangli-akrót جنگلي اكروت (*Hind. and Duk.*) Náttu-
akrótu-kottai நாட்டு அக்ரோடுகொட்டை. (*Tam.*) Nàtu-
akrótu-vittu నాటు అక్రోటువిత్తు. (*Tel.*) Náṭ-akróḍu నాట్
అక్రోడు. (*Can.*) Banglá-ákrót. (*Beng*) Gámṭi-akrót.
(*Guz.*) Kakkuna. (*Cing.*) To-ṣikiya-ṣi. (*Bur.*).

The vernacular names given to this plant in every book
which treats of it, are those properly belong to *Juglans regia*,
(*walnut*), and to convert them into those of *Aleuritis triloba*,
(*Belgaum walnut*), it is necessary the word *country, wild, Indian,*
or *Belgaum*, should be added to them.

32. ALHAGI MAURORUM, *Tourn.*

Ḥáj حاج ; Áqúl عاقول ; Sh-oukul-jamal شوك الجمل.
(*Arab.*) Kháre-shutar خار شتر ; Ushtar-khár اشترخار;
Shutar-khár شتر خار. (*Pers.*) Javásá جوا سا ; Javánsá
جوا نسا. (*Hind.*) Girikarṇika గిరికర్ణిక; Tella-giniya-
chettu తెల్లగినియచెట్టు. (*Tel.*) Javaṣhá; Jávásá. (*Beng.*).

The Hindustani names *Únṭ-kaṭárú* and *Únṭ-kaṭyah*, are
applied to this plant in some books, but they are the names of
another plant, probably *Echinops echinatus*.

33. ALHAGI MAURORUM, *Tourn.* (*Manna of.*)

Turanjabín ترنجبين. (*Arab. and Pers.*)

34. ALLIUM CEPA, *Linn.* (*Bulb of——Onion.*)

Baṣl بصل. (*Arab.*) Piyáz پياز. (*Pers. Hind. and Duk.*)
Veṇgáyam வெங்காயம் ; Írulli ஈருள்ளி ; Íra-veṇgáyam
ஈரவெங்காயம் ; Vella-veṇgáyam வெள்ளைவெங்காயம். (*Tam.*)
Vulli-gaḍḍalu ఉల్లిగడ్డలు ; Tella-vulli-gaḍḍalu తెల్లవుల్లిగడ్డలు ;
Erra-vulli-gaḍḍalu ఎఱ్ఱవుల్లిగడ్డలు ; Nirulli నిరుల్లి. (*Tel.*) Ven-
gáyam വെങ്കായം ; Chokanna-ulli ചൊകന്ന ഉള്ളി ; Íra-ven-
gáyam ഈരവെങ്കായം. (*Malyal.*) Írulli ಈರುಳ್ಳಿ. (*Can.*)
Piyáj. (*Beng.*) Palánḍuhu. (*Sans.*) Kándé. (*Mah.*) Dun-
gaḷi ; Kánda. (*Guz.*) Lúnú. (*Cing.*) Keṣún-ni. (*Bur.*).

In some languages in the Catalogue, same names are
applied to both the *onion* and *garlic*, and they are distinguished
from each other by the words *red* and *white;* while the same distinction in some other languages will only indicate the varieties
of the former. This is a source of confusion, particularly with
reference to the names of the white variety of *onion*, which are
very apt to be confounded with those of the *garlic.* To avoid
this confusion, I have included in the text the names of the

white and red varieties of *onion* in those languages in which the *garlic* has the same names, except the distinction of color.

In Cingalese, the names of the *common salt* and *onion* are sometimes confounded with each other from the great resemblance of their sounds. The slight difference which exists between them is shown in their spelling by an accent over the letter *ú* in the latter.

Kúndú كاندا is properly the Hindustani name of the *Indian squill (Urginea Indica)* and it should be confined to that drug, although misapplied in some books to *Onion;* probably in accordance with the usage of the Mahratti and Guzratti languages, in which the synonyms for the latter are *Kándé* and *Kúndo,* respectively.

35. ALLIUM SATIVUM, *Linn.* (*Bulb of——Garlic.*)

Şóm نوم; Fóm فوم. (*Arab.*) Sír سير. (*Pers.*) Lahsan لهسن. (*Hind.*) Lassan لسن. (*Duk.*) Vellaip-púndu வெள்ளைப்பூண்டு; Vellulli வெல்லுள்ளி. (*Tam.*) Tellagadda తెల్లగడ్డ; Vellulli వెల్లుల్లి. (*Tel.*) Vellulli വെളുള്ളി. (*Malyal.*) Belluli ಬೆಳ್ಳುಳಿ. (*Can.*) Rasun; Laşhan. (*Beng.*) Lasuna. (*Sans.*) Lasaņa. (*Mah.*) Lasan; Şhunam. (*Guz.*) Sudu-lúnú. (*Cing.*) Keşun-phiú. (*Bur.*).

See the remarks on *Allium cepa.*

36. ALOE INDICA, *Roy.*

Nabátuşşibr نبات الصبر; Aalsí علسي. (*Arab.*) Darakhte-şibr د. درخت صبر. (*Pers.*) Ghígavár كهيگوار; Kanvàr كنوار; Kumárí كاى. (*Hind.*) Ghi-kanvár كهي كنوار; Kanvár-pátha كنوار پاتها; Kalbandá كل بندا. (*Duk.*) Katrázh-ai கற்றுழை; Shóttu-katrázh-ai சோற்றுகற்றுழை; Kumari குமரி. (*Tam.*).

Kalabanda కలబంద. *(Tel.)* Katru-vázha കറ്റുവാഴ. *(Malyal.)*
Lóla-sará ಲೋಳೆಸರ. *(Can.)* *Ghirta-kumári* ; Kumári; *Ghirta-*
kanvár. *(Beng.)* Komári ; Kumár. *(Guz.)* Komárika. *(Cing.)*
Tazávon-le-pa or *Shazávn-le-pa. (Bur.).*

Komárika is the Cingalese name of the above plant, but is
often incorrectly applied to *aloes (the drug)* in some books.

37. ALOE LITORALIS. *Koen.*

Chhótá-rákus-pattah چهوٹا راکس پته ; *Chhótá-kanvár*
چهوٹا کنوار. *(Hind. and Duk.)* Shiru-katrázh-ai சிறுகற்
றுழை. *(Tam.)* Chinna-kalabanda చిన్నకలబంద; Chinna-
rákáshi-matta చిన్నరాక్షిమట్ట. *(Tel.)* Cheru-katru-vázha
ചെറുകറ്റുവാഴ. *(Malyal.)* Kattáli ಕತ್ತಾಲಿ; Shíme-kattáli
ಸೀಮೆಕತ್ತಾಲಿ. *(Can.)* Chhóta-jangli-ánanásh. *(Beng.)* Náni-
komári. *(Guz).*

In one or two books ' Koyangali' is found to be the name
of the above plant in Burmese, but it is the name of a small
variety of *Crinum Asiaticum.*

38. ALOES, *(the drug).*

Sibr صبر. *(Arab.)* Sibr صبر ; Bóle-síyáh بول سیاہ. *(Pers.)*
Musabbar مصبر ; Ilvá الوا ; Yalvá یلو. *(Hind.)* Élvá ایلوا,
Musanbar مصنبر. *(Duk.)* Kariya-pólam கரியபோளம்; Irakta-
pólam இரக்தபோளம். *(Tam.)* Múshámbaram మూషాంబరం.
(Tel.) Chenna-náyakam ചെന്നനായകം. *(Malyal.)* Mó-
shabbar. *(Beng.)* Musambarabóla. *(Mah.)* Yéliyo. *(Guz.)*
Kalu-bólam or Kari-bólam *(Cing.)* Mou or Mo. *(Bur.).*

See the remarks under *Aloe Indica* with regard to the
Cingalese name *Komárika.*

39. ALPINIA GALANGA, *Swz.* (*Root of——Greater galangal*).

Ḵhúlanjáne-qaṣbi خولنجان قصبی ; Ḵhúlanjáne-kabír خولنجان كبیر. (*Arab.*)   Ḵhusrave-dárúé-kaláṅ خسروداروئ كلان (*Pers.*) Baṛá-kulanján بڑا كلنجان ; . (*Hind.*) Baṛá-kalíjan بڑا كليجن ; Baṛá-kulanjan بڑا كلنجن . (*Duk.*) Baṛá-ḵhúlanjan بڑا خولنجن . Péra-ṛattai பேரரத்தை (*Tam.*) Pedda-dumpa-ráshṭrakaṃ పెద్దదుంపరాష్ట్రకం (*Tel.*) Péra-ratta പേരരത്ത. (*Malyal.*) Dumpa-rásmí దుంపరాస్మి. (*Can.*) Baṛákalanján. (*Beng.*) Dumparástma. (*Sans.*) Padagoji *or* Padegoji. (*Bur.*).

The *greater* and *lesser galangals* are generally known and sold in the bazaars of India as the roots of the *betle-leaf plant* (*Chavica Betle*). The *greater galangal* is considered to be the *Baṛé* or *Suféd Pún-ki-jaṛ* بڑے یا سفید پان كی جڑ (*root of the large or white variety of Chavica Betle*), and the *lesser galangal*, the Chhóṭé or *Kalé Pún-ki-jaṛ* چھوتے یا كالی پان كی جڑ (*root of the small or black variety of Chavica Betle*). Although this is according to the popular notion among the natives, including many practitioners and druggists, and also according to many medical and other works, yet it is quite contrary to the fact. The root of *Chavica Betle*, however old it may be, is neither a tuberous root, nor bears any resemblance whatever to the *lesser* or *greater galangal*. The greater galangal is the rhizome of *Alpinia galanga*, and I believe the lesser galangal also to be the produce of another species of the same genus, and shall describe it in another place.

From the great similarity of the Hindustani synonymes of the *lesser* and *greater galangals* to those of *Nigella Indica* (*N. sativa*) in the same language, they are generally confounded with each other. The name of the latter is *Kalónji*, not *Kulanjan*, &c., as found in several books.

40. ALSTONIA SCHOLARIS, *R. Br.*

Ézhilaip-pálai எழிலைப்பாலை. (*Tam.*) Éḍákula-pála ఎడాకులపాల ; Pála-garuḍa పాలగరుడ ; Éḍákula-ariṭi ఎడాకులఅరిటి

ఆకు; Édákula-ponna ఏడాకులపొన్న. *(Tel.)* Pála പാല;
Mukkan-pala മുക്കമ്പാല. *(Malyal.)* Chhátin. *(Beng.)*.

' *Rook-attana*' is the Cingalese name found in some books
for *A. scholaris*, but it is very doubtful one and requires to be
avoided, because *attana* is the name of *Datura*, and '*Rook-attana*'
appears, therefore, to be the name of one of its species.

41. ALUMEN. *(Alum.)*

Shib شب ; **Záj** زاج ; **Zájc-abyaz** زاج ابيض .. *(Arab.)*
Zák زاك ; **Zake-suféd** زاك سفيد ; **Zake-bilór** زاك بلور .
(Pers.) **Phiṭkári** پهٹكرى . *(Hind.)* **Phaṭakṛi** پهٹكژي .
(Duk.) **Paṭi-káram** பழிகாரம்; **Shiná-káram** சிணகாரம்.
(Tam.) **Paṭi-káram** పటికారం. *(Tel.)* **Paṭik-káram** പടി
ക്കാരം; **Chinik-káram** ചിനിക്കാരം. *(Malyal.)* **Paṭi-kárá**
ಪಟಿಕಾರ. *(Can.)* **Phiṭkiri.** *(Beng.)* Turaṭi ; Paṭikár.
(Mah.) **Phatakarḍi.** *(Guz.)* Sina-káram *or* Chinna-káram.
(Cing.) Keo-*khin or* Kiyou-*khin*. *(Bur.)*.

Sahinda-lunu is the Cingalese name of another salt, but
incorrectly applied to *alum* in some books.

42. AMARANTHUS SPINOSUS, *Linn.*

Kánṭe-mát كانٹے مات . *(Duk.)* **Mulluk-kírai** முள்ளுக்க
ீரை. *(Tam.)* **Mundla-tóta-kúra** ముండ్లతోటకూర ; **Nalla-**
doggali నల్లడొగ్గలి. *(Tel.)* **Mullan-chíra** ഉള്ളച്ചീര. *(Malyal)*
Mulla-danṭu ముళ్ళదంటు. *(Can.)* **Kánṭá-naṭi ; Kánṭá-maris.**
(Beng.) **Kánṭá-nu-danṭ.** *(Guz.)* Hinkanoe-súbà *or* Hinnoe-
súbá. *(Bur.)*.

43. AMMANNIA VESICATORIA, *Roxb.*

Dád-màri دادمارى *(Hind.)* Agin-búti اگن بوٹی
(Duk.) **Kalluriví** கல்லுரிவி; **Nirumél-neruppu** திரு?மல்

ஒடருப்பு. *(Tam.)* Agni-venḍa-pàku అగ్నివెండపాకు. *(Tel.)* Kallúr-vanchi കള്ളൂർവഞ്ചി. *(Malyal.)*.

44. AMMONIÆ HYDROCHLORAS. *(Hydrochlorate of Ammonia or Sal-ammoniac.)*

Armínà ارمينا ; Milḥunnàr ملح النار . *(Arab.)* Nósh-ádar نوشادر . *(Pers.)* Nousàdar نوسادر . *(Hind.)* Nou-sàgar نوساگر . *(Duk.)* Navàch-chàram நவாச்சாரம் ; Navà-chàram நவாசாரம் ; Chàram சாரம். *(Tam.)* Navá-sàgarain నవాసాగరం : Navà-chàram నవాచారం. *(Tel.)* Nava-sàram നവസാരം. *(Malyal.)* Navà-sàgarà ನವಾಸಾಗರ. *(Can.)* Nóshàgar. *(Beng.)* Navsàgar. *(Guz.)* Navàchàram. *(Cing.)* Zavaṣa. *(Bur.)*.

45. AMMONIACUM. *(Ammoniac or Gum Ammoniac.)*

Ush-shaq أشق ; Ush-shaj اشج . *(Arab.)* Ush-shah اشه ; Kilyàní كلياني . *(Pers.)* Gama-nàyakam கமநாயகம். *(Tam.)* Gama-nàyakam గమనాయకం. *(Tel.)*.

46. AMOMUM. *Sp. of.* *(Capsules of.)*

Qàqilahe-kubàr قاقلة كبار ; Hél-ẕakar هيل ذكر . *(Arab.)* Qàqilahe-kalàṅ قاقلة كلان ; Qàqilahe-ẕakar قاقلة ذكر . *(Pers.)* Baṛi-ilàchí بڑی الاجي . *(Hind.)* Baṛi-ilàyechi بڑی الايچي . *(Duk.)* Periya-yélak-kày பெரியயேலக்காய் ; Kàṭṭu-yélak-kày காட்டுயேலக்காய். *(Tam.)* Pedda-yéla-kàyalu పెద్దయేలకాయలు : Aḍavi-yéla-kàya అడవియేలకాయ. *(Tel.)* Péré-lam പെരേലം ; Periya-élattari പെരിയ ഏലത്തരി. *(Malyal.)* Doḍḍa-yélakki ದೊಡ್ಡಯೇಲಕ್ಕಿ. *(Can.)* Baraalachi. *(Beng.)* Brahata-upakunchikà. *(Sans.)* Thora-vélà. *(Mah.)* Moṭṭo-ilàchi. *(Guz.)*.

The meaning of almost all the above synonyms is *the larger cardamom*, and they are generally applied in India to a kind of *cardamom* which is not the capsule of *the true paradise grains* (although considered to be so in many medical and other works), but may be a variety of it, and it is of very inferior kind. The following is a description of this capsule and its seeds:—

Capsule—Ovate or bluntly triangular, with a tuft of fibres at its smaller end, which is often destroyed in course of time; generally 1 inch in length, and 1½ inches in circumference; ribbed; coriaceous; and reddish brown in color.

Seeds—Small; almost round or bluntly angular; brown; and feebly aromatic in taste and smell, the latter not being distinct until they are bruised or chewed.

Although all the names in the text are synonymous with each other, but the *cardamom* under reference is more easily recognised in Calcutta, Hyderabad, Bombay, and many other places, under the Arabic name *Qiqilahe-kubar* than any other. In Madras, it is also easily obtained under the following names, which signify *the wild cardamom.*

Jangli-ilàchi جنگلي الا چي. *(Duk.)* *Kàṭṭu-élakkáy* காட்டு ஏலக்காய். *(Tam.)* *Aḍavi-élakáya.* అడవియేలకాయ. *(Tel.)*

When other names are used, the druggists generally give the *larger* capsules *picked out* from different varieties of the *lesser cardamom;* and often they sell the same *(wilfully)* under every name in the text. *Hyderabádi-iláyechi* حیدرابادی الایچی is the proper Hindustani name for one very large *(perhaps the largest)* variety of the *lesser cardamom* in India, which differs in no other way from the capsules of *Elettaria cardamomum,* except the size. See the remarks on the following article.

47. AMOMUM. *Sp. of.* *(Seeds of.)*

Ilàyechi-dànah الایچیدانه *or* Ilàyechi-dàné الایچیدانے. *(Hind.)* Ilàchi-dànah الاچیدانه *or* Ilàchi-dàne الاچیدانے. *(Duk.)* Élam ஏலம். *(Tam.)* Élakulu యేలకులు. *(Tel).*

The above seeds are not the produce of India, but are said to be imported from Singapoor, China, and Burmah, and this must be in great abundance, for they are always found in every large bazaar, and are much cheaper than the seeds of *the common or Malabar cardamom*. They are often confounded with the latter and sold under the same names, but can be distinguished from them by the following characters:—

They are angular and very irregular seeds, generally inclining to be triangular, and sometimes compressed or flat; smaller in size than the common cardamom seeds; color pale-brown; odour strongly aromatic and agreeable; and taste aromatic and slightly pungent. Although the smell and taste of these seeds are stronger than those of the common or Malabar cardamom (*Elettaria cardamomum*), yet they are more agreeable; and there is the same difference between the *Tinctures* prepared from these drugs.* The seeds under reference are always brought to India without their capsule or pericarp, and the reason of this I believe is, that when the fruit arrives at a certain maturity, it bursts and the seeds are either scattered or remain loosely in the capsule, which are picked up or taken out, washed, dried, and then sent out to different places for sale.

These seeds may be either a variety of the *paradise grains*, or the produce of the *Amomum xanthioides* of Wallich. The latter is more probable, because the facts of the seeds being confounded with the *Malabar cardamom* and sold without their pericarp, correspond with the remarks on that plant by Mr. Daniel Hanbury in his 'Notes on Chinese Materia Medica,' published in 1862 at London. But, as I never had an opportunity of seeing myself the seeds or capsules of *A. xanthioides*, I cannot be positive on this point, and did not, therefore, place the plant at the heading of this article.

The seeds under consideration are used in India chiefly as a medicine and for preparing one kind of sweet-meat, but are neither chewed with the *betel-leaf*, nor made use of in curries, &c., as is the case with the seeds of the common cardamom.

The meaning of the Hindustani and Dukhni names in the text is simply *the cardamom seeds*, and therefore they can be

---

* By further examinations I find that the easiest and readiest way of distinguishing the above seeds from the common cardamom seeds is by their freeness of the bitterish taste, which is slightly but distinctly felt when the latter are well chewed.

applied to the seeds of any cardamom; but according to the usage of the languages, they are generally restricted to the above seeds, because they are, as already remarked, always found in the bazaar without their capsules.

The Tamil and Telugu names in the text are also confined to these seeds, and in contradistinction of which the following names are used for the seeds of the common cardamom.

Elakáy-virai எலகாய்விரை. *(Tam.)* *Elakúya-vittulu* యెలకాయవిత్తులు. *(Tel.)*

48. AMYGDALA. *(Almond.)*

Louz لوز. *(Arab.)* Bàdàm بادام. *(Pers. and Hind.)* **Bàdam** بادم. *(Duk.)* Vàdam-koṭṭai வாதம்கொட்டை. *(Tam.)* Bádam-vittulu చాదంవిత్తులు. *(Tel.)* Bádam ബാ ദം; Vàtam-kotṭa വാതംകൊട്ട. *(Malyal.)* Bàdàmi ಬಾದಾ ಮಿ. *(Can.)* Bilàti-badàm. *(Beng)* Bádámitte. *(Sans.)* Bàdàm. *(Mah.)* Badàm. *(Guz.)* Raṭa-koṭambà. *(Cing.)* Bàdan. *(Bur.)*.

If necessary, the *sweet* and *bitter varieties* of *almond* should be distinguished as follows:—

a. Sweet almond—*Louzul-ḥaló* لوزالحلو. *(Arab.)* *Bádúme-shírín* بادام شيرين. *(Pers.)* *Miṭhé-bádám* میٹھے بادام. *(Hind. and Duk.)* *Tittippu-vádam-koṭṭai* தித்திப்புவாதம்கொட்டை. *(Tam.)* *Tipu-bádam-vittulu* తీపుచాదంవిత్తులు. *(Tel.)* *Madhura-bádam* മധുരബാദം; *Madhura-vátam-koṭṭa* മധുരവാതംകൊട്ട. *(Malyal.)* *Shíyúda-bádámi* ಶಿಯೂದಬಾದಾಮಿ. *(Can.)* *Miṭhá-ba-dím. (Beng.)* *Madhuryá-bádámitte. (Sans.)* *Guḷachiṭa-bádám. (Mah.)* *Miṭho-badám. (Guz.)* *Peni-raṭu-koṭambú. (Cing.).*

b. Bitter almond—*Louzul-murr* لوزالمر. *(Arab.)* *Bádúmé-talkh* بادام تلخ. *(Pers.)* *Karvé-bádám* کروے بادام. *(Hind. and Duk.)* *Kaṣhappu-vádam-koṭṭai* கசப்புவாதம்கொட்டை. *(Tam.)* *Chédu-bádam-vittulu* చేడుచాదంవిత్తులు. *(Tel.)* *Kaipa-bádam* കൈപ്പബാദം; *Kaipa-vátam-koṭṭu* കൈപവാതംകൊട്ട

Malyal.) *Tikta-bádámi* ತಿ ಕ್ತುಬಾದಾಮಿ. *(Can.)* *Tito-badím.* *(Beng.)* *Tikta-bádámitte.* *(Sans.)* *Kaḍú-bádám.* *(Mah.)* *Kaḍuru-badám.* *(Guz.)* *Titta-raṭu-koṭambú.* *(Cing.).*

The names in the text are often improperly applied to *Terminalia catappa*, the correct names of which will be given under its proper head ·

49. ANACARDIUM OCCIDENTALE, *Linn.* (*Nut of——Cashew nut.*)

Kàjú-ki-guṭli كاجوكي گنٹلي ——*fruit of,* Kájú كاجو . (*Hind and Duk.*) Koṭṭai-mundiri கொட்டைமுந்திரி; Mundiri-koṭṭai· முந்திரிகொட்டை. (*Tam.*) Jiḍi-màmiḍi-vittu జీడిమామిడివిత్తు ; Muntamámiḍi-vittu ముంతమామిడివిత్తు. *(Tel.)* Paranki-máva പറങ്കിമാവ ; Kappal-chérun-kuru കപ്പല് ചെരുകുരു ; Kappa-mávakuru കപ്പമാവകുരു. (*Malyal.*) Gérapoppu ಗೇರಪಪ್ಪು. *(Can.)* Hijli-bádám ; Kájú. (*Beng.*) Kájúcha-bi. (*Mah.*) Kàju. (*Guz.*) Kaju *or* Kaju-aṭṭa. (*Cing.*) Ṣihosaye-si *or* Tihotiya-si. (*Bur.*).

The Canarese name for *cashew-nut* and *marking-nut* is nearly the same. In some languages the same name is often applied to both the *nut* and *fruit* of *A. occidentale.*

50. ANAMIRTA COCCULUS, *W. et A.* (*Seeds of—Cocculus Indicus seeds.*)

Kákmári-ké-binj كاكماري بينج . (*Hind. and Duk.*) Kákkáy-kolli-virai காக்காய்கொல்லிவிரை; Pén-koṭṭai பென்கொட்டை. (*Tam.*) Káka-mári కాకమారి; Káki-champa కాకిచంప. (*Tel.*) Karaṇṭa-kattin-káya കരണ്ടകത്തിന്കായ; Poḷḷak-kàya പൊള്ളക്കായ. (*Malyal.*) Kákamári-bijá ಕಾಕಮಾರಿಬಿಜಾ. (*Can.*) Kàkà-mári. (*Beng.*) Tittaval. *Cing.*).

51. ANANAS SATIVUS, *Mill.* (*Pine apple.*)

Aṣinunnás عين الناس . (*Arab. and Pers.*) Anannás
اناس ; Anánás اناناس . (*Hind.*) Annannas انس :
(*Duk.*) Anáshap-pazham அனாசப்பழம். (*Tam.*) Anása-
paṇḍu అనాసపండు. (*Tel.*) Kaita-chakka കൈതചക്ക ;
Parangi-chakka പറങ്കിചക്ക. (*Malyal.*) Anánasu-haṇṇu
ಅನಾಸುಹಣ್ಣು. (*Can.*) Ánanásh ; Ánanás. (*Beng.*) Anninas;
Anáras. (*Guz.*) Annási. (*Cing.*) Nanna-ṣi. (*Bur.*).

52. ANDROGRAPHIS ECHIOIDES, *Nees.*

Charáyetah چرايته٠. (*Hind.*) Gópuram-tángi கோபுரம்-
தாங்கி. (*Tam.*) Chalava-puri-káḍa చలవపురికాడ ; Gorre-
chimiḍi గొఱ్ఱచిమిడి. (*Tel.*) Mala-kulukki മലകുളുക്കി.
(*Malyal.*).

53. ANDROGRAPHIS PANICULATA, *Wall.* (*Creat or Kreat.*)

Qaṣabuzzarírah قصب الزريره ; Qaṣabbuvá قصب بوا .
(*Arab.*) Nainehávandí ني نهاوندي . (*Pers.*) Charáyetah
چرايته ; Mahá-títá مهاتيتا ;. Kiryát كريات . (*Hind.*)
Charáyetah چرايته ; Kalaf-náth كلفناته . (*Duk.*) Shiraṭ-
kuch-chi ஷிரட்குச்சி ; Nila-vémbu நிலவேம்பு. (*Tam.*) Néla-
vému నేలవేము. (*Tel.*) Nila-véppa നിലവെപ്പ ; Kiriyáttu
കിരിയാത്തു (*Malyal.*)· Nela-bevinágiḍá ನೆಲಬೆವಿನಾಗಿಡಾ.
(*Can.*) Cherota ; Mahá-tita. (*Beng.*) Bhúnimbaha. (*Sans.*)
Chiráyitá. (*Mah.*) Kiryáta ; Kiryáto. (*Guz.*) Binko-
hamba *or* Hinbinko-hamba. (*Cing.*).

Kara-kanniram or ' Cara caniram' is the Malyalim name
found in the Hortus Malabaricus (Vol. IX, Tab. 56), which

means *the black Strychnos nux vomica*. It is neither correct nor safe to be applied to *A. paniculata*.

The Bengali appellation given to this plant in the Hortus Suburbanus Calcuttensis and several other works is ' Kalo-megh.' It is not generally recognisable as the name of any plant. Its literal meaning is *the black cloud*.

' *Sitta rattai*' occurs as the Cingalese designation of *chiretta* in some books, but it is properly the name of the *Lesser galangal*.

54. ANDROPOGON MARTINI, *Roxb.* *Syn.* A. CALAMUS AROMATICUS, *Roy. (Oil of——Rousà-kn-tél.)*

Rousá-kà-tél روساكاتيں ; Rousá-ká-aitr روساكاعطر . (Hind.) Rousá-ká-aatar روساكاعطر . (Duk.).

See the rémarks on the next plant.

55. ANDROPOGON MURICATUS, *Retz. (Khus-khus grass——Roots of.)*

Usír أسير . (*Arab.*) Khas خس . (*Pers.*) Bálah باب or Bálá بالا . (*Hind. and Duk.*) Vetti-vér வெட்டி-வேர் ; Vizhal-vér விழல்வேர் ; Ilàmich-cham-vér இலாமிச்சம்வேர் ; Víraṇam வீரணம். (*Tam.*) Vaṭṭi-véru వట్టివేరు ; Ávvuru-gaḍḍi-véru ఆవ్వురుగడ్డివేరు ; Làmajjakamu-véru లామజ్జకమువేరు ; Viḍavali-véru విడవలివేరు ; Ouru-véru ఔరువేరు. (*Tel.*) Veṭṭi-vér വെട്ടിവേര ; Rámach-cham-vér രാമച്ചംവേര. (*Malyal.*) Lávanchá ಲಾವಂಚಾ. (*Can.*) Bálá ; Shandalér-jar. (*Beng.*) Uṣhíram. (*Sans.*) Válá. (*Mah.*) Válo. (*Guz.*) Savandra-múl. (*Cing.*) Miya-móe. (*Bur.*).

In Madras and all other parts of Southern India, the lowest part of the culms of this grass (*A. muricatus*) with or without a portion of its roots, is cut out and sold under the

Arabic name *Izkhïr* اذخر while the same name is used for the roots of *A. Schœnanthus* in Hyderabad, Calcutta, &c. I am informed by a few persons that have seen the *Izkhir* in Arabia, that this grass resembles the *Rousá-ká-ghás* of upper India, but it is not the same. *Rousá-ká-ghás* is the name of *A. Martini.*

The true *Izkhir* does not exist in India, and the best substitute for it is the root of *A. muricatus*, which is correctly designated *Izkhire-hindi* اذخرهندي (*Indian Izkhir*) in some books.

The meaning of the Bengali name Shandlér-jar is *the root of sandle*, and it is applied to the roots of *A. muricatus* from the resemblance of their smell to that of the *sandle-wood*. 'Khus-khus' is the English name (probably from the Persian *khas*) of the grass, and its meaning in Bengali is *the poppy-seeds*. In some books, however, it is converted into 'Khuskhus-ghas' and applied to the grass under reference as a Bengali name, which is not correct.

56. ANDROPOGON NARDUS, *Linn.* (*Oil of.*)

Ganjní-ká-aitr كنجني كاعطر. (*Hind.*) **Ganjní-ka-aatar** كنجني كاعطر. (*Duk.*) **Kámákshi-pullu-yenney** காமாகூஷிபுல் லுயென்னெய்; **Mándap-pullu-yenney** மாந்தப்புலலுயென் னெய்; **Kávattam-pullu-yenney** ; காவட்டம்புல்லுயென்னெய்; **Shunnárip-pullu-yenney** சுன்னுரிப்புல்லுயென்னெய். (*Tam.*) **Kámákshi-kasuvu-núne** ; **Kámanchi-gaddi-núne** . (*Tel.*) **Kámákshi-pulla-enna** ; **Chóra-pulla-enna** . (*Malyal.*) **Ganda-hanchi-khaddi-yanne** . (*Can.*) **Ká-má-khér-tail.** (*Beng.*) **Sinng-ou-miá-Si.** (*Bur.*).

57. ANDROPOGON SCHŒNANTHUS, *Linn.* *Syn.*

A. CITRATUS, *D. C. (Oil of——Lemon-grass oil.*)

Róghane-cháe-kashmíri روغن چاءكشميري. (*Pers.*) **Ak-yá-ghás-ka-aitr** اكياگھاسكاعطر. (*Hind.*) **Hazár-masáleh-ká-**

a̤aṭar اِزخر مصالح کا عطر. *(Duk.)* Vásh*a*nap-pullu-yeṇṇcy வாசனைப் புல்லுவெண்ணெய்; Karpúra-pullu-yeṇṇey கர்ப்பூரபுல்லுவெண்ணெய். *(Ṭam.)* Nimma-gaḍḍi-núne నిమ్మగడ్డినూనె; Ch*i*ppa-gaḍ-ḍi-núne చిప్పగడ్డినూనె. *(Tel.)* Vásanap-pulla-eṇṇa വാസനപ്പുല്ലെണ്ണ; Samb*h*àra-pulla-eṇṇa സംഭാരപ്പുല്ലെണ്ണ. *(Malyal.)* Púrvaḷi-hullú-yaṇṇe ಪೂರ್ವಳಿಹುಲ್ಲುಯಣ್ಣೆ; Vásane-hullú-yaṇṇe ವಾಸನೆಹುಲ್ಲುಯಣ್ಣೆ. *(Can.)* Agya-*gh*áṅs-t*a*il. *(Beng.)* Dévajag*dh*aka-t*a*ilam. *(Sans.)* Lilli-*ch*áya-tél. *(Guz.)* Pengrimá-tel. *(Cing.)* Sabaleṉ-Ṣ̤i. *(Bur.)*.

In the Hortus Malabaricus, where this grass is correctly figured (Vol. XII, Tab. 72) *Rámach-cham* രാമച്ചം is the Malyalim name assigned to it, whereas it is undoubtedly the name of *A. muricatus*. There is a much greater confusion in several other works (Materia Indica, Hortus Suburbanus Calcuttensis, Flora Andhrica, and Shakespear, Forbes, Bailey, Reeve, Rottler and Winslow's Dictionaries, &c.,) in which the names of this grass, as well as of several others, are confounded with each other. As it is rather tedious to explain all these confusions separately, I shall not enter upon their explanation, and think it sufficient to state that the species of grasses included in this Catalogue are generally and correctly recognisable, at present, only by the names inserted in the text under each of their heads.

Pengrimá-tel is the proper Cingalese name for the *Lemon-grass oil* and not '*Saira-tel*' as found in some books.

See the remarks on *A. muricatus.*

58. ANETHUM SOWA, *Roxb.* *(Fruits of——Dill seeds.)*

*Sh*ibbit شبت. *(Arab.)* Vàlàne-*k̤h*urd والان خرد; Shód شود. *(Pers.)* Suvà سوا; Sóyah سويه. *(Hind.)* Sóyí سوئي. *(Duk.)* Ṣ*h*atakuppi-vir*a*i சதகுப்பிவிரை; Ṣ*h*óyi-kír*a*i-vir*a*i சோயிக்கீரைவிரை. *(Tam.)* Ṣ*h*atakuppi-vittulu శతకుప్పవిత్తులు;

Pedda-sadápara-vittulu పెద్దసాదాపరవిత్తులు; Sóyikúra-vittulu సోయికూరవిత్తులు. *(Tel.)* Ṣhatakuppa ശതകുപ്പ. *(Malyal.)* Sabbasagi సబ్బసగి. *(Can.)* Ṣhulphá; Ṣhónvá or Ṣhóvá. *(Beng.)* Suvá; Suvá-nu-bí. *(Guz.)* Sada-kuppa; Sata-kuppi. *(Cing.)* Samíṅ. *(Bur.)*.

The Burmese names of the seeds of *Anethum sowa* and *Ptychotis ajwain* are mistaken for each other in some books in consequence of the analogy of their sounds. *Sópu* is the Telugu name of *aniseed*, but is incorrectly applied to the seeds of *Anethum sowa* in Flora Andhrica and some other books.

59. ANISOCHILUS CARNOSUS, *Wall.*

Panjirí-ká-pát پنجيري كا پات; Sitá-ki-panjírí پنجيري كا پتا; سيتاكي پنجيري. *(Hind.)* Panjirí-ká-pattá پنجيري كا پتا; Ajván-ká-pattá اجوان كا پتا. *(Duk.)* Karppúra-vaḷḷi கர்ப்பூர வல்லி. *(Tam.)* Karpúra-valli కర్పూరవల్లి; Ómamu-áku ఓమముఆకు; Róga-cheṭṭu రోగచెట్టు. *(Tel.)* Chómara ചൊമര; Káṭṭu-kúrkká കാട്ടുക്കൂക്ക; Kúrkká കൂക്ക; Paṭu-kúrkká പടുക്കൂക്ക. *(Malyal.)* Doḍḍa-patri ದೊಡ್ಡಪತ್ರಿ. *(Can.)* Kapúrli. *(Mah.)* Ájmu-nu-pátro. *(Guz.)*.

In Flora Andhrica, *Karpúra-valli* is applied to *Coleus amboinicus (C. aromaticus)*, and its application to *Anisochilus carnosus* is considered to be incorrect. The names given to the latter plant in that work are *Róga-cheṭṭu* and *Piṇḍi-boṇḍa*. This may be the case in some parts of the Northern Circars; but, if the plant figured in the Hortus Malabaricus (Vol. X, Tab. 90) is *A. carnosus (which I have no doubt it is)*, *Karpúra-valli* is more in use for that plant in most parts of Southern India, both in Telugu and Tamil, than any other name. The next name frequently in use in Telugu is *Ómamu-áku.*

The literal meaning of the Dukhni, Telugu, and Guzeratti names *Ajván-ká-pattá*, *Ómamu-áku,* and *Ajmu-nu-pátro* is *the leaf of Ptychotis Aiwain,* and they are applied to *A. carnosus* simply on account of the resemblance of the smell of its leaves with that of the seeds of the former.

60. ANISODUS LURIDUS, *Link.*

61. ANISOMELES MALABARICA, *R. Br. (Malabar Cat-mint.)*

Mogbiré-kà-pattà مگبیریکاپتا (*Duk.*) Péya-veruṭṭi பேய வெருட்டி; Péy-maruṭṭi பேய்மருட்டி; Iraṭṭai-péy-maruṭṭi இரட்டைபேய்மருட்டி. (*Tam.*) Moga-bira ముగబీర; Màbhéri మాభేరి; China-raṇa-bhéri చీనరణభేరి; Maga-bira మగబీర. (*Tel.*) Péyi-meraṭṭi പെയിമെരട്ടി; Peruntumba പെരുന്തുമ്പ; Karintumba കരിംതുമ്പ. (*Malyal.*).

62. ANTHEMIS. (*Chamomile flowers.*)

Bábúnaj بابونج . (*Arab.*) Bábúnah بابونه ; Gule-bábúnàh گل بابونه . (*Pers.*) Bábúné-ké-phúl بابونے کے پهول . (*Hind. and Duk.*) Shimai-chámantippú ஷிமைசாமந்திப்பூ. (*Tam.*) Sima-chámanti-pushpamu సీమచామంతిపుష్పము. (*Tel.*) Shima-jevanti-pushpam ശീമജെവന്തിപൂഷ്പം. (*Malyal.*) Shime-shyámantigé ಶೀಮೆಶ್ಯಾಮಂತಿಗೆ. (*Can.*)

63. ANTIARIS SACCIDORA, *Dalz.*

Neṭṭávil-maram நெட்டாவில்மரம். (*Tam.*) Neṭṭávil നെട്ടാവില്. (*Malyal.*).

64. ANTIMONII SULPHURETUM. *Syn.* ANTIMONIUM SULPHURATUM. (*Sulphuret or Tersulphuret of Antimony.*)

Iṣmad اثمد ; Koḥal کحل. (*Arab.*) Surmah سرمه ; Sange-surmah سنگ سرمه. (*Pers.*) Surmah سرمه ; Surmé-ká-

patthar سرمے کا پتهر . (*Hind.*) Anjan انجن; Anjan-ká-patthar
انجن کا پتهر (*Duk.*) Aṇjanak-kallu
(*Tam.*) Anjana-ráyi (*Tel.*) Aṇjanak-kalla
(*Malyal.*) Anjená (*Can.*) Ṣhurmá
or Surmá. (*Beng.*) Anjanam. (*Sans.*) Surmo; Surmo-nu-
phatro. (*Guz.*) Shurma-khiyia *or* Súrma-khiyo. (*Bur.*).

65. AQUA. (*Water.*)

Máa ماء . (*Arab.*) Áb آب . (*Pers.*) Páni پاني .
(*Hind. and Duk.*) Taṇṇi ; Jalam ; Nir .
(*Tam.*) Jalam ; Niḷḷu . (*Tel.*) Veḷḷam .
(*Malyal.*) Niru . (*Can.*) Jal; Páni. (*Beng.*)
Jalam. (*Sans.*) Páṇi. (*Mah.*) Páni. (*Guz.*) Vaturu.
(*Cing.*) Yé. (*Bur.*).

The following are the names of the *rain* and *distilled* waters,
which are often required for pharmaceutical purposes:—

a. Rain-water——*Múe-matar* ماءمطر . (*Arab.*) *Ábe-*
búrún آب باران . (*Pers.*) *Ménh-ká-páni* مينهـکا پاني; *Barsát-ká-*
páni برسات کا پاني . (*Hind.*) *Méhún-ká-páni* ميهون کا پاني . (*Duk.*)
Mazh-ait-taṇṇi . (*Tam.*) *Vúna-níḷḷu* .
(*Tel.*) *Mazha-veḷḷam* . (*Malyal.*) *Maḷe-niru*
. (*Can.*) *Brishti-páni; Brishti-jal.* (*Beng.*) *Mégha-*
jalam. (*Sans.*) *Mégha-púṇi.* (*Mah.*) *Barsát-nu-púni.* (*Guz.*)
Vahín-vaturu. (*Cing.*) *Mó-yé.* (*Bur.*).

b. Distilled-water——*Múe-moqattar* ماءمقطر . (*Arab.*)
Ábe-mo-qattar آب مقطر . (*Pers.*) *Tapkáyá-huvá-páni* ٹپکایاهواپاني .
(*Hind.*) *Moqattar-páni* مقطر پاني . (*Duk.*) *Ti-nir* . (*Tam.*).

66. ARACHIS HYPOGÆA, *Linn.* (*Nut of——*
Ground-nut.)

Vilávetí-múng ولايتي مونگ . (*Hind. and Duk.*)
Vérk-kadalai ; Nilak-kadalai . (*Tam.*)

Véruṣhanaga ವೆಊಷಗಸಕ; Véruṣhanaga-káya ವೆಊಷಸಕ ಕಾಯ.
(*Tel.*) Nelak-kaṭalá നെലക്കടലാ; Vérk-kaṭalá പെക്ക
ലാ. (*Malyal.*) Nelagalc-káyi ನೆಲಗಳ ಕಾಯಿ. (*Can.*) Chíná-
bádám; Biláti-mun*g*. (*Beng.*) Bhói-cha*n*é. (*Mah.*)
Bhóya-che*n*á. (*Guz.*) Raṭa-kaju. (*Cing.*) Míbé. (*Bur.*).

67. ARECA CATECHU, *Linn.* (*Nut of——Betel-*
nut.)

Fófal فوفل *or* Foufal فوفل. (*Arab.*) Gird-cḥób
گردچوب; Pópal پوپل. (*Pers.*) Supyári سپياري. (*Hind.*)
Supári سپاري. (*Duk.*) Kamugu கமுகு; Pákku பாக்கு;
Koṭṭai-pákku கொட்டைப்பாக்கு. (*Tam.*) Póka-vakka పోక
వక్క; Vakka వక్క. (*Tel.*) Aṭakka അടക്ക. (*Malyal.*)
Aḍike ಅಡಿಕೆ. (*Can.*) Gu*n*á; Supári; Ṣhupári. (*Beng.*)
Púgi-*ph*alam. (*Sans.*) Suppári. (*Mah.*) Sopári; Hopári.
(*Guz.*) Puvák *or* Puvákka. (*Cing.*) Kún-si. (*Bur.*).

68. ARGEMONE MEXICANA, *Linn.*

Bharbhánḍ بهربهانڈ; Pilá-*dh*atúrá پيلادهتورا; Farangí-
*dh*atúrá فرنگيدهتورا; *Shí*yál-kánṭá شيالكانٹا. (*Hind.*)
Bharamdandí بهرمدنڈي; Pilá-*dh*atúrá پيلادهتورا. (*Duk.*)
Birama-daṇḍu பிரமதண்டு; Kurukkam-*ch*eḍi குருக்கம்செடி.
(*Tam.*) Bramha-danḍi-cheṭṭu బ్రహ్మదండిచెట్టు. (*Tel.*) Brahma-
danti ബ്രഹ്മദന്തി. (*Malyal.*) Ṣiel-káṭá; Ṣhéaál-kánṭá.
(*Beng.*) Khyàà. (*Bur.*).

Datturí ದತ್ತೂರಿ *or Datturí-giḍá* ದತ್ತೂರಿಗಿಡಾ is the Canarese appellation under which the above plant is generally
known in many districts of Mysore, Bangalore, and Bellary;
but as this name is very liable to be confounded with that of
Datura alba in several other languages on account of the similarity of the word *Datturí*, I have not included it in the text.

69. ARGENTUM. *(Silver——Leaf of.)*

Varqul-fizah ورق الفضه . *(Arab.)* Varqe-nuqrah ورق نقره
Varqe-sim ورق سيم . *(Pers.)* Rupehrá-varaq روپهرا ورق
(Hind.) Rupéri-tagat روپيري تگت . *(Duk.)* Velli-rékku
வெள்ளிஇரக்கு. *(Tam.)* Vendi-réku వెండిౌేకు. *(Tel.)*
Vellit-takita പെള്ളിത്തകിട. *(Malyal.)* Belli-rékhu
ಬೆಳ್ಳಿರೇಖು. *(Can.)* Ruppécha-varakh. *(Mah.)* Rupéri-
varakh. *(Guz.)* Ridi-tahadu; Ridi-tagadu. *(Cing.)* Noye-
saku. *(Bur.)*.

70. ARGYREIA SPECIOSA, *Swt.* *(Leaves of)*

Samandar-ká-pát سمندركاپات;   Samandar-sóf
سمندرسوف; Samandar-sókh سمندرسوكه. *(Hind.)* Sa-
mandar-ká-pattá سمندركاپتا. *(Duk.)* Shamuddirap-pach-ch-ai
சமுத்திரப்பச்சை; Kadal-pálai கடல்பாலை. *(Tam.)* Samu-
dra-pála సముద్రపాల; *Chandra-poda* చంద్రపోడ; Kokkita
కొక్కిట; Pála-samudra పాలసముద్ర; Kokkiti కొక్కిటి. *(Tel.)*
Samudra-pach-cha സമുദ്രപച്ച; Samudra-yógam സമുദ്ര
യോഗം; Samudrap-pala സമുദ്രപ്പല *(Malyal.)* Bicho-
tárok. *(Beng.)* Samudracha-pána. *(Mah.)*.

The above plant, which is generally known in Hindustani
and Dukhni by the name of its leaf (*Samandar-ká-pát or Saman-
dar-ká-pattá*) is quite different from the one named, *Samandar-
phal*, in the same languages, although the literal meaning of
both names is almost the same, one signifying *the leaf of Saman-
dar*, and the other *the fruit.* The latter is the name of the fruit
of *Baringtonia acutangula.*

71. ARISTOLOCHIA BRACTEATA, *Retz.*

Gandán گندان; Kírá-már كيرامار. *(Hind. and Duk.)*
Ádu-tinná-pálai ஆடுதிண்ணைபாலை. *(Tam.)* Gádide-gada-

para-áku గాండెగపరఅకు; Kaḍapara కడపర. (Tel.) Aṭu-
tiṇṭáp-paḷa ആടതിണ്ടാപ്പള. (Malyl.).

72. ARISTOLOCHIA INDICA, *Linn.* (Root of.)

Zarávande-hindi زراوندهندي. (*Arab.* and *Pers.*)
Isharmul اشرمل; Isharmul-ki-jar اشرمل کي جڑ. (*Hind.*)
Isharmúl اشرمول; Isharmúl-ki-jar اشرمول کي جڑ. (*Duk.*)
Ich-chura-múli ஈச்சுரமூலி; Peru-marindu பெருமரிந்து;
Perum-kizhaṇgu பெரும்கிழங்கு. (*Tam.*) Íṣhvara-véru
ఈశ్వరవేరు; Dúla-góvela దూలగోవెల; Góvila గోవిల. (*Tel.*)
Karaḷekam കരളെകം; Karukap-pulla കരുകപ്പുല്ല; Karaḷ-
vékam കരംവേകം; Iṣhvarámúri ഈശ്വരാമൂരി. (*Mal-
yal.*) Íṣhveri-bérú ಈಶ್ವರಿಬೇರು. (*Can.*) Íshor-mul or
Íṣhur--múl. (*Beng.*) Sassanda. (*Cing.*).

73. ARRACK. (*Indian Spirituous Liquor.*)*

Khamarul-hind خمر الهند. (*Arab.*)   Maié-hindí
مئي هندي. (*Pers.*)   Sharáb شراب. (*Hind.*)   Dáru
دارو. (*Duk*)   Ṣháṛáyam சாருயம். (*Tam.*) Sáráyi సారాయి.
(*Tel.*)   Cháráyam ചാരായം; Tákaram താകരം. (*Malyal.*)
Sáráyi ಸಾರಾಯಿ. (*Can.*)   Mad; Suráp. (*Beng*)   Surá;
Madyam. (*Sans.*)   Dáru; Saráph. (*Mah.*)   Dáru. (*Guz.*)
Arak *or* Araku. (*Cing.*)   Aye. (*Bur.*).

74. ARSENICUM ALBUM. *Syn.* ACIDUM ARSENIOSUM.
(*Arsenious acid, White Arsenic, or White oxide of
Arsenic.*).

Shuk شک; Turábul-hálik تراب الهالك; Sammulfár
سم الفار. (*Arab*) Marge-mósh مرگ موش *or* Marg-mósh

مرگ‌موش. *(Pers.)* Sunbul-*khár* سنبل‌کھار; Suféd-sunbul سفیدسنبل; Sankhyâ-sunbul سنکھاسنبل *or* Sakhyâ-sunbul سکھیاسنبل. *(Hind. and Duk.)* Vellai-pásháṇam ெவள்ளை பாஷாணம். *(Tam.)* Tella-pásháṇam తెల్లపాషాణం; Shen-ku-páshánam శెంకుపాషాణం. *(Tel.)* Vellap-pásháṇam വെള്ളപ്പാഷാണം. *(Malyal.)* Pháshání ಫಾಷಾಣ *(Can.)* Sumbul-*khàr*; Sammal-*khár.* *(Beng.)* Sómal-*khár.* *(Guz.)* Sudu-pásánam. *(Cing.).*

The word Sunbul سنبل by itself is commonly applied in Dukhni to the *white arsenic*, while the same is frequently used in Arabic and Persian for *Nardostychis jatamansi* (Indian spikenard). To avoid any serious error that might result from the above confusion, I have omitted the word from the text under both medicines, which are well recognised by all other names inserted.

75. ARSENICUM TERSULPHURETUM. *(Yellow Sulphuret of Arsenic or Yellow Orpiment.)*

Zarní*khe*-aṣfar زرنیخ‌اصفر; Arsáníqún ارسانیقون. *(Arab.)* Zarní*khe*-zard زرنیخ‌زرد. *(Pers.)* Harṭál هرتال. *(Hind. and Duk.)* Tàram தாரம்; Ari-táram அரிதாரம்; Ponnari-tárakam பொன்னரிதாரகம்; Tálakam தாளகம். *(Tam.)* Haridaḷam హరిదళం; Tálakamu తాళకము. *(Tel.)* Ponnari-táram പൊന്നരിതാരം; Cháliyam ചാലിയം. *(Malyal.)* Aridaḷá ಅರಿದಳ. *(Can.)* Horitál. *(Beng.)* Hari-tálakam. *(Sans.)* Haritála. *(Mah.)* Artál. *(Guz.)*

76. ARTABOTRYS ODORATISSIMA, *R. Br.*

Madmántí مدن‌مانتی. *(Hind.)* Madan-mast مدن‌مست. *(Duk.)* Manó-raṇjitam மனோரஞ்சிதம். *(Tam.)* Manóranjitam మనోరంజితం; *Phala-sampenga* ఫలసంపెంగ; Sakala-phala-sampenga సకలఫలసంపెంగ. *(Tel.)* Madura-káméṣhvari മധുരാകാമേശ്വരി; Manóranjitam മനോരഞ്ജിതം. *(Malyal.).*

Madan-mast and *Madan-mast-ka-*phúl are the Dukhni names of the above plant and its flower, and their use is confined only in Southern India. In all other parts; such as Hyderabad, Bombay, &c., *Madan-mast* is applied to a root, which will be found described in the remarks on *Curcuma aromatica.*

The Malyalim name *Mótira-valli* മോതിരവള്ളി is found applied to *A. odoratissima* in the Hortus Malabaricus (Vol. VII, Tab. 46), but as it implies *a creeper,* which is not the case with the plant, nor is so figured in that work itself, it is a very doubtful one. See the remarks on the word *Madan-mast* under ' Aconitum. *sp. of.* (*Judvar*).'

77. ARTEMESIA INDICA, *Willd.*

Afsantine-hindí افسنتين هندي. *(Arab.)* Barinjásife-kóhí برنجاسف كوهي *or* Balinjásefe-kóhí بلنجاسف كوهي *(Pers.)* Majtari مجتري; Mastáru مستارو. *(Hind.)* Máchi-pattiri மாசிபத்திரி. *(Tam.)* Máchi-patri మాచిపత్రి. *(Tel.)* Tiru-niṭripach-cha തിരുനിറവിപച്ച. *(Malyal.)* Mancha-patri ಮಂಚಪತ್ರಿ; Máchi-patri ಮಾಚಿಪತ್ರಿ. *(Can.)* Mastaru. *(Beng.)* Granthiparni. *(Sans.)* Walkotondu. *(Cing.).*

78. ARTICHOKE GUM.

Kankarzad كنكرزد; Turábul-qai تراب القي. *(Arab.)* Kankari كنكرى; Ṣamaghe-ḥarshaf صمغ حرشف; Kankarzhad كنكرزد. *(Pers.).*

Kankarzad and *Kankarzhad* are corruptions of, and synonymous with, each other, but the latter is incorrectly applied to *Mastic* in some Dictionaries.

79. ASCLEPIAS CURASSAVICA, *Linn.*

80. ASPARAGUS ASCENDENS, *Roxb.* *(Root of.)*

Shaqáqule-hindi شقائل هندي. *(Arab. and Pers.)*
Sufèd-músli سفيدموسلي *or* Sufèd-muṣli سفيدوصلي. *(Hind.)*
Shqáqule-hindi شقائل هندي. *(Duk.)* Saféda-musali. *(Mah.)*
Saphèd-musli ; Ujli-musli. *(Guz.).*

There is a great confusion about the nature of the medicines known as *Sufèd-musli* and *Káli-musli* in India. Among some curious notions about them there is one in some native and other medical works to the effect that both are the produce of one and the same plant, the difference being that the *Sufèd musli* is the root of it before it begins to flower, and the *Káli musli* the root after that period. The plant in question is *Bombax Malobaricus.* In a few other books, the former is considered to be the root of *Asparagus sarmentosus*, and the latter that of *Curculigo orchioides.*

On procuring the medicines known under these names from many places, including Calcutta, Bombay, and Hyderabad, I have found that there are two kinds of *Sufèd musli*, the one obtained from almost all the Indian bazaars except those in Southern India; and the other sold in the latter place.

a. The *Sufèd-musli* of Southern India is the dried and splitted root of *Asparagus sarmentosus.* It occurs in thin and long pieces like strings, curled upon itself once or twice, varies in length from three or four inches to a span or more, of pale-grey or dirty-white color, and devoid of any particular taste or smell. When the fresh root is splitted or torn longitudinally in three or four pieces and dried, it acquires the above condition. Although the dried root is often used by native practitioners, it is almost useless as a medicine. But when fresh, it is a nutrient and demulcent. In this state, it is very fleshy and succulent, about a foot or foot and a half in length, generally of the thickness of a finger, smooth and round, tapering to a very narrow and long point at both ends, of dull white or pale grey color, no smell, and taste slightly demulcent. When a plant is dug out with these roots, it has a very singular appearance as though a great number of large round worms attached to it, and their number is often very great, amounting sometimes to about a hundred. The fresh root is distinguished in many parts of India, including Southern India, as Shaqáqul شقاقل, and its preserve, which is generally imported from China, is named *Murabbahe-shaqáqul* مربهٔشقاقل or *Shaqáqul-ká-murabbah* شقاقل‌کامربه . The above name is applied in Arabia, Egypt, and Persia, to some similar root, which is considered there to be the *wild carrot* or *turnip.* From its description in some books, I believe it to be a species of *Asparagus.*

b. The *Suféd-muslí* of all other parts of India is the real drug to which that name is properly applicable, and it is the root of *Asparagus ascendens.* It is also procurable in Southern India, but under a different name, which is *Shaqáqule-hindí* شقاقل‌هندي or *Indian* Shaqáqul. It is a useful medicine, and a very good substitute* for *Salep.* It bears the following characters.

When new or not very old, this root looks like a thin cylindrical piece of gum; partially translucent; very hard, whitish or yellowish-grey; from one to two or three inches long; generally crooked, some times bent upon itself, and occasionally knotty; and of bland and mucilaginous taste. If some pieces be carefully examined, one of their ends will be found thinner and more pointed than the other, indicating their original tapering form. A few pieces are also flat or compressed, forming a kind of small irregular plates. When the root is very old, it is opaque and of light-brown color.

With regard to the *Kálí-muslí,* it is correctly the root of *Curculigo orchidioides* as is mentioned and described in several books.

The roots or rootlets of *Bombax Malabaricus* (which is a very large tree), bear no resemblance whatever to any of the varieties of the *muslí.* When dried, they are as nearly useless as the dried root of *Asparagus sarmentosus.*

---

* By subsequent trials I have found that it is a *better* substitute for *Salep* for medicinal purposes.

81. ASPARAGUS RACEMOSUS, *Willd. (Root of.)*

Shaqáqul شقاقل . (*Arab. Pers. Hind. and Duk.)——dry root of,* Shaqáqule-miṣrí شقاقل مصري . (*Duk.*) Taṇṇir-muṭṭán-kizhaṇgu தண்ணீர்முட்டான்கிழங்கு; Shadávari சதாவரி. (*Tam.*) Challa-gaḍḍalu చల్లగడ్డలు; Pilli-pichara పిల్లిపిచర; Pilli-téga పిల్లితేగ; Shatávari శతావరి. (*Tel.*) Shatávali ശതാവലി. (*Malyal.*) Majjige-gaḍḍe ಮಜ್ಜಿಗೆಗಡ್ಡೆ. (*Can.*) Sat-mulí. (*Beng.*) Satávari-muli. (*Mah.*) Hatávari. (*Cing.*).

82. ASPARAGUS SARMENTOSUS, *Linn. (Root of.)*

Shaqáqul شقاقل . (*Arab. Pers. Hind. and Duk.)——dry root of,* Safèd-músli سفيد موصلي (*Duk.*) Kiḷavari இளவரி; Taṇṇir-viṭṭán-kizhaṇgu தண்ணீர்விட்டான் இழங்கு; Taṇṇi-muṭṭán-kizhaṇgu தண்ணிமுட்டான்கிழங்கு. (*Tam.*) Challa-gaḍḍalu చల్లగడ్డలు ; Pilli-pichara పిల్లిపిచర. (*Tel.*) Shatávari-kizhaṇṇa ശതാവരികിഴങ്ങ; Shatávali ശതാവലി. (*Malyal.*) Majjige-gaḍḍe ಮಜ್ಜಿಗೆಗಡ್ಡೆ. (*Can.*) Sat-múli. (*Beng.*) Satávari-muli. (*Mah.*) Hatávari. (*Cing.*) Kaṇyo-mi. (*Bur.*).

In several languages the same names are applied to both the root of *A. racemosis* and *A. sarmentosis*. See the remarks on *A. ascendens*.

83. ASSAFŒTIDA.

Hiltit حلتيت . (*Arab.*) Angózah انگوزه; Angusht-gandah انگشت گنده. (*Pers.*) Hing هينگ . (*Hind.*) Hing هنگ. (*Duk.*) Káyam காயம்; Peruṇgáyam பெருங் காயம்.. (*Tam.*) Inguva ఇంగువ. (*Tel.*) Perun-gáyam

പെരുങ്കായം; Káyam കായം. (*Malyal.*) Ingu ಇಂಗು.
(*Can.*) Hing. (*Beng.*) Hinguhu; Rámaṭham. (*Sans.*) Hing.
(*Mah.*) Hing; Vagárni. (*Guz.*) Perunkayam *or* Perrungá-
yam. (*Cing.*) *Shinkhu or Shingu.* (*Bur.*).

84. ASTERACANTHA LONGIFOLIA, *Nees.*

Tál-ma*kh*ánè-ká-pèṛ تال مكھانے کا پیڑ; Tál-ma*kh*árè-ká-
pèṛ تال مكھارے کا پیڑ. (*Hind.*) Tál-ma*kh*ánè-ká-*j*háṛ
تال مكھانے کا جھاڑ. (*Duk.*) Nìr-
mulli நீர்முள்ளி. (*Tam.*) Nìrugobbi నీరుగొబ్బి; Gobbi గొబ్బి.
(*Tel.*) Vayal-chuḷḷi വയൽച്ചുളളി. (*Malyal.*) Koḷava-
like ಕೊಳವಲಿಕೆ. (*Can.*) Káṅṭa-koliká. (*Beng.*) Ikshu-
gand*h*aha. (*Sans.*) Tál-ma*kh*áná. (*Mah.*) Ikkiri *or* Ikkiri-
gahá. (*Cing.*) Ṣúpadáṇ. (*Bur.*).

The Dukhni name of the above plant, *Kőlsé-ká-*jháṛ, is
incorrectly applied in some books to *Solanum Indicum.*

85. AURUM. (*Gold——Leaf of.*)

Varqu*zz*ahab ورق الذهب. (*Arab.*) Varqe-zar ورق زر;
Varqe-ṭilá ورق طلا. (*Pers.*) Sónèrì-varaq سونیری ورق; Su-
nehrì-varaq سنھری ورق. (*Hind.*) Sunehrì-tagaṭ سنھری تگٹ.
(*Duk.*) Tanga-rèkku தங்கரேக்கு. (*Tam.*) Kundanapu-
rèku కుందనపు-రేకు; Bangáru-rèku బంగారు-రేకు. (*Tel.*)
Tangarè*kh*á തങ്കരേഖാ; Sornṇatakaṭa സൊണ്ണതകട.
(*Malyal.*) Bangárada-ré*kh*u ಬಂಗಾರದ ರೇಕು. (*Can.*) Sónár-
pát; Sónár-orak. (*Beng.*) Suvarna-patram. (*Sans.*) Sónè-
cha-vara*kh*. (*Mah.*) Sunèri-vara*kh*; Sunáni. (*Guz.*)
Ran-ta-haḍu; Ran-tagaḍu. (*Cing.*) Shue-saku; *Shue-*
zaiṅ. (*Bur.*).

86. AVERRHOA BILIMBI, *Linn.* (*Blimbi tree—Fruit of.*)

Belambú بلمبو. (*Hind. and Duk.*) Koch-chit-tamarttai கொச்சித்தமர்த்தை; Pulich-chakkáy புளிச்சக்காய். (*Tam.*) Pulusu-káyalu పులుసుకాయలు; Bili-bili-káyalu బిలిబిలికాయలు. (*Tel.*) Vilunbikká വിളുമ്പിക്കാ; Vilimbi വിലിമ്പി; Karichakka കരിചക്ക. (*Malyal.*) Blimbi. (*Beng.*) Blimbu. (*Guz.*) Kála-zoun-si; Kala-zoun-ya-si. (*Bur.*).

87. AVERRHOA CARAMBOLA, *Adans.* (*Fruit of.*)

Khamrak خمرک. (*Hind.*) Khamra خمرق. (*Duk.*) Tamarttam-káy தமர்த்தம்காய். (*Tam.*) Támarta-káya తమర్తకాయ. (*Tel.*) Tamarat-túka താമരത്തൂക. (*Malyal.*) Kamarak ಕಮರಕ. (*Can.*) Kamarangá; Kamarak. (*Beng.*) Tamarak. (*Guz.*) Zoun-si; Zoun-ya-si. (*Bur.*).

88. AVICENNIA TOMENTOSA, *Linn.*

Nalla-mada నల్లమడ; Mada-chettu మడచెట్టు. (*Tel.*) Upputti ഉപ്പുത്തി. (*Malyal.*) Biná. (*Beng.*).

89. AZADIRACHTA INDICA, *Juss.* (*Neem or Margosa tree.*)

Ázád-darakhte-hindì آزاد درخت هندي; Nib نيب. (*Pers.*) Ninb نينب; Nimb نيمب. (*Hind.*) Nim نيم. (*Duk.*) Vémbu வேம்பு; Véppam வேப்பம்; Véppa-maram வேப்பமரம். (*Tam.*) Vépa-chettu వేపచెట్టు; Nim-bamu నింబము. (*Tel.*) Véppa വെപ്പ; Ariya-véppa ആരിയ വെപ്പ. (*Malyal.*) Béviná-mará ಬೇವಿನಾಮರಾ. (*Can.*) Nim; Nim-gáchh. (*Beng.*) Nimba-vrikshaha. (*Sans.*)

Limbácha-*jháda. (Mah.)* Limbdánu-*jháda. (Guz.)* Kohumba;
Nimba-gahá. *(Cing.)* Tama-biṇ; *Thamákhá or Thamágá;*
Kamákhá *or Khamákhá. (Bur.).*

The Burmese names of *Azadirachta Indica* and *Melia azadarach* are often confounded with each other. For example, in Mason's Natural Productions of Burmah the names of the former will be found applied to the latter, and *vice versa.*

B

90 BACCHARIS ILLINITA, *D. C.*

91. BALANITES ÆGYPTIACA, *Delile.*

Hingan-ká-péṛ هنگن کاپیڙ. *(Hind.)* Hingan-ká-*jháṛ* هنگن کا جهاڙ. *(Duk.)* Naṇjuṇdán நஞ்சுண்டான். *(Tam.)* Gárn-cheṭṭu గార్ఞ్చెట్టు. *(Tel.)* Nanchunṭa നഞ്ചുണ്ട. *(Malyal.)* Hingon. *(Beng.)* Inguḍi-vrikshaha. *(Sans.)* Hing-aṇa. *(Mah.).*

92. BALSAMODENDRON AGALLOCHA, *W. et A.*
(Resin of——Bdellium.)

Moql مقل ; Moqle-arzaq مقل ارزق ; Aflátạan افلاطن. *(Arab.)* Boé-jahúdáṅ بوئ جهودان. *(Pers.)* Gogil گوگل. *(Hind.)* Gugal گوگل. *(Duk.)* Mai-ṣhákshi மைசாக்ஷி ; Gukkal குக்கல் ; Gukkulu குக்குலு. *(Tam.)* Mahi-sákshi మహిసాక్షి ; Mại-sákshi మైసాక్షి. *(Tel.)* Guggaḷá ಗುಗ್ಗುಳ. *(Can.)* Gúgul. *(Beng.)* Kou-ṣhikaha. *(Sans.)* Gugguḷa. *(Mah.)* Gúgal. *(Guz.)* Gugula; Jaṭayu or Javáyu; Raṭa-dummula. *(Cing.).*

93. BALSAMUM. *Var. of.* *(Balsam of Mecca or Balm of Gilead.)*

Aqovoyalásamún دهن البلسان ; Dohnul-balsán اقوبلاسمون (*Arab.*) Roghane-balsán روغن بلسان. (*Pers.*) Balsán-kátél بلسان كاتيل. (*Hind. and Duk.*).

The above are properly the synonymes of the *Balsam of Mecca*, but are also applied to the oil of *Copaiva* in India.

94. BAMBUSA ARUNDINACEA, *Sch.* *(Siliceous concretion of——Tabashir.)*

Tabáshír طباشير. (*Arab.*) Tabáshír تباشير. (*Pers.*) Bans-lóchan بنس لوچن ; Bans-kapúr بنس كپور. (*Hind. and Duk.*) Múnga-luppu முங்கலுப்பு. (*Tam.*) Veduruppu వెదురుప్పు. (*Tel.*) Mole-uppa മോളെ‌ഉപ്പ. (*Malyal.*) Bidaruppu ಬಿದರುಪ್ಪ ; Tavakshírá ತವಕ್ಷೀರಾ. (*Can.*) Báns-kápúr. (*Beng.*) Vénu-lavanam. (*Sans.*) Banasa-lóchana ; Banasa-mítha. (*Mah.*) Váns-kapúr ; Vás-nu-mítha. (*Guz.*) Una-lunu ; Una-kapuru. (*Cing.*) Vá-chhá ; Váthegá-kiyo ; Vathegasá or Vádegá-sá ; Vasan or Vasan. (*Bur.*).

The two varieties of *Tabashír* found in the bazaars are distinguished by their color; viz., *Kabúdi* كبودي (*blue*), and *Suféd* سفيد (*white*). The first named variety is not quite blue, but *pale-blue* or *bluish-white.*

95. BASSIA BUTYRACEA. *Roxb.*

Phalvara پهلوارا. (*Hind.*).

96. BASSIA LATIFOLIA, *Roxb.*

Darakhte-gulchakáne-sahrái درخت گل چكان صحرائي. (*Pers.*) Jangli-mohá جنگلي مها ; Jangli-mohvá جنگلي مهنو ا. (*Hind.*) Jangli-móhá جنگلي موها. (*Duk.*) Káttu-iluppai

காட்டு இலுப்பை; Káṭṭu-iruppai காட்டு இருப்பை. *(Tam.)* Aḍavi-ippe-chettu అడవి ఇప్పేచెట్టు. *(Tel.)* Káṭṭirippa കാട്ടിരിപ്പ. *(Malyal.)* Kádu-ippe-giḍá ಕಾಡುಇಪ್ಪೆಗಿಡಾ. *(Can.)* Bon-mohuvá. *(Beng)* Aṭavi-maḍhúka-vrikshaha. *(Sans.)* Rúṇácha-móhácha-jháḍa; Rúṇácha-ippécha-jháḍa. *(Mah.)*.

97. BASSIA LONGIFOLIA, *Linn.* *(Mowa or Mahwah tree.)*

Daraḳhte-gulchakáñ درخت گل چکان. *(Pers.)* Mohá مہا; Mohvá مهوا. *(Hind.)* Móhá موہا. *(Duk.)* Iluppai இலுப்பை; Iruppai இருப்பை. *(Tam.)* Ippe-chettu ఇప్పేచెట్టు; Pinna-ippa పిన్నఇప్ప; Ippa-chettu ఇప్పచెట్టు. *(Tel.)* Irippa ഇരിപ്പ. *(Malyal.)* Ippe-giḍá ಇಪ್ಪೆಗಿಡಾ. *(Can.)* Mohuvá. *(Beng.)* Maḍhúka-vrikshaha. *(Sans.)* Móhácha-jháḍa; Ippicha-jháḍa. *(Mah.)* Mová-nu-jháḍa. *(Guz.)* Kánsó. *(Bur.)*.

See the remarks under *Liquor Spirituous*.

98. BENZOINUM. *(Benzoin.)*

Lubán لبان; Ḥaṣi-lubán حصي لبان. *(Arab.)* Ḥasn-lubah حسن لبه. *(Pers.)* Lóbán لوبان; Áúd عود. *(Hind.)* Áúd عود. *(Duk.)* Shámbiṛáṇi சாம்பிராணி; Dúpam தூபம். *(Tam.)* Sámbráṇi సాంబ్రాణి. *(Tel.)* Sámbráṇi സാമ്പ്രാണി. *(Malyal.)* Sámbráṇi ಸಾಂಬ್ರಾಣಿ. *(Can.)* Lóbán. *(Beng.)* Déva-dhúpaha. *(Sans.)* Sámbráṇi. *(Mah.)* Lubán; Sámbráṇi. *(Guz.)* Sámbráni; Kaṭakumanchal. *(Cing.)* Lobáñ. *(Bur.)*.

The above Arabic and Cingalese names *Lubán* and *Kaṭaku-manchal* are properly applicable only to *Benzoin*, but are also often applied to the Resin of *Boswellia thurifera (Olibanum).*

The best variety of *Benzoin* is known by the following names in the bazaars of Southern India.

Lóbáni-gúd لو بانی عود . *(Duk.) Palingi-shámbiráni* பளிங்கு சாம்பிரானி. *(Tam.) Palingu-sámbráni* పళింగు సాంబ్రాణి. *(Tel.).*

The above Tamil and Telugu words, *Palingi* and *Palingu*, are quite different from, and must not be confounded with, those which will be found under *Boswellia glabra*, and *B. thurifera*, viz., *Parangi* and *Parangi*.

99. BERBERIS ARISTATA, *D. C.*
Syn. B. TINCTORIA, *Lesch.*

100. BERBERIS ASIATICA, *D. C.*

101. BERBERIS LYCIUM, *Roy.*

Indian Barberry.

The dry berries, extract, and wood or root of all the above plants have the same names, and they are as follows:—

Berries————*Anbar-búrís* انبربا ريس ; *Ambar-búrís* امبربا ريس . *(Arab.)* Zarishk زر شك . *(Pers. and Hind.)* *Zarish* زر ش . *(Duk.).*

Extract————*Huzuze-hindí* حضض هند ي ; *Fíl-zahraj* فيل زهرج . *(Arab.)* *Fíl-zahrah* فيل زهره ; *Píl-zahrah* پيل زهره . *(Pers.)* *Rasvat* رسوت . *(Hind.).*

Wood or Root————*Dár-hald* دارهلد. *(Arab.)* *Dár-hald* دارهلد ; *Dár-chób* دارچوب . *(Pers. and Hind.).*

The dry berries of the above and some other species of *Berberis* are a very popular medicine, and found plentifully in many large bazaars of India, including those of South India. They are the principal ingredients in many useful prescriptions which are frequently used by the Hakeems. They can be easily recognised by the following characters.

Berries shrivelled and much compressed; dark-brown or black in color; pleasantly acid in taste; about ⅓rd of an inch long, and ⅛th broad; smooth, soft, and moist; pedunculate; contain a little dark-brown pulp; and generally contain no seeds, but sometimes one small, hard, and oblong seed is to be found in each. I have examined the berries chemically and found them to contain *Tartaric* and *Malic Acids*, to which they owe their acid taste.

These berries are called *Vilάyati-amli* ولايتي املي in Hyderabad, whereas the same name is applied to the legume of *Inga dulcis* in many places of Southern India. *Zarishk* is the surest name to obtain these berries from any part of India.

The meaning of *Dárhald* is *turmeric-wood* or *yellow-wood*, and it is therefore applied in some native and other works to several kinds of yellow root or wood, such as that of *Curcuma aromatica, C. longa,* and *Coscinium fenestratum*; but as it is very frequently used for the wood or root of the above species of *Berberis* in Central and Northern India, it must be restricted to them.

102. BERTHELOTIA LANCEOLATA, *var.* Indica, D. C. (*Leaves of.*);

Rái-sanά را ني سنا . (*Hind.*).

103. BEZOAR. (*A mineral variety of——Silicate of Magnesia and Iron.*)

Fádaje-maadani فاد ج معدني ; Bádzahre-maadani بادزهر معدني ; Hajrussam حجرالسم . (*Arab.*) Fádzahre-kάni فاد زهر كا ني ; Pάdzahre-kάni پاد زهر كا ني . (*Pers.*) Kάni-zahr-mohrah كاني زهر مهره . (*Hind.*) Kάni-páv-zahar كاني پاو زهر . (*Duk.*).

Two kinds of *Bezoar* are commonly sold in the native medicine-shops of India, and they are well known as *Pάdzahre-kάni* پاد زهر كاني (*Mineral Bezoar*) and *Pάdzahre-hnivάni* پاد زهر حيواني (*Animal Bezoar*). The former is not obtained from any animal, but is the *natural* and *mineral produce* of India, Persia, Tartary, and many other places. There is no medicine in this country so frequently resorted to by native practitioners, especially the Hakeems, in cholera, as the *Mineral Bezoar*, and I believe this is not without sufficient reason.

In all the English works on Native medicines, which I have access to, the term *bezoar* is confined either to a concretion found in one of the stomachs of an animal of the goat-kind, or to all the concretions produced in the body of animals. Although a great deal of information on the subject appears to have been gathered from native works and from the examination of the varieties of the drug in India, and even the very word *bezoar* is apparently derived from *Bádzahr (Arab.)* or *Pádzahr (Pers.):* yet, there is no mention made at all of its mineral variety, which is so commonly known in the bazaar, and so frequently noticed in books. Whatever may be the cause of this, it is enough for my purpose to say that the *Mineral Bezoar* is more useful in medicine than the *Animal,* and deserves some attention.

Besides the difference in their source, they differ a great deal from one another, as follows :—

Mineral variety.	*Animal variety.*
1. Form not defined ; it occurs in very irregular and angular pieces of various shape, like pieces of *Marble* or any other stone.	1. Form defined and regular ; oval, oblong, ovate, globular, or flat and circular.
2. Size unlimited, often as large as a fist, and sometimes much larger.	2. Seldom of the size of an egg, but generally of various sizes below that.
3. Surface generally rough, but smooth when covered with clay, which is the case sometimes.	3. Surface very smooth and glossy.
4. Of various colors between white and green or yellowish-green, but generally pale green with one or two shades of yellow.	4. Color various, generally dark green, marbled, or bluish-brown.
5. Structure amorphous.	5. Structure laminated and concentric.

There are several varieties of the *Mineral Bezoar*, but the variety I have just described is the one generally found in the bazaar and in the possession of Hakeems. The best variety sought for to be used in Cholera is of pale green color, and easily ground with water on a stone. The paste thus obtained, is white and slightly odorous, the smell being often very feeble and somewhat like that of the prepared Pipe-clay. This stone is a variety of *Steatite* or *Soap-stone*, and its greenish hue depends upon the presence of *Protoxide of Iron*. So, chemically, it is a *Silicate of Magnesia and Iron*. (See Fownes' Chemisary, Ninth Edition, page 313.)

It is necessary to be aware that the above stone is often cut out or rubbed out into different forms, generally oblong or oval, so as to resemble the shape of the *Animal Bezoar*, and sold as rare varieties of *Bezoar* brought from foreign countries, as Arabia, Persia, &c. The price asked for them is enormous, and sometimes more than a hundred Rupees. This deception is, however, easily detected by rubbing or breaking a portion of the stone, when it will be found that it is nothing else but the same variety of *Bezoar* which I have just described, and that it is *amorphous* in structure, and *not laminated* or *concentric*.

Whether the stone under discussion, is properly a *Bezoar* or not, I have given it under that head as its mineral variety according to the meaning of all its native names.

With regard to the *Animal Bezoar*, its varieties are very numerous, and they are named after the animal from which it is obtained ; as, *Hajruttis* حجر التيس *(Goat-bezoar)*, *Hajrul-jamal* حجرالجمل *(Camel-bezoar)*, *Hajrul-hút* حجرالحوت *(Fish-bezoar)*, *Hajrul-haiah* حجرالحيه *(Snake-bezoar)*, &c. The last named *Bezoar* is supposed to be the produce of some large species of snake, and is quite different from the *Bezoar* known as *Tiryáqul-haiyah* ترياق الحيه *(antidote to Snake)*, the *Snake-stone*. The list of these *Bezoars* has been much augmented since the modern writers have extended that term to all the Concretions in the body of animals. The substances of the latter kind, however, are very different in some of their essential characters from those which have been hitherto known as *Bezoars*.

104. BEZOAR. *(A variety of Animal Bezoar——Gall-stone or Biliary concretion of a Cow or Bullock).*

Hajrul-baqar حجرالبقر . *(Arab.)* Gáv-zahrah گاوزهره. *(Pers.)* Gáiróhan گاني روهن. *(Hind.)* Góróchaná

چنا گوروچنا ; Gáirón گا ني روون . (*Duk.*) Górójanai கோ ரோ சணை. (*Tam.*) Górójanam గోరోజనం. (*Tel.*) Góróchanam ഗോരോചനം. (*Malyal.*) Góróchaná ಗೋಚೂಜನಾ. (*Can.*) Gáerún. (*Beng.*) Goróchanam. (*Sans.*) Góróchan. (*Mah.*) Gáirón. (*Guz.*) Górocha. (*Cing.*) Goyázin. (*Bur.*).

The above medicine is not considered as a variety of *Bezoar* by native practitioners, nor is it mentioned so in any of their works. But, as all the concretions in the body of animals are now included among the varieties of *Bezoar* in several recent works in the English language, I have given it under that head. It is the only variety of *Animal Bezoar*, which deserves an attention as a medicine.

It occurs in more or less spherical form, brown externally, very smooth and glossy, varies in size from a Soap-nut to a large Nutmeg, very light and easily broken with hands. When broken, its structure is laminated and concentric ; and of deep, bright, or reddish yellow color. If not for the particular arrangement of its structure, it would be difficult to say that it is not made of *Rhubarb*. Its taste is bitterish, slightly sweetish, and occasionally aromatic. See the remarks in the preceding article, with regard to the *Mineral* and *Animal* varieties of *Bezoar* and other facts connected with it, as well as the native names of some of the latter varieties.

105. BIT-LOBAN. (*Black salt.*)

Milhe-nifti ملح نفطي ; Milhe-asvad ملح اسود . (*Arab.*) Namake-siyáh نمك سياه . (*Pers.*) Bid-lón بد لون ; Kálá-lón كالا لون ; Kálá-namak كالا نمك ; Pádá-lón پادا لون ; Pádá-namak پادا نمك . (*Hind.*) Bit-lóbán بت لوبان ; (*Duk.*) Karuppuppu கருப்புப்பு : Gendaka-vuppu கெந்தகவுப்பு. (*Tam.*) Nalla-uppu నల్ల ఉప్పు ; Gendhaka-uppu గెంధకఉప్పు. (*Tel.*) Karutta-uppa കരുത്ത ഉപ്പ. (*Malyal.*) Karéuppu ಕರೆಉಪ್ಪು. (*Can.*) Kálá-nún ; Kálá-nimak. (*Beng.*) Krishtna-lavanam. (*Sans.*) Kála-mitha. (*Mah.*) Kalu-lunu. (*Cing.*) Şá-me *or* Şá-me. (*Bur.*).

Some of the above names *(Milhe-niṭṭi, Púdá-lón, Púdá-namak, Púdrá-nimak, Genduka-vuppu, &c.,)* signify a bad smell, and are correctly applicable only to that variety of *Bitloban*, which possesses a smell something like that of rotten eggs. It is this variety which is in great vogue in India as a useful Carminative, Stomachic and Tonic medicine in Dyspepsia and some other diseases of the chylo-poietic viscera.

The meaning of all other names is *black salt*, and they are generally in use for another variety, which is more common, but very inferior and chiefly consists of *Chloride of Sodium* and *Carbon.* It is said to be prepared in Nugree, a village in the central Carnatic, by melting the *Common Salt* with *Emblic Myrobalans* in a close vessel. It occurs in very rough and irregular masses of brown color, which look like the pieces of a black brick; and has a strong saline taste.

The first variety appears to be manufactured in two different ways: at Azeemabad, by melting together the *Sajji-khár* of the bazaar *(Crude Carbonate of Soda)* and *Emblic Myrobalans;* and at another place, by the same process, but with an addition of other ingredients, viz., *Chloride of Sodium, Sulphur,* and the *Rust of Iron.* The smell of this variety, which is strong at the commencement, is lost in time in proportion to its oldness, till it becomes so feeble that it can only be felt when the salt is recently broken and a bit of it well chewed. In the bazaars of Madras, it is found in large and round masses or balls, weighing from 1 to 2 or more lbs.; and when broken, it is either grey, whitish-grey, or pale-brown in color, and more or less crystalline. It is much harder and heavier than the other variety, and contains a large quantity of *Chloride of Sodium* and *Carbonate of Soda,* some *Carbon, Iron* and *Sulphur,* and a trace of *Hydrosulphuric acid (Sulphuretted Hydrogen).*

If this salt is new, the presence of *Sulphuretted Hydrogen* is easily known; but if it is old, its detection is rather difficult. In a few old specimens, however, I have found out its existence in the following way :—

A large piece of the salt was broken, and a piece of paper moistened with the solution of *Acetate of Lead* was kept on a broken surface. After a minute or two, the paper was found to be slightly but distinctly blackened.

This test, together with the offensive smell of the salt, leaves no doubt in my mind as to the·presence of the *gas.* however small in quantity it may be.*

106. BLUMEA AURITA, *D. C.*

Kamáfiṭús كا فيطو س . *(Arab.)* Kakróṅdá ككر و ند ا *(Hind.)* Jangli-kásni جنگلي كا سني ; Jangli-múli جنگلي مولي *(Duk.)* Nárak-karandai நாரக்கரந்தை ; Káṭṭu-muḷḷáṇgi காட்டுமுள்ளாங்கி. *(Tam.)* Káru-pógáku రుపొగాకు ; Aḍavi-mullangi అడవిముల్లంగి. *(Tel.)* Mai-yagán. *(Bur.)*.

This is an annual herbaceous or somewhat shrubby plant found in every creek and corner, particularly along the walls in old and ruinous buildings, and in grave yards. Its appearance when young, differs so much from that when old, that it is considered by those that are not acquainted with this fact as two different plants in those periods, and often recognised accordingly by different names. The size of the leaves is the chief cause of the difference, which are comparatively very large when the plant is young, and resemble the leaves of *Radish.* From this and from the plant being generally found along the walls, it is often named in Tamil Ṣhevuru-muḷḷáṇgi செவுருமுள்ளாங்கி, in Telugu Góḍa-mullangi గోడముల్లంగి, and in Hindustani and Dukhni Díwárí-múlí د يواری مولي . These names, however, properly belong to another plant of the same Natural Order, Compositæ, which generally grows on the top of the walls. When *B. aurita* is in flower, the leaves, except a few old ones near the root, become very small and quite sessile with many auricles or leafy appendages near their base, and the plant

---

* Although this Salt contains a trace of *Sulphuretted Hydrogen,* yet it is not only used by native practitioners internally ; but is also a domestic medicine all over India, and frequently resorted to by women in some dyspeptic complaints.

itself is much altered from numerous branches. In this condition
it is generally recognised by the names in the text, which correctly belong, and should always be applied, to it, whether
young or old.

The meaning of the Dukhni, Tamil and Telugu synonymes
Jangli-múli, Káttu-mullángi and *Adri-mullangi* is *the wild Radish,*
and this is partly from the appearance of the leaves of the plant
when young, as already explained, and partly from the occasional resemblance of its root to a small or abortive Radish.

As this plant is often known under the Telugu name *Káru-
pógáku* in Madras, it is probably the same intended by that
name in Flora Andhrica, to which no botanical name is assigned.
Sir Walter Elliot says, that it is ' A composite plant not found
in flower.' The *Káru-pógáku* of Madras is also a composite
plant, and found here in flower soon after the rainy season
(January, February, and March). It quite corresponds with
the characters of *Conyza aurita* described in Dr. Roxburgh's
Flora Indica, Vol. III, page 428, and of *Blumea aurita* in
Dr. Wight's Contributions to the Botany of India, page 16;
except the size and color of flowers which are not mentioned in
those works. The flowers are generally about the size of a large
pea, and of pale white color.

107. **BLUMEA GRANDIS.** *D. C.*

Phúm-masiñ. (Bur.).

108. **BOLUS ARMENIA RUBRA.** *(Red Arme-
nian bole.)*

‌Ṭéne-armaní طين ارمني ; Hajare-armaní حجرا ارمني‎.
(Arab.) Gile-armaní گل ارمني‎. *(Pers. and Hind.)*
Gile-armaní گل ارمنی ; *Phúl-gérú* پهول گيرو‎ . *(Duk.)*
Ṣḥimai-kávi சீமைகாவி ; Púk-kávi புக்காவி ; *Shimai-kávi-
kallu* சீமைகாவிகல்லு. *(Tam.)* Ṣḥima-kávuráyi சீமாகாவு
ராயி ; Púk-kávi పూక్కావి ; Ṣḥima-kávi సీమాకావి. *(Tel.)*

109. BOLUS ARMENIA RUBRA. *(Indian variety of.)*

Maghrah مغره ; Tine-maghar طين مغر . *(Arab.)* Gile-surkh گل سرخ . *(Pers.)* Géru گيرو . *(Hind. and Duk.)* Kávi காவி ; Kávi-kallu காவிகல்லு. *(Tam.)* Kávi కావి ; Kávu-ráyi కావురాయి. *(Tel.)*.

110. BOMBAX MALABARICUM, *D. C. (Red cotton-tree.)*

Ragat-sénbal رگت سينبل ; Ragat-sémal رگت سيمل ; Kánti-sénbal كانتي سينبل . *(Hind.)* Kántón-ká-khatyán كا نتون كا ختيان ; Kántón-ká-sémal كا نتون كا سيمل . *(Duk.)* Muḷ-ilava-maram முள் இலவமரம் ; Muḷ-ilavu முள் இலவு. *(Tam.)* Mundla-búraga-cheṭṭu ముండ్లబూరగచెట్టు. *(Tel.)* Púla-maram പൂളമരം ; Muḷ-ḷilava മുള്ളിലവു. *(Malyal.)* Muḷḷu-búraga-mará ಮುಳ್ಳುಬೂರಗಮರಾ. *(Can.)* Rokto-simul. *(Beng.)* Kaṭṭu-imbul. *(Cing.)* Lepán-biṇ *or* Lephánbiṇ. *(Bur.)*.

There are two varieties of the gum sold in the Indian bazaars under the name of *Mócharas* موچرس . Both occur in very irregular, nodular, smooth, and shell-like pieces, opaque and dark-brown in color; the difference being, one is very hard and broken with difficulty; and the other is brittle and easily broken, and less astringent in taste. The latter is the inferior of the two, and is the produce of Bombax Malabaricum. No gum is produced from this tree on making incisions (however deep), but occasionally a very small quantity of it is exuded spontaneously. It is of a yellowish red or flesh color at the beginning for some days, and then becomes deep brown. After some months, it gradually and occasionally acquires the form I have just described.

Kaṭṭu-imbul is the Cingalese name for *B. Malabaricum* and not *Imbul* as marked in some books. The latter is the name of *Eriodendron anfractuosum.*

See the remarks on *Asparagus ascendens* with respect to the roots of *B. Malabaricum* being confounded with the *Suféd* and *Kálimuṣli* of the bazaar.

111. BORASSUS FLABELLIFORMIS, *Linn.* (*Palmyra-tree.*)

Darakhtc-tári درخت تاري . (*Pers.*) **Tár** تاڙ . (*Hind.*) **Tár-ká-***jhár* تاڙ كاجهاڙ . (*Duk.*) **Panai-maram** பனைமரம். (*Tam.*) **Táti-chettu** తాటిచెట్టు. (*Tel.*) **Paná** പന. (*Malyal.*) **Pané-mará** ತಾಳೆಮರ. (*Can.*) **Tálgáchh.** (*Beng.*) **Tála-vrikshaha.** (*Sans.*) **Táticha-***jháda.* (*Mah.*) **Tád-nu-***jháda.* (*Guz.*) **Tál** or **Tál-gahá.** (*Cing.*) **Thán-bin.** (*Bur.*).

The Cingalese names *Tál* and *Tal* or *Talla* are some times confounded with each other from the similarity of their pronunciation. The former is the name of *B. flabelliformis*, and the two latter of *Sesamum Indicum*.

For the names of the *vinegar, arrack, jaggery,* and *toddy* of this plant see the remarks under *Acetum, Liquor Spirituous, Saccharum,* and *Toddy.*

112. BOSWELLIA GLABRA, *Roxb.,* (*Resin of——Indian Frankincense.*)

Kundur كندر . (*Arab. Pers. and Hind.*) **Farangí-aúd** فرنگي عود . (*Duk.*) **Parangi-ṣhámbiráni** பறங்கி சாம்பிராணி ; **Kundurukam-piṣhin** குந்துருகம்பிஷின். (*Tam.*) **Parangi-sámbráni** పరంగిసాంబ్రాణి ; **Anduga-pisunu** అందుగ పిసును. (*Tel.*) **Manna-kungiliyam** മന്നാകുങ്കിലിയം ; **Valanku-chámbráni** വളങ്കുചാമ്പ്രാണി. (*Malyal.*) **Bringi-lobán.** (*Bur.*).

Kundur is more properly the Arabic, Persian, Hindustani, and Dukhni name of *Olibanum*, but is also often applied to the Resin of *B. glabra*, particularly when it occurs in tears, so as to resemble the former. See the remarks under *B. thurifera.*

113. BOSWELLIA THURIFERA, *Roxb.,* *(Resin of——Olibanum.)*

Bastaj بستج ; Kundur كندر ; Lubán لبان . *(Arab.)* Kundur كندر . *(Pers.)* Sél-gónd سیل گوند ; Kundur كندر .. *(Hind.)* Kundur كندر . *(Duk.)* Parangi-ṣhámbi-ráni பறங்கிசாம்பிரானி ; Kundurukkam-piṣhin குந்துருக்கம் பிஷின். *(Tam.)* Parangi-sámbráṇi ఖరంగిసాంబ్రాణి ; Anduga-pisunu అందుగపిసును. *(Tel.)* Veḷḷa-kundirukkam വെള്ള കുന്തിരുക്കം. *(Malyal.)* Kundro ; Salai ; Salai-gún. *(Beng.)* Salasi-niryásam. *(Sans.)* Kundrikam. *(Cing.).*

When the Resin of *B. thurifera* and *B. glabra,* &c., occurs in *tears*, it is recognised as *Kundur* ; but when it is found in *soft masses*, it is generally called *Gandah-férozah* گند ه فیر وز ه . The latter is, however, more properly the name of different varieties of *Turpentine.*

The tears of *Kundur* have different names according to their shape and color. If they are circular and reddish-yellow, they are called *Kundur-ẕakar* كندر ن كر ; if yellowish-white and transulent, *Kundur-unṣá* كندرانثى and *Ánval-kundur* آنول كندر ; and if spherical, *Kundur-madháraj* كندر مدحرج . If the Resin, again, occurs in flat and scaly pieces, it is named *Qishár-kundur* قشار كندر ; and if in powder, *Daqáq-kundur* دقاق كندر .

See the remarks under *Benzoinum,* and *B. glabra.*

114. BRYONIA CALLOSA, *Rott.* *(Seeds of.)*

Jangli-kakṛi-ké-bínj جنگلي ككڑ يكے بيذج . *(Hind.)* Jangli-kankṛi-ké-bínj جنگلي كنكڑي كے بيذج ; Buṛamkái-ké-bínj بڑم كا ئي كي بيذج . *(Duk.)* Shukkaṇkáy-virai சுக்கண் காய்விரை ; Komaṭṭi-virai கொமட்டி விரை. *(Tam.)* Nakka-dósakáya-vittulu నక్కదోసకాయవిత్తులు ; Buḍamakáya-vittulu బుడమకాయవిత్తులు. *(Tel.)* Karumattan-vitta കരുമത്തൻ വിത്ത. *(Malyal.)* Buḍamakáyi-bijá ಬುಡಮಕಾಯಿಬೀಜ. *(Can.)*

See the remarks under *Citrullus colocynthis.*

115. BRYONIA EPIGÆA, *Rott.*

Ákás-gaddah آکاس گدّه; Rákas-gaddah راکس گدّه.
(*Hind.*) Ákas-gaddah آکس گدّه; Rakkas-gaddah رکس گدّه;
Garaj-*phal* گرج پهل. (*Duk.*) Gollan-kóvaik-kizhangu கொல்
லன்கோவைக்கிழங்கு; Ákásha-garudan ஆகாசகருடன்; Garu-
dan கருடன். (*Tam.*) Ákásha-garuda-gaddalu ఆకాశగరుడ
గడ్డలు; Nágadonda నాగదొండ; Murudonda మురుదొండ. (*Tel.*)
Kollam-kóva-kizhanna കൊല്ലം കോവകിഴങ്ങ. (*Malyal.*)
Ákásha-garuda-gadde ಆಕಾಶಗರುಡಗಡ್ಡೆ. (*Can.*).

116. BUTEA FRONDOSA, *Roxb.*

Darakhte-palah درخت پله; Palah پله. (*Pers.*) *Dhák*
داک; *Dhák* ڈهاک; Palás پلاس. (*Hind.*) Palás-
ká-*jhár* پلاس کا جهاڑ. (*Duk.*) Murukkan-maram முருக்கன்
மரம்; Puraishu புணாசு; Purashu புரசு; Palásham பலாசம்.
(*Tam.*) Móduga-chettu మోదుగచెట్టు; Paláshamu పలాశము;
Kimshukamu కింశుకము. (*Tel.*) Plách-cha പ്ലാച്ച; Murukka-
maram മുരുക്കമരം. (*Malyal.*) Muttaga-mará ಮುತ್ತಗಮರಾ;
Muttuga-gidá ಮುತ್ತುಗಗಿಡಾ. (*Can.*) Pálásh. (*Beng.*) Palásha-
vrikshaha. (*Sans.*) Phalásácha-*jhá*da; Kakrácha-*jhá*da.
(*Mah.*) Khákar-nu-*jhá*da. (*Guz.*) Káliya. (*Cing.*) Páv.
(*Bur.*).

117. BUTEA FRONDOSA, *Roxb..* (*Seeds of.*)

Tukhme-palah تخم پله. (*Pers.*) Palás-ké-bínj
پلاس کی بیدنج. (*Hind.*) Palás-páprá پلاس پا پڑا. (*Duk.*)
Murukkam-virai முருக்கம்விரை. (*Tam.*) Móduga-vittulu
మోదుగవిత్తులు; Kimshukamu కింశుకము; Palásha-vittulu పలాశ
విత్తులు. (*Tel.*) Plách cham-kuru പ്ലാച്ചംകുരു Murukka-vitta
മുരുക്കവിത്ത; Plashu പ്ലാശു. (*Malyal.*) Muttaga-bijá

ముడుగవిత్తు. *(Can.)* Palásha-bíjam. *(Sans.)* *Phalásá-*
cha-bí ; Kakrácha-bí. *(Mah.)* *Khákar-nu-biyán* ; Palás-
páparo. *(Guz.)* Kaliya-atta. *(Cing.)* Páv-si. *(Bur.).*

118. **BUTEA FRONDOSA,** *Roxb.*⎱ *(Gum of ——*
                                    ⎰ *Butea or Ben-*
119. **BUTEA SUPERBA,** *Roxb.*⎰ *gal Kino.)*

Ṣamagẖc-palah صمغ پله . *(Pers.)* Palás-ki-gónd
پلاس کی گوند . *(Hind.)* Ċhinyá-gónd چنیا گوند ; Kinyá-
gónd کنیا گوند ; Palás-ká-gond پلا س کا گوند . *(Duk.)*
Murukkan-piṣhin முருக்கன்பிஷின் ; Palásha-piṣhin பலாச
பிஷின். *(Tam.)* Móduga-banka మొదుగబంక ; Palasha-banka
పలాశబంక. *(Tel.)* Plách-cha-paṣha വാത്തുവശ ; Murukkin-
paṣha ഒരുക്കിൻവശ. *(Malyal.)* Muttaga-góndu ముత్తగ
గోండు. *(Can.)* Pálásh-gun. *(Beng.)* Palásha-niryásam.
(Sans.) Kakrácha-gónda ; *Phalásácha-gónda.* *(Mah.)*
Khákar-nu-gún. *(Guz.)* Káliya-melliyam. *(Cing)* Páv-si.
(Bur.).

See the remarks under *Kino.*

120. **BUTEA SUPERBA,** *Roxb.*

Bél-palás بیل پلا س . *(Duk.)* Koḍi-murukkam கொடி
முருக்கம் ; Koḍi-palásham கொடிபலாசம். *(Tam.)* Tíge-
móduga తీగమొదుగ ; Tíge-paláshamu తీగపలాశము. *(Tel.)*
Vaḷḷiplách-cha വള്ളിപ്ലാച്ച Valli-murukka വള്ളിമുരുക്ക.
(Malyal.) Baḷḷi-muttaga ബള്ളിముత്തగ. *(Can.)* Latá-pálásh.
(Beng.) Latá-palásha. *(Sans.)* Vél-khákar. *(Guz.).*

C.

121. CACALIA KLEINIA. *Linn.*

The leaves of *Cacalia kleinia* are considered in several books to be the *Gáv-zabán* of bazaar, but the latter is neither the produce of that plant, nor of any other species of the Nat. Ord. to which it belongs, viz., *Compositæ*. *It is the produce of a species of Boraginaceæ.* See the remarks under *Echium*.

122. CÆSALPINIA CORIARIA. *Willd. (Dividivi or American Sumach).*

Sumáqe-amríqah سماق امريقه . (*Arab. and Pers.*) Amríqe-ká-sumáq کا سماق امریقے (*Duk.*) Shúmak சுமக். (*Tam.*).

123. CÆSALPINIA (GUILANDINA) BONDU-CELLA, *Linn. (Nut of——Bonduc-nut.)*

Akitmakit ا. كتمكت (*Arab.*) Kháyahe-iblis خايه ابليس. (*Pers.*) Katkaranj كتكرنج ; Karanjo كرنجو ; Karanjavá كرنجوا ; Kat-kalijí كت كليجي ; Katklijá كت كليجا ; Ságar-ghólah ساگر گهوله. (*Hind.*) Gajgá گجگا. (*Duk.*) Kazhar-shikkáy கழறிச்சிக்காய் ; Gech-chakkáy கெச்சக்காய். (*Tam.*) Gach-chakáya గచ్చకాయ. (*Tel.*) Kazhanchik-kuru കഴഞ്ചിക്കുരു ; Kalanchik-kuru കളഞ്ചിക്കുരു. (*Malyal.*) Gajaga-káyi ಗಜಗ ಕಾಯಿ. (*Can.*) Jhagrá-gúlá; Sétán-gúlá ; Nátá ; Nátú-koranjá. (*Beng.*) Kubérákshí-phalam. (*Sans.*) Gajaga. (*Mah.*) Gájgá ; Gajga. (*Guz*) Kumburu-atta. (*Cing.*) Kalain-si or Kalén-zi. (*Bur.*).

The Hindustani names *Katkaranj, Karanjó,* and *Karanjavá* are confounded in some books with *Karanj* کرنج or *Karanjh* کرنجه , which is the name of *Pongamia glabra*.

124. CÆSALPINIA SAPPAN, *Linn.* (*Wood of*
———*Sappan wood.*)

Baqam بقم. (*Arab.*) Bakam بكم. (*Pers.*) Patang بتنگ;
Patang-ki-lakṛi بتنگ كي لكڑي . (*Hind. and Duk.*)
Vattáṇgi வத்தாங்கி; Vattékku வத்தெக்கு; Vartaṇgi வர்தங்கி.
(*Tam.*) Okánu-katṭa ఒకానుకట్ట; Patanga-katṭa పటంగకట్ట;
Bakánu-chekka బకానుచెక్క; Bukkapu-chekka బుక్కపుచెక్క.
(*Tel.*) Chappaṇṇam ചപ്പണ്ണം. (*Malyal.*) Patanga-chekke.
ಚಟ್ಟಂಗಚೆಕ್ಕೆ. (*Can.*) Bokom. (*Beng.*) Patang. (*Mah.*)
Patang-nu-lákḍo. (*Guz.*) Patangi. (*Cing.*) Tainṇiya or
Tainngiya. (*Bur.*).

125. CAJANUS INDICUS, *Spr.* (*Seeds of.*)

Sháẓ شاض. (*Arab.*) Tuvvar تور; Arhar ارهر. (*Hind.*)
Tuvvar تور. (*Duk.*) Tuvarai துவரை. (*Tam.*) Kandulu
కందులు. (*Tel.*) Tuvara തുവര. (*Malyal.*) Togari ತೊಗರಿ.
(*Can.*) Oror; Orol. (*Beng.*) Turí. (*Mah.*) Tuvéro. (*Guz.*).

126. CAJUPUTI OLEUM. (*Cajuput Oil.*)

Kái-putí-ká-tél كائي پتي كا تيل; Kái-búṭi-ká-tél
كائي بوٹي كا تيل. (*Hind. and Duk.*) Kaiyáp-puḍai-tailam
கையாப்புடைதைலம். (*Tam.*) Káyaputí-tail. (*Beng.*) Káy-
putí-nu-tél. (*Guz.*).

127. CALOPHYLLUM SPURIUM, *Choisy.*

128. CALOPHYLLUM INOPHYLLUM, *Linn.*
(*Alexandrian-laurel.*)

Surpan سرپن; Sulṭánah-champá سلطانه چمپا. (*Hind.*)
Surfan سرفن. (*Duk.*) Punnai புன்னை; Punnai-maram
புன்னைமரம் Punnágam புன்னாகம் (*Tam.*) Punnágamu
పున్నాగము; Ponna-chettu పొన్నచెట్టు. (*Tel.*) Punna പുന്ന

(Malyal.) Suragonne-mará సురగొన్నెమరా. *(Can.)* Sultáná-champá. *(Beng.)* Punnága-vrikshaha. *(Sans.)* Domba-gahá. *(Cing.)* Phoun-ṇiya. *(Bur.).*

129. CALOTROPIS GIGANTEA, *R. Br.* ⎫
130. CALOTROPIS PROCERA, *R. Br.* ⎬ *Mudar.*
⎭

Aushar عشر or Aush-shar عشر. *(Arab.)* K'karak خرک. *(Pers.)* Ák آک; Madár مدار; Akond اکوند or Akan اکن. *(Hind)* Ák آک; Ákṛá آکڑا. *(Duk.)* Erukku எருக்கு; Erukkam எருக்கம். *(Tam.)* Jillédu-cheṭṭu జిల్లేదుచెట్టు; Mandáramu మందారము. *(Tel.)* Erukka എരുക്ക. *(Malyal.)* Yakkeda-giḍá ಯಕ್ಕೆಡಗಿಡಾ. *(Can.)* Ákondo; Ák. *(Beng.)* Arka-vrikshaha. *(Sans.)* Ákḍa-cha-jháḍa. *(Mah.)* Ákḍa-nu-jháḍa. *(Guz.)* Vará or Vará-gahá. *(Cing)* Mayo-biṇ. *(Bur.).*

Sukkarul-gushar سكر العشر is the name of the *Manna* or *Saccharine substance* produced by *C. procera* or some other species allied to it, in Arabia and Persia, which was formerly imported into India; but it is not found at all now in any bazaar, nor is it ever produced here, as far as my knowledge extends, by any species of *Calotropis.*

131. CALUMBÆ RADIX, *(Calumbo or Calumbo Root.)*

Biḳhe-kalambah بيخ كلمبه. *(Pers.)* Kalambé-ki-jaṛ کلمبی کی جڑ. *(Hind. and Duk.)* Kalambá-vér கலம்பாவேர். *(Tam.)* Kalambá-véru కలంబావేరు. *(Tel.).*

132. CALX, *(Lime or Quick-lime.)*

Kils كلس. *(Arab.)* Áhak آهک; Núrah نوره. *(Pers.)* Chúná چونا; Chúnah چونه. *(Hind.)* Chunnah چنه. *(Duk.)* Shunṇámbu சுண்ணாம்பு. *(Tam)* Sunnam సున్నం.

(Tel.) Núra ನೂರ. *(Malyal.)* Suṇṇá സുണ്ണ. *(Can.)* Chúṅ;
Chúná. *(Beng.)* Sudhá. *(Sans.)* Chunná. *(Mah.)* Chúno
(Guz.) Hunu. *(Cing.)* Thónpkiyu. *(Bur.).*

The above are the general names for *Lime,* whether *slaked*
or *unslaked,* but the former is generally meant by them. If the
latter *(unslaked)* is intended, it may be particularized as
follows :—

Kali-ká-chúná كلّى كا چو نا . *(Hind.)* *Kalli-ká-chunnah*
كلّى كا چنه . *(Duk.)* *Kaṛ-ṣhuṇṇámbu* கற்சுண்ணும்பு. *(Tam.)*
Rálla-sunnamu రాళ్ళ సున్నము. *(Tel.).*

133. CAMBOGIA. *(Gamboge.)*

Rubbe-révand رب ريو ند ; **Auṣárahe-révand**
غوتا غنبا عصا رأ ريو ند . *(Arab. and Pers.)* **Ghótághanbá**
عصار أ ريون . *(Hind.)* **Auṣárahe-révan** گو تا گنبا
(Duk.) **Makki** மக்கி; **Iréval-chinip-pál** இரேவல்சினிப்பால்.
(Tam.) **Révalchini-pál** రేవల్చిని-పాల్. *(Tel.)* **Révachinni-
sirá.** *(Mah.)* **Gokatu; Gokatu-melliyam.** *(Cing.)* **Ṣanato-
si, Tanato-asi** *or* **Ṣanatho-asi.** *(Bur.).*

The literal meaning of the above Arabic, Persian, Hindustani, Dukhni, Telugu, and Mahratti synonymes is *the juice* or
extract of Rhubarb, but they are, according to the usage of the
languages, the correct names of *Gamboge,* and should be restricted
to it, though misapplied in some books to Rhubarb. In some
other books, again, not only the names of the above drugs
(Gamboge and Rhuburb), but also those of the *yellow Orpiment*
are confounded with each other. Whatever may be the cause
of this confusion, it will be avoided by recognising those drugs
by the names inserted in this Catalogue under each of their
respective heads.

134. CAMPHORA. *(Camphor.)*

Káfúr كا فور . *(Arab. Pers. and Hind.)* **Kápúr** كاپور.
(Duk.) **Karuppúram** கருப்பூரம்; **Karppúram** கர்ப்பூரம்;

Shúḍan சூடன். (*Tam.*) Karpúram కర్పూరం. (*Tel.*) Karp-púram കപൂരം. (*Malyal.*) Karpúra ಕರ್ಪೂರ. (*Can.*) Kápúr; Káphúr. (*Beng.*) Karpúraha. (*Sans.*) Kápúra. (*Mah.*) Kapúr; Karpúr. (*Guz.*) Kapuru. (*Cing.*) Payo or Piyo. (*Bur.*).

From their close resemblance, the words *Kápúr* كاپور and *Kapúr* كپور are often confounded with each other in many books, and considered to be corruptions of *Káfúr* كافور. The Dukhni name *Kápúr* is correctly a corruption of the latter (*Káfúr*); but *Kapúr* كپور is a distinct name and only applicable to Amber.

The following are the names of the varieties of *Camphor* generally met with in the bazaars of Southern India:—

a. *Káfúre-qaiṣúrí* كا فور قيصري. (*Pers. Hind. and Duk.*) Pach-ch-ai-karup-púram பச்சைகருப்பூரம். (*Tam.*) Pach-cha-karpúramu పచ్చకర్పూరము. (*Tel.*).

b. *Súratt-káfúr* صورتي كافور. (*Hind. and Duk.*) Shúrattu-karup-púram சூரத்துகருப்பூரம். (*Tam.*) Súratu-karpúramu సూరతుకర్పూరము. (*Tel.*).

c. *Chíní-káfúr* چيني كا فور. (*Hind. and Duk.*). Shíná-karup-púram சீனகருப்பூரம். (*Tam.*) Chíná-karpúramu చీనకర్పూరము. (*Tel.*).

d. *Batái-kúfúr* بتا ئي كا فور. (*Hind. and Duk.*) Battáyi-karup-púram பத்தாயிகருப்பூரம். (*Tam.*) Battáyi-karpúramu బత్తాయికర్పూరము. (*Tel.*).

The Dukhni, Tamil, and Telugu names, *Ras-kápúr* رس كاپور *Raṣha-karup-púram* ரசகருப்பூரம் and *Rasa-karpúramu* రసకర్పూరము, though somewhat analogous to the above names, should not be confounded with them, for they are the names of an impure *Sub-chloride of Mercury*, not of any variety of Camphor.

135. CAMPHORA GLANDULIFERA. *Nees.* (*Sassafras of Nepaul.*)

136. CANARIUM COMMUNE, *Linn.* *(Elemi Tree.)*

137. CANARIUM STRICTUM, *Roxb. (Resin of—— Black-dammer).*

Kálá-ḍámar كالا ڈامر . *(Hind. and Duk.)* Karuppu-ḍámar அருப்படாமர். *(Tam.)* Nalla-rójan నల్లరోజన్. *(Tel.)* Kálá-ḍámar. *(Beng.)* Kálo-ḍámar. *(Guz.).*

138. CANNABIS SATIVA, *Linn.* *(Indian Hemp plant.)*

Nabátul-qinnab نبات القنب ; Nabátul-qunnab نبات القنب . *(Arab.)* Darakhte-bang درخت بنگ ; Da-rakhte-kinnab درخت كنب . *(Pers.)* Gánjé-ká-péṛ گانجے كا پیڑ . *(Hind.)* Gánjé-ká-jhaṛ گانجے كا جهاڑ . *(Duk.)* Ganjá-cheḍi கஞ்சாசெடி Kórkkar-múli கோர்க்கர்முல். *(Tam.)* Ganjávi-cheṭṭu గంజావిచెట్టు ; Kalpam-cheṭṭu కల్పంచెట్టు. *(Tel.)* Kancháva-cheṭi കഞ്ഞാവചെടി. *(Malyal.)* Bhangi-giḍá ಭಂಗಿಗಿಡ. *(Can.)* Gánjár-gáchh. *(Beng.)* Vajradru-vriksha-ha. *(Sans.)* Bhángácha-jháḍa. *(Mah.)* Bháng-nu-jháḍa ; Gánjá-nu-jháḍa. *(Guz.)* Ganjá-gahú ; Kansá-gahú. *(Cing.)* Bhén-bin ; Séjáv-bin. *(Bur.).*

Almost every part of the above plant is a useful medicine, and there is a different name for each in India. The names are as follows :—

Flowering-tops.

Qinnab قنب , or Qunnab قنب . *(Arab.)* Kinnab كنب . *(Pers.)* Gánjá گانجا . *(Hind. and Duk.)* Kór-kkar-múli கோர்க்கர்முல் ; Kalpam கல்பம் ; Ganjá கஞ்சா. *(Tam.)* Ganjá గంజా ; Bangi బంగి. *(Tel.)* Kanchá കഞ്ഞാ *(Malyal.)* Bhangi ಭಂಗಿ. *(Can.)* Gánjá. *(Beng.)* Vaj-radru. *(Sans.)* Ganjá. *(Mah.)* Gánjá. *(Guz.)* Kansá ; Ganjá. *(Cing.)* Sigiyo or Ségiyáv. *(Bur.).*

Leaves.

Ḥashish حشيش ; Qinnab قنب or Qunnab قنب . (*Arab.*) Bang بنگ . (*Pers.*) Bhang بهنگ ; Siddhí سدهي ; Sabzí سبزي . (*Hind. and Duk.*) Gaṇjá-ilai சஞ்சாஇலை ; Baṇgi-ilai பங்கிஇலை. (*Tam*) Ganjá-áku గంజాఆకు ; Bangi-áku బంగిఆకు. (*Tel.*) Kancháva-ela കഞ്ഞാവഎല. (*Malyal.*) Bhangi ಭಂಗಿ. (*Can.*) Bháng. (*Beng.*) Vajradru. (*Sans.*) Bhángá-cha-pána. (*Mah.*) Bháng. (*Guz.*) Ganjá-kola ; Kansá-kolá. (*Cing*) Bhéṅ. (*Bur.*).

Resin.

Charas چرس . (*Hind. and Duk.*) Gaṇjá-pál சஞ்சா பால் ; Gaṇjá-raṣham சஞ்சாரஷம். (*Tam.*) Ganjá-rasam గంజారసం ; Ganjá-pálu గంజాపాలు. (*Tel.*) Kanchách-cheṭip-paṣhá കഞ്ഞാചെടിപ്പശാ ; Kancháva-pála കഞ്ഞാവപാല. (*Malyal.*) Choros. (*Beng.*) Bháng-nu-ras ; Charas. (*Guz.*) Kansa-kiri ; Ganja-látu. (*Cing.*) Ṣégiyáv-así. (*Bur.*).

Seeds.

Shahdánaj شهدانج ; Bazrul-qinnab بزرالقنب . (*Arab.*) Shahdánah شهدانه ; Tuḳhme-kinnab تخمكنب ; Tuḳhme-bang تخم بنگ . (*Pers.*) Bhang-ké-bínj بهنگ كي بينج ; Gáṅjé-ké-bínj گانجي كي بينج . (*Hind. and Duk.*) Gaṇjá-virai சஞ்சாவிரை. (*Tam.*) Ganjá-vittulu గంజావిత్తులు. (*Tel.*) Kancháva-vitta കഞ്ഞാവവിത്ത. (*Malyal.*) Bhangi-bíjá ಭಂಗಿಬೀಜಾ. (*Can.*) Gáṅjár-bij. (*Beng.*) Vajradru-bíjam. (*Sans.*) Bhángácha-bí. (*Mah.*) Bháng-nu-bi ; Ganjá-nu-bí. (*Guz.*) Ganjá-aṭṭa ; Kansá-aṭṭa. (*Cing.*) Bhéṇ-si ; Séjáv-si. (*Bur.*).

Maʾjùn معجون is a general name for *Confection* or *Electuary* of any kind, but it is familiarly used for the *Confection of Indian Hemp*, which is commonly sold in the bazaar.

Subzi and *Bang* or *Bhang* are properly the names of the leaves of *C. sativa*, but they are also often used for an intoxicating drink made from them.

The Burmese names of the leaves of *Indian Hemp* (Bhén), and of Opium (Bh-ain *or* Bhín) are occasionally confounded with each other on account of the close resemblance of their pronunciation.

139. CAPPARIS APHYLLA, *Roxb.* (Oil of.)

Karél-ká-tél كريلكاتيل ; Karér-ká-tél كريرکاتيل . (*Hind.*) Karyal-ká-tél كريل كاتيل . (*Duk.*).

140. CAPSICUM FASTIGIATUM, *Blume, Syn.* CAPSICUM ANNUUM, *Linn.* (*Fruit of——Chillies.*)

Filfile-aḥmar فلفل احمر . (*Arab.*) Fifile-sur*kh* فنفل سرخ ; Pilpile-sur*kh* پلپل سرخ . (*Pers.*) Mirch مرچ ; Lál-mirch لال مرچ ; Gâch-mirch گاچ مرچ . (*Hind.*) Mirch*í* مرچي ; Lál-mirch*í* لال مرچي . (*Duk.*) Miḷagáy மிளகாய் ; Muḷagáy முளகாய். (*Tam.*) Mirapa-káya మిరపకాయ. (*Tel.*) Kappal-meḷaka കപ്പൽമെളക. (*Malyal*) Méṇaṣhiná-káyi ಮೆಣಸಿನಕಾಯಿ. (*Can.*) Lál-morich ; Lanká-morich. (*Beng.*) Marichi-phalam. (*Sans.*) Mir-singá. (*Mah.*) Lál-mirich ; Marchu. (*Guz.*) Miris. (*Cing.*) Náyu-ṣi. (*Bur.*).

141. CARBON. (*Charcoal.*)

Faḥm فحم or Faḥam فحم . (*Arab.*) Zug*h*ál زغال. (*Pers.*) Kóyelah كويله . (*Hind.*) Kólsá كولسا . (*Duk.*) Kari கரி. (*Tam.*) Boggu బొగ్గు. (*Tel.*) Kari കരി. (*Malyal.*) Iddallu ಇದ್ದಲು. (*Can.*) Kóyalá. (*Beng.*) Angá-raha. (*Sans.*) Kóḷasé. (*Mah.*) Kóelo ; Kólso. (*Guz.*) Anguru. (*Cing.*) Miṣu-e or Mídu-ye. (*Bur.*).

The wood and animal charcoals are distinguished as follows:—

Wood-charcoal (Carbo Ligni)————*Faḥmul-khashab*
فحم الخشب . (*Arab.*)   *Zughále-chóbi* زغال چوبي . (*Pers.*)
Lakri-ká-kóyclah لكڑى كا كويله . (*Hind.*) *Lakri-ká-kólsá*
(*Duk.*)   *Aḍuppu-kari* அடுப்புகரி; *Kaṭṭai-kari* சட்டைகரி. (*Tam.*)
Kaṭṭa-boggu కట్టబొగ్గు. (*Tel.*)   *Aṭuppa-kari* അടുപ്പുകരി; *Muṭṭi-*
kari ഒട്ടികരി. (*Malyal.*)   *Kaṭṭige-iddallu* ಕಟ್ಟಿಗೆಇದ್ದಲು.
(*Can.*) *Kúsh-tha-kóyalú.* (*Beng.*) *Kúshṭa-angúraha.* (*Sans.*) *Láka-*
ḍúcha-kóḻasé. (*Mah.*) *Lákḍu-kóelo.* (*Guz.*) **Thén-miṣu-e.** (*Bur.*).

Animal-charcoal (Carbo Animalis).——

Faḥmul-ḥaiván فحم الحيوان ,; *Faḥmul-gaẓm* فحم العظم . (*Arab.*)   *Zughále-ḥaiváni* زغال حيواني ;   *Zughále-ustakhán*
زغال استخوان . (*Pers.*)   *Haḍḍi-ká-kóyelah* هڈّي كا كويله . (*Hind.*)
Huḍ-ká-kólsú هڈّكا كولسا . (*Duk.*)   *Elumbu-kari* எலும்புகரி.
(*Tam.*)   *Emika-boggu* ఎమికబొగ్గు. (*Tel.*)   *Astí-kari* അസ്തികരി.
(*Malyal.*)   *Eluvu-iddallu* ಎಲುವುಇದ್ದಲು. (*Can.*)   *Asti-angúraha.*
(*Sans.*)   *Haḍa-kóḻasé.* (*Mah.*)   *Ayu-miṣu-e.* (*Bur.*).

The Cingalese name in the text, *Anguru*, is confounded in some books, with *Inguru*, which is the name of *Ginger*.

142. CARCHARIAS GLAUCUS, ——.
143. CARCHARIAS VULGARIS, ——.

} *Oil of* ——
Fish oil.

See the names under *Oleum Piscis.*

144. CARDAMOMUM. (*Cardamoms or Lesser Cardamoms.*)

Qáqilah قاقله ; *Qaqilahe-ṣighár* قاقلهصغار ; *Hél* هيل ;
Hél-bavá هيل بوا; *Kh-air-bavá* خير بوا ; *Shóshmír* شو شمير .
(*Arab.*)   *Qaqilahe-khurd* قا قلهخرد . (*Pers.*)   *Iláyechí*
الايچي ; *Chhóṭí-iláyechí* چهوٹي الايچي . (*Hind.*)   *Ilághí*
الاچي ; *Chhóṭí-iláchí* چهوٹي الاچي . (*Duk.*)   *Ela-ká* எலகா ;
Ela-káy எலகாய்; *Elakáy-virai* எலகாய்விரை. (*Tam.*)   *Ela-*
káya ఎలకాయ; *Elakáya-vittulu* ఎలకాయవిత్తులు. (*Tel.*) *Elat-*
tari എലത്തരി. (*Malyal.*)   *Yálakki* ಯಾಲಕ್ಕಿ. (*Can.*)

Elàchi. *(Beng.)* Upakunchikà. *(Sans.)* Vélà. *(Mah.)* Ilàchí. *(Guz.)* Ensal *or* Enasal. *(Cing.)* Phàlà *or* Bhàlà. *(Bur.)*.

The above are properly the names of the *Capsule*, but are generally used for both the *capsule* and *seeds*. If necessary to indicate the former particularly, the Hindustani and Dukhni names *Ilàyechí-dóré* الاچی‌توری and *Ilàchi-búndé* الاچی‌بوندے are employed.

See the remarks under the heads of ' *Amomum. Sp. of*,' with regard to the names of *Cardamom seeds*, &c.

145. CARICA PAPAYA, *Linn.* *(Fruit of.)*

Aanabahe-hindí عنبۀهندي . *(Arab. and Pers.)* Popaiyà پپیا *or* Popaiyah پپیه . *(Hind.)* Popài پپائی . *(Duk.)* Pappàyi பப்பாயி ; Pappáyi-pazham பப்பாயிபழம் ; Pappáli-pazham பப்பாளிபழம். *(Tam.)* Boppáyi-pandu బొప్పాయిపండు ; Madana-anapakáya మదనఅనపకాయ ; Madhurnakam మధుర్నకం. *(Tel.)* Pappáya-pazham പപ്പായപഴം ; Ápap-páya-pazham ആപപ്പായപഴം. *(Malyal.)* Boppáyi-hannu ಬೊಪ್ಪಾಯಿಹಣ್ಣು ; Pharangi-hannu ಫರಂಗಿಹಣ್ಣು. *(Can.)* Pappaiyà ; Pópoyiàà. *(Beng.)* Pópnyà. *(Mah.)* Papyo ; Papáyi. *(Guz.)* Pepolká. *(Cing.)* Ṣimbo-ṣi *or* Ṭimbo-ṣi. *(Bur.)*.

146. CARTHAMUS TINCTORIUS, *Linn.* *(Seeds of)*

Qurtum قرطم *or* Qirtum قرطم . *(Arab.)* Ḳhasakdánah خسکدانه ; Kájírah کاجیره ; Kázhírah کاژیره . *(Pers.)* Kaṛ کڑ ; Karaṛ-ké-bíj کڑرکے بیج . *(Hind.)* Kusam-ké-bínj کسم کے بینج . *(Duk.)* Kuṣhumbá-virai குசும்பாவிரை. *(Tam.)* Kusumbà-vittulu కుసుంబావిత్తులు ; Kusumba-vittulu కుసుంబవిత్తులు. *(Tel.)* Kusambi-bíjà కుసంబిబీజా. *(Can.)* Kusum-bíchi. *(Beng.)* Kusamba-bíjam. *(Sans.)* Ṣupán *or* Subán. *(Bur.)*.

147. CARUI FRUCTUS. *(Caraway fruits or Cara-*
way seeds.)

Karoyá كرويا ; Kamúne-armani كمون‌ارمني ; Kamúne-
rúmi كمون‌رومي . *(Arab.)* Karóyah كرويه ; Zirahe-rúmi
زيره‌رومي ; Zirahe-armani زيره‌ارمني . *(Pers.)* Viláyati-
zírah ولايتي‌زيره . *(Hind.)* Karóyah كرويه . *(Duk.)* Kékku-
virai கேக்குவிரை ; Shímai-shómbu சீமைசோம்பு . *(Tam.)*
Kéku-vittulu కేకువిత్తులు ; Shíma-sópu శీమసోపు . *(Tel.)* Bilá-
ti-jirá. *(Beng.)* Raṭa-duru. *(Cing.).*

The English and Arabic words *Caraway* and *Karóyá* being
somewhat analogous in their pronunciation, they are used
synonymously in Southern India; while in many other parts
of India, they are considered to be two distinct fruits. In
the latter places, *Caraway seeds* are named *Viláyati-zírah*, and no
Arabic and Persian names assigned to it.

The Cingalese name *Mahá-duru*, which occurs in some
books for Caraway seeds, is correctly the name of *Ani-seeds.*

148. CARUM NIGRUM,———(Fruit of.)

Kamúne-kirmáni كمون‌كرماني . *(Arab.)* Zirahe-síyáh
سياه‌زيره ; Zirahe-kirmáni زيره‌كرماني ; Síyáh-zírah سياه‌زيره .
(Pers.) Shúh-zírah شادزيرا or Shah-zirá شه‌زيره . *(Hind.*
and Duk.) Shímai-shíragam சீமைசீரகம் ; Piḷappu-shíra-
gam பிளப்புசீரகம் . *(Tam.)* Síma-jilakara సీమజీలకఱ . *(Tel.)*
Shíma-jirakam ശീമജീരകം . *(Malyal.)* Shíme-jirage
ಶೀಮೆಜೀರಗೆ . *(Con.)* Viláyati-jiré. *(Mah.).*

149. CARUM (PTYCHOTIS) AJOWAN. D. C.
(Fruit of—Ajowan fruit.)

Kamúne-mulúkí كمون‌ملوكي . *(Arab.)* Nánkháh
نانخواه ; Zinyán زنيان . *(Pers.)* Ajváyan اجواين . *(Hind.)*
Ajván اجوان . *(Duk.)* Ómam ஓமம் . *(Tam.)* Ómamu

ఓమము ; Vámamu వామము. *(Tel.)* Ayamódakam അയമോ
ദകം ; Hómam ഹോമം. *(Malyal.)* Vóma ವೋಮ. *(Can.)*
Ájvain ; Ajván. *(Beng.)* Vóva-sádá ; Vóvá. *(Mah.)*
Ajwán. *(Guz.)* Assamodaguṇ *or* Assamodagam ; Omam.
(Cing.) Samhúm. *(Bur.)*.

The *Ajowan* or *Ómam water (Aqua Ptychotis)* is known in
the bazaar by the following names:—

Aarqe-ajván عرق اجوان. *(Hind. and Duk.)* Ómat-ti-nir
இமத்தி நீர். *(Tam.)* Óma-drávakam ఓమ ద్రావకం. *(Tel.)*.

150. CARUM (PTYCHOTIS) ROXBURGHIANUM.

Benth. Syn. APIUM. INVOLUCRATUM, *Roxb. (Fruit of.)*

Bazrul-karafs بزرالكرفس. *(Arab.)* Tukhme-karafs
تخم كرفس. *(Pers.)* Ájmúd آجمود ; Ájmúdá آجمودا
(Hind.) Ájmúdah آجمودہ ; Ájmúdah-ajván آجمودہ اجوان.
(Duk.) Asham-tágam அசம்தாகம் ; Ashamtá-ómam அசம்
தாஓமம். *(Tam.)* Ajumóda-vómam అజుమోదవ్యోమం ; Ashu-
madága-vómam అశుమదాగవ్యోమం. *(Tel.)* Ájamodá-vómá
ಲಾಜಮೊದಾವೋಮಾ. *(Can.)* Rán-dhoni ; Ájmúd. *(Beng.)*
Ajamódá-vóvá. *(Mah.)*.

Karafs كرفس is in use in Arabia and Persia for the common *Celery*, but in India generally applied to the above plant.

Ájmúd, Ájmúdá, and *Ájmudah-ajván* are the Hindustani
and Dukhni synonymes of the fruit of *Carum Roxburghianum*,
but are misapplied to 'Henbane-seeds' and other drugs in
Shakespears' and other Dictionaries.

151. CARYOPHYLLUM. *(Cloves.)*

Qaranful قرنفل. *(Arab.)* Mekhak ميخک. *(Pers.)*
Lóng لونگ. *(Hind.)* Lavang لونگ. *(Duk.)* Kirámbu
கிராம்பு ; Ilavangap-pú இலவங்கப்பூ ; Karuváp-pú சுருவாப்பூ.

(*Tam.*) Lavangálu எசொ௱ய ; Lavanga-pú எசொ௰ழ. (*Tel.*)
Karámpu கராம்பு. (*Malyal.*) Lavangá எசொ௰. (*Can.*)
Lóng. (*Beng.*) Lavanga*ha*. (*Sans.*) Lavanga. (*Mah.*)
Lavang. (*Guz.*) Krábu-naṭi *or* Krámbu-naṭi. (*Cing.*) Le-
ŋiah-poén *or* Lengaṅ-poén. (*Bur.*).

152. CARYOTA URENS, *Linn.* (*Bastard Sago Tree.*)

Máṛi مازي. (*Hind.*) Máṛi-ká-*j*haṛ مازيكاجهار. (*Duk.*)
Kúndal-panai கந்தல்பணை. (*Tam.*) Chúṇṭap-pana ஜூண்ட
பன ; Íṛan-pana ௰ற௰௰ம்பன. (*Malyal.*).

153. CASSIA ABSUS, *Linn.* (*Seeds of.*)

Tashmízaj تشميزج ; *Chashmízaj* چشميزج. (*Arab.*)
Chashmízak چشميزک ; *Chashúm* چشوم. (*Pers.*) *Cháksú*
چا کسو ; *Chákút* چاکوت. (*Hind. and Duk.*) Karuṇká-
ṇam கருங்காணம் ; Káṭṭukkoḷ காட்டுக்கொள் ; Iḍikkoḷ இடிக்
கொள் ; Mulaippál-virai முலைப்பால்விளை. (*Tam.*) Chanu-
pála-vittulu சனுபாலவித்துலு. (*Tel.*) Karin-koḷḷa கரிங்கொள்ள.
(*Malyal.*) Kan-kuṭi. (*Mah.*) Chinól. (*Guz.*) Kalu-koḷḷu ;
Bú-tóra. (*Cing.*).

The meaning of some of the above names (*Karin-koḷḷa, Kalu-koḷḷu, &c.,*) is *black Horse-gram*, and they are applied to the seeds of *C. absus*, because they are black and bear a resemblance to the *Horse-gram*. But some black seeds are often found in the *Horse-gram* itself, and also used for medicinal purposes, and they are, therefore, sometimes confounded with the former.

154. CASSIA ALATA, *Linn.*

Dádmurdan دادمردن ; Dát-ká-pát داتکاپات. (*Hind.*)
Dát-ká-pattá داتکاپتا ; Viláyati-agtí ولايتی اکتی. (*Duk.*)
Shimai-agatti சீமையகத்தி ; Vaṇḍukolli வண்டுகொல்லி.

(Tam.) Shima-avishi-chettu ல. *(Tel.)* Shima-akatti ೦. *(Malyal.)* Shime-agase ಾ. *(Can.)* Dád-murdan; Dádmári. *(Beng.)* Attóra. *(Cing.)* Timbó-mezali or Simbo-maizali; Maizali-gi. *(Bur.).*

155. CASSIA AURICULATA, *Linn.*

Tarvar تَرْوَر. *(Hind. and Duk.)* Ávirai ந; Ávárai ந. *(Tam.)* Tangédu ೎. *(Tel.)* Ávára ೪; Ponnáviram ക. *(Malyal.)* Tángádi-gidá ಕ; Ávara-gidá ಕ; Taravada-gidá ಕ. *(Can.)* Taravada. *(Mah.)* Rana-vará. *(Cing.).*

156. CASSIA (CATHARTOCARPUS) FISTULA.
Linn. *(Purging Cassia—Pod or Legume of.)*

Khiyár-shanbar خيارشنبر. *(Arab.)* Khiyár-chanbar خيارچنبر. *(Pers.)* Amaltás املتاس; Amaltás-ki-*phalli* املتاس كي پهلي; Girmálah گرمالہ. *(Hind. and Duk.)* Konraik-káy க; Sharak-konraik-káy க. *(Tam.)* Réla-káyalu ర; Suvarnam స. *(Tel.)* Kounak-káya ക. *(Malyal.)* Kakke-káyi ಕ. *(Can.)* Hónálu; Shónálu; Bánor-láti. *(Beng.)* Suvarnaka. *(Sans.)* Bhávachi-séngé. *(Mah.)* Gar-málu. *(Guz.)* Áhalla or Ahilla. *(Cing.)* Nusi. *(Bur.).*

The following are the names of the *Cassia-pulp (Cassiæ pulpa)*, which is often sold in the bazaars of S. India, separately:—

Maghze-khiyár-shanbar مغز خيار شنبر. *(Arab. and Pers.)* Maghze-amaltás مغز املتاس. *(Hind. and Duk.)* Shara-konrai-puli ச. *(Tam.)* Réla-gozzu ర; Réla-gonzu ర. *(Tel.).*

157. CASSIA LIGNEA. *Syn.* **CORTEX CASSIÆ.**
(Cassia-bark).

Qirfah قرفه . *(Arab.)* Salikhah سليخه . *(Pers.)*
Taj تج . *(Hind.)* Móti-dár-chíni موتي دارچيني . *(Duk.)*
Periya-lavanga-pattai பெரியலவங்கபட்டை. *(Tam.)* Moddu-
lavanga-patta మొద్దులవంగపట్ట. *(Tel.)* Élavannap-pattá എല
വണ്ണപ്പട്ട. *(Malyal.)* Taj. *(Guz.).*

158. CASSIA LANCEOLATA, *Forsk.* } *Leaves of—*
Country, Indian,
or   Tinnevelly
159. CASSIA OBOVATA, *Colladon.* } *Senna.*

Sanáe-hindí سنا ' هندي . *(Arab. and Pers.)*   Hindí-
saná هندى سنا ; Hindí-saná-ká-pát هندي سناكاپات . *(Hind.)*
Nát ki-saná نات كي سنا ; Nat-kí-saná-ká-pattá نات كي سناكاپتا .
(Duk.)   Náttu-nilá-virai நாட்டுநிலாவிரை ; Nilávirai நிலா
விரை ; Nila-vákai நிலவாகை. *(Tam.)*   Néla-tangédu నేలతం
గేదు. *(Tel.)*   Níla-váká നിലവാക. *(Malyal.)* Nelávarike
ನೆಲಾವರಿಕೆ. *(Can.)*   Shón-pát *or* Són-pát. *(Beng.)*   Bhúí-
taravada ; Mulkácha-shóná-makhi. *(Mah.)*   Sana-kola ;
Nilávari *or* Nelávari. *(Cing.)* Puve-kain-yoe. *(Bur.).*

From the prefixes *nil, níl, nel,* and *nél,* in the Tamil, Telugu,
Canarese, Malyalim, and Cingalese names of *Senna leaves (country or otherwise)* they are misapplied sometimes to the *Indigo
plant,* and occasionally to *Indigo* itself. The proper names for
the latter are given under its respective head.

160. CASSIA OCCIDENTALIS, *Linn.*

Kasóndi كسوندي ; Bari-kasóndi بڑى كسوندي . *(Hind.*
and Duk.) Náttam-takarai நாத்தம்தகரை. *(Tam.)* Kasindha
ర్గొండ. *(Tel.)* Nátram-takara നാറ്റംതകര. *(Malyal.)*
Peni-tóra. *(Cing.)* Mezali *or* Maizali. *(Bur.).*

161. CASSIA SOPHORA, *Linn.*

Bás-kí-kasóndí باسكيكسوندي . *(Hind.)* Saṛi-kasóndí سڑ بكسوندي . *(Duk.)* Ponná-virai பொன்னைவிளை; Periya-takarai பெரியதகரை; Péṛá-virai பேறாவிளை. *(Tam.)* Kása-mardhakamu కాసమర్దకము; Tagara-cheṭṭu తగరచెట్టు; Paiḍi-tangéḍu పైడితంగేడు; Núti-kaṣhindha నూతికషింధ. *(Tel.)* Pon-nám-takara പൊന്നാംതകര. *(Malyal.)* Kál-kosandi. *(Beng.)* Úru-tora. *(Cing.).*

162. CASSIA TORA, *Linn.*

Sanjsabóyah سنجسبويه . *(Arab.)* Sangsabóyah سنگسبويه . *(Pers.)* Chakóndá چكوندا; Chakóṇḍ چكوند; Chakónṛ چكونڙ; Paṅvár پنوار . *(Hind.)* Taróṭá تروٹا or Taróṭah تروٹه . *(Duk.)* Úṣhit-tagarai ஊசித்தகரை; Tagarai தகரை. *(Tam.)* Tanṭepu-cheṭṭu తంటెపుచెట్టు; Tagiriṣha-cheṭṭu తగిరిషచెట్టు. *(Tel.)* Takara തകര. *(Malyal.)* Çhakondá. *(Beng.)* Ṭánklí. *(Mah.)* Tóra. *(Cing.)* Kiyn-e. *(Bur.).*

Qilqil قلقل or Quiqul قلقل , and *Dajrul-akbar* دجرالاكبر are found in some books (*Materia Indica, &c.,*) among the synonymes of the above seeds, but they are correctly the names of two other drugs.

163. CASTOREUM. *(Castor.)*

Jund جند ; Jande-bédastar جندبيدستر ; Quṣyatul-kalbul-baḥr قصيتالكلبالبحر . *(Arab.)* Kunde-bédastar كندبيدستر ; Áshbachagán آشبجگان ; Ḳháyahe-sage-ábí خايةسگ آبى . *(Pers.)* Jund جند . *(Hind.)* Jun جن . *(Duk.)* Junnu జున్ను; Nír-náy-virai நீர்நாய்விளை. *(Tam.)* Zunnu జున్ను; Níru-kukka-bíjam నీరుకుక్కబీజం. *(Tel.).*

164. CASUARINA MURICATA, *Roxb.* *(Casua-rina or Tinian Pine.)*

Jangli-sarv جنگلي‌سرو . *(Hind.)* Jangli-*jháú* جنگلي‌جهاؤ ; Jangli-sarú جنگلي‌سرو . *(Duk.)* Ṣhavuku-maram சவுகுமரம். *(Tam.)* Çhavuku-mánu చవుకుమాను. *(Tel.)* Chavaka-maram ചവുകമരം. *(Malyal.).*

Jangli-sarv is misapplied to *Ailanthus excelsa* in some Diction-aries, &c.

165. CATECHU *(the drug.)*

Kat کت ; Kát کات ; Kath کتهه ; Katthá کتها . *(Hind.)* Katthah کتهه . *(Duk.)* Káṣhu காசு ; Kattakámbu கத்தகாம்பு ; Káṣhukaṭṭi காசகட்டி . *(Tam.)* Kánçhu కాంచు. *(Tel.)* Káṣhikaṭṭi കാശികട്ടി ; Kátta കാത്ത. *(Malyal.)* Káchu కాచు. *(Can.)* Kat ; Kát. *(Beng.)* Kát ; Káncha. *(Mah.)* Kath-tho. *(Guz.)* Kaipu. *(Cing.)* Shází. *(Bur.).*

Besides the three usual varieties of Catechu, *black,* *red,* and *pale,* there is another in the bazaars of Southern India, which is called *Suféd-katthah* سفيدكتهه (*white catechu*). It occurs in round masses of various size, grey or pale-brown externally and white internally, and astringent in taste. It is not the produce of any particular plant, but is supposed to be prepared from the Decoction of several astringent barks. It is brought here from Hyderabad, and therefore known also as *Hyderabádi-katthah* حيدرابادي‌كتهه (*Hyderabad catechu*).

166. CAVALLIUM URENS, *Schott.*

Kavile ಕವಿಲೆ ; Errapuniki-cheṭṭu ఎఱ్ఱపునికిచెట్టు ; Tabasi తబసి ; Taṇuku-mánu తనుకుమాను. *(Tel).*

167. CEDRELA TOONA, *Roxb.*

Tún-ká-*jhár* تون‌كا‌جهار . *(Hind.)* Túṇu-maram தூணுமரம். *(Tam.)* Nandi-cheṭṭu నందిచెట్టు. *(Tel.)* Araṇa-maram അരണമരം. *(Malyal.)* Tún. *(Beng.)*

168. CELASTRUS PANICULATA, *Willd.* *(Seeds of.)*

Mál-kangni مال كنگني ; Mál-kangni-ké-binj مال كنگني كے بينج . *(Hind.)* Váluluvai வாலுளுவை ; Atiparich-cham அதிபரிச்சம். *(Tam.)* Málkanguni-vittulu కూరగంచపవిత్తులు ; Gunḍumcḍa గుండుమెడ. *(Tel.)* Váluzhuvá വാലുഴുവാ. *(Malyal.)* Málkangni. *(Beng.)* Málkángéni. *(Mah.).*

169. CELSIA COROMANDELIANA, *Vahl.*
Kúkshima. *(Beng.).*

170. CERA. *(Wax.)*

Shama شمع . *(Arab.)* Móm موم . *(Pers. Hind. and Duk.)* Mozhukku மொழுக்கு. *(Tam.)* Mainam మైనం. *(Tel.)* Mezhuka മെഴുക. *(Malyal.)* Ména మేన. *(Can.)* Móm. *(Beng.)* Madhujam. *(Sans.)* Ména. *(Mah.)* Míṇ. *(Guz.)* Iṭṭi. *(Cing.)* Phayouñ. *(Bur.).*

171. CETACEUM. *(Spermaceti.)*

Shaḥmussamak شحم السمك . *(Arab.)* Paiyahe-máhí پيئة ماي . *(Pers.)* Machhli-ki-charbi مچھلي كى چربي . *(Hind.)* Mach-chhi-ki-charbi مچھي كي چربي . *(Duk.)* Mín-kozhuppu மீன்கொழுப்பு. *(Tam.)* Chépa-kovvu చేపకొవ్వు. *(Tel.).*

172. CHAVICA (PIPER) BETLE, *Miq. (Leaf of— Betel leaf).*

Tanból تنبول . *(Arab.)* Barge-tanból برگ تنبول ; Tamból تمبول . *(Pers.)* Pán پان . *(Hind. and Duk.)* Vettilai வெத்திலை. *(Tam.)* Tamalapáku తమలపాకు ; Nága-valli నాగవల్లి. *(Tel.)* Veṭṛila വെറ്റില. *(Malyal.)* Víle-

dele ಎಲೆ ಬೆಲ. *(Can.)*   Pán. *(Beng.)*   Nágávallí. *(Sans.)*
Víḍecha-pána. *(Mah.)* Pán. *(Guz.)*   Balát. *(Cing.)*   Kún-
yoe. *(Bur.).*

See the remarks on *Alpinia galanga*, with reference to the
Greater and *Lesser Galangals* being erroneously considered to be
the roots of *Chavica Betle*.

173. CHAVICA OFFICINARUM, *Miq. Syn.* PIPER

CHABA, *Hemter.*

    Cháb چا ب ——— *fruit of*, Gaj-phal گج پھل . *(Hind.).*

174. CHAVICA ROXBURGHII, *Miq. Syn.* PIPER

LONGUM, *Linn.* *(Berries of——Long-pepper).*

    Dár-filfil فلفل د را ز . *(Arab.)* Filfile-daráz دارفلفل
(Pers.) Piplí ببلي *or* Piplíyáṅ ببليان . *(Hind. and Duk.)*
Tippili திப்பிலி. *(Tam.)* Pippaḷḷu పిప్పళ్ళు. *(Tel.)* Tippili
തിപ്പലി. *(Malyal.)* Yippali ಯಿಪ್ಪಲಿ. *(Can.)* Piplí.
(Beng.) Pippali. *(Sans.)* Pimpḷi. *(Mah.)* Pipli ; Pipér.
(Guz.) Tippili. *(Cing.)* Paikhiṅ *or* Pakhén ; Peziṅ-
ng-ouṅ. *(Bur.).*

Krishna means *black* in Sanscrit, but by some mistake it is
given as the name of *Long Pepper* in some books.

Instead of *Tippili, Káṭ-tippili* is found in the Hortus Malabaricus. The latter means *the wild Long Pepper.*

In a few books, the *Long Pepper* is confounded with *Cubebs;*
and in a few more, the Hindustani names *Piplí* and *Pippal* are
used synonymously. The latter is, however, the name of *Ficus
religiosa.*

175. CHAVICA ROXBURGHII, *Miq. (Root of.)*

    Filfile-móyah فلفل مويه . *(Arab. and Pers.)* Piplá-
mór ببلامور . *(Hind.)* Piplá-mól ببلامول . *(Duk.)*
Tippili-kaṭṭai திப்பிலிகட்டை; Tippili-vér திப்பிலிவேர்; Tippili-

múlam திப்பிலிமூலம். (*Tam.*) Módi ఠువ-2; Pippili-katta ఇప్పొరజు. (*Tel.*) Tippili-vér தിப്പിലിവെര; Kátta-tippili ಾಟ್ಟ ತಿಪ್ಪಿಲಿ. (*Malyal.*) Pipli-múl. (*Beng.*) Pimpli-múla. (*Mah.*) Pipli-múl. (*Guz.*) Tippili-múl. (*Cing.*).

176. CHICORIA ENDIVIA, *Linn.* (*Endive—Seeds of.*)

Bazrul-hindabá با الهند بزر. (*Arab.*) Tukhme-kásní (*Pers.*) Kásní-ké-binj کے بیذج کاسنی. (*Hind. and Duk.*) Káshini-virai காசിനിவിரൈ. (*Tam.*) Kásini-vittulu కాసినివిత్తులు. (*Tel.*) Káchani. (*Mah.*).

177. CHIRONIA CENTAURIOIDES, *Roxb.* Syn. ERYTHRÆA ROXBURGHII, *G. Don.*

Charáyatah چرایته. (*Hind.*) Gimá. (*Beng.*).

178. CHRYSANTHENUM ROXBURGHII, *Desv.* (*Flowers of.*)

Gule-dáúdi داؤدی گل. (*Pers.*) Gul-chíní چینی گل; Gul-chíní-ká-phúl پھول کا چینی گل. (*Hind. and Duk.*) Shámantip-pú சாமந்திப்பூ. (*Tam.*) Chámanti చామంతి; Chémanti చేమంతి. (*Tel.*) Jévanti-púva ജെവന്തിപ്പൂവ. (*Malyal.*) Shyávantige-huvu ಶ್ಯಾವಂತಿಗೆಹೂವು. (*Can.*) Gul-dáúdi. (*Beng.*) Shévantiká-pushpam. (*Sans.*) Shévanti-cha-phúla. (*Mah.*) Guldáúdi. (*Guz.*).

Gul-chíní or *Gule-chíní* is applied to the above plant in South India, but in Calcutta and many other places to *Plumiera acuminata.*

179. CICER ARIETINUM, *Linn.* (*Acidulated water or Exudation of.*)

Khallul-himmaṣ الحمص خل. (*Arab.*) Sirkahe-nakhúd نخود سرکه. (*Pers.*) Chané-ká-sirkah سرکہ کا چنے

Búnṭ-ká-sirkah بونٹ کاسرکه . *(Hind.)* Búṭ-ká-sirká بونٹ کا سرکا ; Harbare-ká-sirká هربرے کا سرکا . *(Duk.)* Kaḍalai-puḷippu கடலைபுளிப்பு; Kaḍalai-káḍi கடலைகாடி. *(Tam.)* Ṣhanaga-pulusu శనగపులుసు; Ṣhanaga-káḍi శనగకాడి. *(Tel.)* Kaḍale-káḍi കടലെകാടി. *(Malyal.)* Kaḍale-káḍi ಕಡಲೆಕಾಡಿ. *(Can.)* Chanér-sirka. *(Beng.)* Búnṭ-nu-sirko. *(Guz.)*.

The above liquid, as I have already remarked under *Acetum,* is held in the highest repute as a useful vinegar amongst the natives, and used by them frequently in many diseases. It is very cheap in those places where it is produced; such as, Mysore, Bangalore, Baigun Pully, but in great many parts of India, including Madras, its price is generally 3 or 4 times more than that of the *Wine* or *Grape Vinegar.*

Although it is commonly called a vinegar, and considered to be really so by the native practitioners and druggists; yet it is not a *vinegar* in the strictest sense of that word, for the following reasons :—

First, it is not a product of *acetous fermentation* or *destructive distillation,* which is the case with all the liquids known as vinegars. Secondly, it consists almost wholly of *Water, Oxalic Acid,* and *Acid Oxalates.* Thirdly, if *genuine,* it does not contain *Acetic Acid,* at least, to any appreciable extent. I say, *genuine,* because on account of its high price and scarcity, it is generally adulterated with the common Vinegar, and this adulteration, if slight, cannot be detected, except by testing for Acetic Acid.

The specimens I have examined for *Acetic Acid,* were of undoubted genuineness, from Baigun Pully and Bangalore, and the usual tests for that acid were applied after the *Oxalic Acid* was completely removed by *Lime,* and the liquid filtered.

The article under examination is a secretion or exudation of the *Bengal-gram* plant (*Cicer arietinum*), and is collected from it during the season of dew, when it becomes mixed with the latter, is easily taken up or absorbed by cloth, and wrung out in a vessel. The following are the two ways adopted for this purpose :—

1. In great many parts of India, where *Cicer arietinum* is cultivated, a piece of thin and clean cloth is tied to one of the ends of a stick, and the plants are touched with it early in the morning so as to absorb the dew on them, which is squeezed out in a vessel.

2. In a few places, particularly in Southern India, the plants are covered with a thin and clean cloth during the whole or last part of the night, which becomes quite wet in the morning, and is wrung out or rinsed out in a vessel.

The latter is not only the more expensive and troublesome plan, but also the liquid produced by it is much weaker ; therefore, it is not extensively employed.

It will be seen from the above explanation, that our present article is simply *an acidulated water or dew*, whose acidity almost wholly depends upon the presence of *Oxalic Acid* and *Acid Oxalates*. It is the best, cheapest, and readiest *natural* source of Oxalic Acid, and as it is, is quite fit to be administered internally all cases where the use of that acid is indicated. This liquid varies in color from pale brown to reddish brown ; and has an intense and sharp acid taste, the characterestic of Oxalic Acid, and a slight and peculiar odour which is different from that of vinegar. Its specific gravity is generally between 1,008 and 1,020.

180. **CINCHONA CALISAYA,** *Wedd.*

181. **CINCHONA CONDAMINEA,** *D. C.*

182. **CINCHONA SUCCIRUBA,** *Pavon,*

and other Sp. of Quinine-yielding CINCHONA.

} *Bark of.*

Bárak بارک . (*Duk.*) Ṣhurap-paṭṭai சரப்பட்டை. (*Tam.*) Jvarap-paṭṭa జ్వరప్పట్ట. (*Tel.*).

Quinine is known amongst the native druggists, practitioners, and other educated persons in India, as follows :—

Kinákin کناکن . (*Hind. and Duk.*) Ṣhurap-paṭṭai-ṣhattu சரப்பட்டைசத்து. (*Tam.*) Jvarap-paṭṭa-sattu జ్వరప్పట్టசత్తు. (*Tel.*).

183. CINNAMOMUM AROMATICUM, *Nees. Syn.*

C. cassia, *Blume. (Bark of——Cassia ?)*

See the names under *Cassia Lignea.*

184. CINNAMOMUM EUCALYPTOI-
DES, *Nees. Syn.* C. nitidum, *Hooker.*
185. CINNAMOMUM TAMALA, *Nees.*

} *Leaves of.*

Zarnab زرنب . (*Arab.*)   Tálispatar تا ليسپتر ؛
Talispatri تا ليسپتری ؛ Barahmí برهمي . (*Hind.*)   Taj-pát
تج پات ؛ Barmí برمي . (*Duk.*)   Tálisha-pattiri தாலிசுபத்
திரி. (*Tam.*)   Tálisha-patri తాలిశపత్రి. (*Tel.*).

Taj-pát means *Cassia-leaves*, and it is applied to the above
leaves, for they were once considered to be the leaves of the plant
which produced the *Cassia-bark.*   The name is, however, in-
correcty used in some books synonymously with *Taj*, which is
the name of *Cassia-bark*, and not of any leaves.

186. CINNAMOMUM INERS, *Rein. (Bark of ?—*
Wild Cinnamon).

Jangli-dár-chiní جنگلي دارچيني . (*Hind.*)   Janglí-
dál-chiní جنگلي دال چيني . (*Duk.*)   Káttu-karuváp-pattai
காட்டுகருவாப்பட்டை. (*Tam.*)   Adavi-lavanga-patta అడవిలవంగ
పట్ట. (*Tel.*)   Káttu-karuvátoli കാട്ടുകരുവാത്തൊലി. (*Malyal.*)
Adavi-lavanga-patte ಅಡವಿ ಲವಂಗ ಪಟ್ಟೆ. (*Can.*)   Ránácha-
dála-chinní. (*Mah.*)   Sikiyabo *or* Tikyobo. (*Bur.*).

The bark known by the above names, which is generally
supposed to be the produce of *C. iners*, is frequently substituted
in the bazaars for *Cassia Lignea*. The distinction, however,
between them is very great, though it has almost the same color.
It is a much larger and thicker bark; generally curved, but seldom completely quilled; and above all its smell and taste are
slightly aromatic, but *quite different* from those of *Cassia* or *Cinna-*

mon. So any one acquainted with *Cassia-bark*, will not easily confound the one with the other.

187. CINNAMOMUM PARTHENOXYLON, *Meissner.*

Kayo-gadis. (*Malays*).

188. CINNAMOMUM ZEYLANICUM, *Nees.* (*Bark of———Cinnamon*).

Qirfahe-sailáníyah قرفۀ سيلا نيه ; Dár-ṣíní دارصيني . (*Arab.*) Salikhahe-sailáníyah سليخۀسيلانيه ; Dár-chíní دارچيني . (*Pers.*) Qalamí-dár-*chí*ní قلمي‌دارچيني ; Dár-chíní تلمي‌دال‌چيني ; (*Hind.*) Qalamí-dal-*chí*ní تلمي‌دال‌چيني ; Dál-chíní دال‌چيني . (*Duk.*) Lavaṇgap-paṭṭai லவங்கப் படடை ; Karuváp-paṭṭai கருவாப்படடை. (*Tam.*) Lavanga-paṭṭa ల‌వ‌ంగ‌ప‌ట్ట ; Sanna-lavangapaṭṭa సన్న‌ల‌వ‌ంగ‌ప‌ట్ట. (*Tel.*) Cheriya-ela-vaṇṇa-toli ചെറിയഎല വണ്ണതൊലി ; Lavan-ga-paṭṭ വലങ്കപട. (*Malyal.*) Lavanga-paṭṭe ಲವಂಗ ಪಟ್ಟೆ ; Dála-chinni ದಾಲ ಚಿನ್ನಿ. (*Can.*) Dál-chinni. (*Beng.*) Dála-chinní. (*Mah.*) Dálchíní. (*Guz.*) Kurundu. (*Cing.*) Ṣimbo-ṣikiyabo *or* Ṭimbo-tikyobo. (*Bur.*).

Sikiyabo or *Tikyabo* is the Burmese name generally found in books for *Cinnamon*. It is not, however, the name of *true Cinnamon*, but of that produced by *Cinnamomum iners*. To distinguish the former (*Cinnamomum Zeylanicum*) the prefix *Simbo* or *Timbo* should always be added to that name.

189. CISSAMPELAS HERNANDIFOLIA, *Wall.*

Nimúka. (*Beng.*).

190. CITRULLUS COLOCYNTHIS, *Schrad.* (*Fruit of—Colocynth.*)

Hanẓal حنظل ; Aulqam علقم . (*Arab.*) Hindavánahe-talkh هندوانۀتلخ ; Kharbuzahe-talkh خربزۀ تلخ ; Kabiste-

talḳh كبست تلخ ; Ḳhar-buzahe-rúbáh خربزۀ روباه ;
(Pers.) Indáráyan اندرایین . (Hind.) Indaráven
اندراون . (Duk.) Péy-komaṭṭi பேய்கொமட்டி ; Tumaṭṭi
துமட்டி ; Péyt-tumaṭṭi பேய்த்துமட்டி ; Varit-tumaṭṭi வரித்து
மட்டி. (Tam.) Éṭi-puçh-çha పెక్కుచ్చ ; Verri-puçh-çha వెఱ్
ఱుచ్చ ; Chiṭṭi-pápara చిట్టిపాపర. (Tel.) Háva-mekke-káyi
ಹಾವಮೆಕ್ಕೆಕಾಯಿ. (Can.) Indrávan ; Múkhál. (Beng.) Indra-
varuṇí. (Sans.) Indravaṇa. (Mah.) Yakkamadu. (Cing.)
Kiyá-ṣi, Ḳhiá-ṣi or Ḳhiá-ti. (Bur.).

In Madras and a few other places, *Colocynth* is generally
named in Tamil *Komaṭṭi* while the same name in many other
parts of South India is applied to the fruit of *Bryonia callosa.*

191. CITRUS AURANTIUM, *Linn.* (*Fruit of—Orange.*)

Náranj نارنج . (*Arab.*) Nárang نارنگ . (*Pers.*) Nárangí
نارنگی . (*Hind. and Duk.*) Kich-chilip-pazham இச்சிலிப்
பழம் ; Kozhuṇjip-pazham கொழுஞ்சிப்பழம். (*Tam.*) Kich-
chili-panḍu కిచ్చిలిపండు Nárija-panḍu నారిజపండు ; Kittaḷi-panḍu
కిత్తళిపండు ; Náranga-panḍu నారంగపండు. (*Tel.*) Madhura-
náraṇṇá മധുരനാരങ്ങാ ; Kóḷánji-nárakam കൊളാഞ്ചിനാരകം
(*Malyal.*) Kittaḷe-haṇṇu ಕಿತ್ತಳೆಹಣ್ಣು. (*Can.*) Komolá-
nébu ; Nárungi. (*Beng.*) Nágaranga-*ph*alam. (*Sans.*) Ná-
ringa. (*Mah.*) Nárangi. (*Guz.*) Doḍang ; Nárang-ká.
(*Cing.*) Sh-on-ṣi. (*Bur.*).

192. CITRUS BERGAMIA. *Risso.* (*Fruit of—Lime.*)

Límúe-ḥámiẓ ليموۀ حامض ; Límú ليمو . (*Arab.*)
Límúe-tursh ليموۀ ترش ; Límú ليمو . (*Pers.*) Límúṅ
ليمون ; Níbú نيبو ; Niṅbú نينبو ; Límú ليمو . (*Hind. and
Duk.*) Elumich-cham-pazham எலுமிச்சம்பழம். (*Tam.*)

Nimma-pandu నిమ్మపండు. *(Tel.)* Cheru-náranná ചെറു നാരങ്ങാ; Jonakam-náranná ജോനകംനാരങ്ങാ. *(Malyal.)* Nimbe-hannu ನಿಂಬೆಹಣ್ಣು. *(Can.)* Nébu. *(Beng.)* Jambira-phalam. *(Sans.)* Limbu. *(Mah.)* Limbu; Nimbu. *(Guz.)* Dehi. *(Cing.)* Șámyá-și or Ṭámbiyá-si. *(Bur.)*.

There are numerous varieties of the fruit known as Nímbú *(Lime)* in India, and except the Mițhá-nímbú *(Sweet-lime)* all others, which are more or less sour in taste, are a perfect substitute for each other. The best and more juicy *Lime*, which is generally sought for by the Hakeems, when *Citron* is not to be obtained, has the following names :—

Kághazi-nímbú کاغذی نینبو *Patti-nímbú* پتي نینبو. *(Hind. and Duk.)* *Kágji-nébu; Pati-nébu. (Beng.)*.

The meaning of the above names is *Paper-lime* and *Leaf-lime*, because its rind is very thin like a *paper* or *leaf*.

193. CITRUS LIMONUM, *Risso. (Fruit of—— Lemon).*

Qalambak قلمبک *(Arab.)* **Kalanbak** کلنبک. *(Pers.)* **Bará-nímbú** بڑا نینبو *(Hind. and Duk.)* Periya-elumich-cham-pazham பெரியஎலுமிச்சம்பழம். *(Tam.)* . Pedda-nimma-pandu పెద్దనిమ్మ పండు. *(Tel.)* Valiya-cheru-náranná വലിയചെറുനാരങ്ങാ. *(Malyal.)* Doddá-nimbe-hannu ದೊಡ್ಡನಿಂಬೆಹಣ್ಣು. *(Can.)* Bara-nébu; Karná-nébú. *(Beng.)* Mahá-jambíra-phalam. *(Sans.)* Thóra-limbu. *(Mah.)* Móțu-limbu; Móțu-nimbu. *(Guz.)* Lokka-dehi. *(Cing.)* Kigı-șámya-șí. *(Bur.)*.

The natives of India do not recognise *Lemon* as a distinct fruit, but consider it a mere variety of *Lime*. It is therefore generally known by the same names or with an addition of the word *large*, as *Bará-nímbú*, &c. In Hyderabad and few other places, however, *Qalambak* or *Kalanbak* seems to be a more familiar name for it than any other.

There is a species of *Citrus* in the gardens of Madras, which I consider as a variety of *C. Limonum*; it has the following characters :—

A large shrub or small tree; much branched; leaves oval or oblong-oval, alternate in young branches and opposite in young shoots, margin slightly toothed, petiole very short and broadly margined; spines axillary, solitary and short; flowers terminal and single, white and middle-sized, stamens 20—30 or more and formed into 4 or 5 bundles, anthers oblong and yellow, petals generally 5 and purely white, calyx cup-shaped with 4 or 5 indistinct clefts; fruit about the size of a small Citron, ovate with a more or less knob at the end, pale yellow when quite ripe, rind thin with numerous vesicles of oil, and pulp acid.

This plant and fruit correspond so much with the *Fig.* in Royle and Headland's Materia Medica, page 325, that the latter looks as if it were originally taken from them. On comparing the above description with that of *C. Limonum* in Wight and Arnott's Prodromus Floræ Peninsulæ Indiæ Orientalis, page 98, I find the plant under examination is deficient only in *red tinge* of flowers, which I believe is not sufficient to consider it a distinct species instead of a variety.

Besides the above variety of *Lemon*, the fruits generally known as *Lemons* in other parts of India, are also some times, though very rarely, met with in the market of Madras. I have obtained them twice from the market, but was not able to trace out their source. On one occasion (20th September 1867), I shewed them to Dr. H. King, and he immediately recognised them to be the fruits known as *Lemons* in Europe.

These fruits were about the size of a small orange; obovate; of a greenish yellow colour; dotted with numerous vesicles of oil; terminated in an obtuse elevation or indistinct knob; and marked with 9 or 10 longitudinal depressions, which corresponded with the division of the cells inside.

194. CITRUS MEDICA, *Linn. (Fruit of—Citron).*

Utraj اترج . *(Arab.)* Turanj ترنج . *(Pers. Hind. and Duk)* Nárttam-pazham நார்த்தம்பழம். *(Tam.)* Nára-

dabba నారదబ్బ ; Dabba దబ్బ; Mádhipala-paṇḍu మాధిపలకండు ;
Bija-púra బిజపూర ; Pulla-dabba పుల్లదబ్బ ; Lungamu లుంగము.
(Tel.) Gaṇapati-náraṇṇá ഗണപതിനാരങ്ങാ. (Malyal.)
Máda-ḷada-haṇṇu మాడళదహణ్ణు. (Can.) Turanj ; Hóüsá-
nébu. (Beng.) Phalapúrá. (Sans.) Turanj ; Bijóra ;
Bálank. (Guz.) Sh-onṣakhavá or Sh-on-takhavá. (Bur.).

195. CLAY. (*A variety of—Pipe-clay.*)

Kadí كدي . (*Pers.*) **K͟harí** كهري . (*Hind. and Duk.*)
Námam நாமம். (*Tam.*) Námam నామం. (*Tel.*) Námam
നാമം. (*Malyal.*) Náma ನಾಮ. (*Can.*).

The above Hindustani and Dukhni name K͟harí should not
be confounded with K͟harí-miṭṭí, which is the name of *Chalk* in
the same languages.

The prepared *Pipe-clay*, fit to be used medicinally, is sold
under the names of *Kadíye-shustah* كدي شسته (*Pers.*) and
Dhói-huri-khaṛí دهوئي هوئي كهڑي (*Hind. and Duk.*).

The following are the names of a few other varieties of *Clay*,
used frequently in medicine by the native practitioners, and
these are in addition to *Armenian Bole* and its *Indian variety*,
which are already given under different heads.

a. *Salájit* سلاجيت . (*Hind.*) *Shilájittu* ஷிலாஜித்து.
(*Tam.*) *Salájittu* సలాజిత్తు. (*Tel.*).

b. *Gile-multání* گل ملتاني . (*Pers. and Hind.*) *Gópi* கோபி.
(*Tam.*) *Gópi* గోపి. (*Tel.*).

c. *Pakán-béd* پكان بيد . (*Hind.*).

Salájit is the *Alum Earth of Nepal; Gile-multání,* a clay
supposed to be exported from Mooltan at one time, and it is of
different color and consistence, generally yellow or pale-yellow;
and *Pakán-béd* occurs in heavy lumps of brown or brownish
blue color, and ferruginous in nature.

In some Indian bazaars, the last name, *Pakán-béd* is also
applied, with a slight alteration (*Pakhán-béd*), to a root (*Gentian*).

196. CLERODENDRON INERME, *Gærtn.*

Sang-kuppi سنگ کوپي ; Sang-kúpi سنگ کوپي ـ
(*Hind.*) Isamdhári اسمدهاري . (*Duk.*) Shengaṇ-kuppi
செங்கங்குப்பி ; Pínú-shengam-kuppi பீனூசெங்கம்குப்பி. (*Tam.*)
Piṣhinika పిషినిక ; Úṭi-cheṭṭu ఊటిచెట్టు ; Pisangi పిసంగి ; Tak-
kólapu-cheṭṭu తక్కోలపుచెట్టు. (*Tel.*) Shangam-kuppi ശങ്കം.
കുപ്പി. (*Malyal*) Bon-joí. (*Beng.*) Kundali. (*Sans.*).

Nír-noch-chi is the Tamil and Malyalim name of *Vitex
trifolia*, but it is erroneously applied to *C. inerme* in the Hortus
Malabaricus (Vol. V, Tab. 49).

197. CLERODENDRON INFORTUNATUM, *Linn.*

Ghantú ; Bhánt. (*Beng.*).

198. CLERODENDRON SERRATUM, *Blume.*
(*Root of.*)

Ganṭ-bahárangi گنت بهارنگي . (*Hind.*) Ganḍ-bahá-
rangi گنڈ بهارنگي . (*Duk.*) Shiruték சிருதேக். (*Tam.*)
Ganḍu-*bhárangi* గండుభారంగి ; Bhárangi భారంగి. (*Tel.*) Cheṛu-
tékka ചെറുതെക്ക ; Núpálu നാപാലു ; Kanṭa-*bháraṇṇí*
കണ്ടഭാരങ്ങി. (*Malyal.*) Barbará. (*Sans.*) Bháranga-
mula. (*Mah.*).

199. CLITOREA TERNATEA, *Linn.*

Mázariyúne-hindi مازريون هندى . (*Arab.*) Nabáte-
biḵhe-ḥayát ; نبات بيج حيات Darakhte-bíḵhe-ḥayát
درخت بيج حيات . (*Pers.*) Aprájitá اپراجنا ; Kavá-ṭhénthi
كواتهينتي ; Phíki-ki-jaṛ-ká-*jhár* پهيكى كى جڑ كا جهاڑ. (*Hind.*)
Ghuṭṭi-ki-jaṛ-ká-*jhár* گهټي كى جڑ كا جهاڑ . (*Hind. and
Duk.*) Kákkaṇaṇ-koḍi காக்கணங்கொடி. (*Tam.*) Dinṭana
డింటన. (*Tel.*) Shanga-puṣhpam ശങ്കപുഷ്പം ; Kákkaṇam-

koṭi കാക്കണംകൊടി; Káka-valli കാകവള്ളി. *(Malyal.)*
Aprájitá. *(Beng.)* Kattarodu. *(Cing.)*.

The two varieties of this plant are distinguished by the
color of their flowers, *white* and *blue*, in most of the languages
in the Catalogue.   In some, such as Malyalim, each variety has
a distinct name.   According to this, the name of the blue variety
in the last named language is *Káka-valli*, which means *the Crow-
creeper* in allusion to the resemblance of the color of its flowers to
that of a crow.   But this name is applied to *Mucuna gigantea*
in the Hortus Malabaricus and some other works.

The meaning of the Arabic name *Múzaríyúne-hindí*[1] is
Indian Mezereon, and this name is in use at Madras for *C. ternatea*
from the supposed resemblance of the action of its root with that
of *Mezereon root.*

The Dukhni names *Kálí-zirkí* كالي زركي or *Kálí-zirkí-ké-bínj*
كالي زركي کے بيذج, and *Suféd-zirkí* سفيد زركى or *Suféd-
zirkí-ké-bínj* سفيد زركي کے بيذج are occasionally applied to the
seeds of *C. ternatea* not only in some books, but also in some
bazaars; but these are undoubtedly the correct names of the
seeds of *Pharbitis nil* and its *red variety*, to which they should
be confined.

The Tamil names *Kákkanáṇ* காக்கணந் or *Kákkaṭáṇ*
காக்கடாந் are as frequently used for *C. ternatea* as for *Pharbitis
nil*, but they are more properly the names of the former, and
should be restricted to it.   The seeds of *Pharbitis nil* are easily
distinguished by other names given under that head.

200. CLITOREA TERNATEA, *Linn.* *(Seeds of.)*

Bazrul-mázaríyúne-hindí   بزرالمازريون هندى . *(Arab.)*
Tukhme-bikhe-ḥayát تخم بيج حيات . *(Pers.)* Aprájite-ké-
binj اپراجتی کے بيج; Kaváthénthi-ké-binj كواتهينتهي کے بيج
(Hind.) Phíki-ki-jar-ké-bínj پهيکي کى جرک بيج; Ghuṭṭi-
ki-jar-ké-bínj کهني کى جرک بيج . *(Duk.)* Kákkaṇaṇkoḍi-virai
காக்கணங்கொடிவிரை. *(Tam.)* Dintana-vittulu దింటనవిత్తులు.
(Tel.) Shanga-vitta ശംഖവിത്ത; Kákkaṇam-vitta കാക്കണംവിത്ത

വിത; Káka-vitta കാകവിത (*Malyal.*) Aprájitár-bíj. (*Beng.*) Kattarodu-bija. (*Cing.*).

See the remarks in the preceding No. with regard to the correct application of some Dukhni and Tamil synonymes to the above seeds and to the seeds of *Pharbitis nil.*

201. CNIDIUM DIFFUSUM, *D. C.* (*Seeds of.*)

Kirminji-ajván كرمنجي اجوان. (*Duk.*) Kirumiṇji-vómam இருமிஞ்சிவோமம். (*Tam.*) Kurinji-vómamu కురింజి వ్యోమము. (*Tel.*) Ban-ajvain. (*Beng.*).

See the remarks on *Hyoscyamus nigrum.*

202. OOCCINIA INDICA, *W. et A.*

Kabare-hindi كبر هندي. (*Arab. and Pers.*) Kanduri-ki-bél كندري كي بيل. (*Hind.*) Kandúri-ki-bél كندا پنڌ وكي بيل. (*Hind.*) Ḍundá-panḍú-ki-bél كند وري كي بيل; (*Duk.*) Kóvai கோவை. (*Tam.*) Doṇḍa దొండ; Káki-doṇḍa కాకిదొండ; Bimká బింక; Bimbiká బింబిక. (*Tel.*) Kóva കോവ. (*Malyal.*) Toṇḍe-baḷḷi ತೊಂಡೆ ಬಳ್ಳಿ. (*Can.*) Gorap-phal-lata; Tilá-shúrá; Tilá-kúchá. (*Beng.*) Bimbika. (*Sans.*) Gluru; Galédu. (*Guz.*) Kóvaká. (*Cing.*) Kenbh-oun-biṇ. (*Bur.*).

In the bazaars of Southern India, the root of the above plant is sold as *Bikhc-kabar* بيخ كبر which is correctly the name of the root of *Capparis spinosa.*

203. COCCULUS VILLOSUS, *D. C.*

Jamti-ki-bél جمتي كي بيل; Jamti-ká-pattá جمتي كاپتا. (*Hind. and Duk.*) Káṭṭuk-koḍi காட்டுக்கொடி. (*Tam.*) Dúsari-tige దూసరితీగ; Chípuru-tige చీపురుతీగ; Kaṭle-tige కట్లెతీగ. (*Tel.*) Haér. (*Beng*).

Faríd-búṭí فريد بوٹی is properly the name of *Pedalium murex*, which was so named in remembrance of the fact that ' Shaik Fareed Shakar-gunj' had lived for a long period solely upon the water rendered thick and mucilaginous by shaking its leaves in it. But the name is applied in some books to *Cocculus villosus*, probably from it possessing also the same property when its leaves are bruised in water.

204. COCCUS CACTI, *Linn.* *(Cochineal).*

Qirmiz قرمز ; Dúdussabbág̲h̲ín دودالصباغين . *(Arab.)* Qirmiz-dánah قرمزدانه ; Qirmize-farangí قرمز فرنگي ; Kirme-rangrézán كرم رنگر يزان . *(Pers.)* Qirmiz-dánah قرمزدانه . *(Hind.)* Kirumiṇchi-puzhuvu இருமிஞ்சிபுழுவு ; *Chappátti*-puzhuvu சப்பாத்திபுழுவு. *(Tam.)* Kiruminchi-purugu కిరుమింఛీపురుగు ; *Chappáti*-purugu చప్పాఛీపురుగు. *(Tel.).*

205. COCHLOSPERMUM GOSSYPIUM, *D. C.*
(Yellow-flowered Cotton-tree.)

Píli-kapás پيلي كپاس ; Píli-kapás-ká-*jháṛ* پيلي كپاس كا جهاڑ . *(Hind. and Duk.)* Tanaku தனகு. *(Tam.)* Konḍa-gógu కొండగోగు. *(Tel.)* S̲hima-paṇṇi-maram. ശിമപണ്ണിമരം. *(Malyal.).*

206. COCHLOSPERMUM GOSSYPIUM. *D. C.*
(Gum of—Indian Tragacanth).

Kaṣéráé-hindí كثيرائ هندى ; Samag̲h̲ul-qatáde-hindí صمغ القتادهندي . *(Arab.)* Katéráé-hindí كتيرائهندي . *(Pers.)* Hindí-katérá-gónd هندى كتيراگوند . *(Hind. and Duk.).*

Although the above gum is generally known in the Indian bazaars by the same names which are applied to *the true Tragacanth;* yet to render them applicable correctly to the former, the prefix *Indian* or *Country* should be added to them, as is the case in the text.

By some mistake, *the Tragacanth gum* is considered in some bazaars of Southern India to be the produce of the *Almond Tree*, and named accordingly in Tamil and Telugu, *Bádam-pishin* பாதம்பிஷின், and *Bádam-pisunu* బాదంపిసును. These names are, however, not in much use, being generally superseded by the Hindustani name *Katérá*.

207. COCOS NUCIFERA, *Linn.* (*Cocoanut Tree*).

Shajratun-nárjíl شجرة النارجيل ; *Shajratul-jouze-hindí* شجرة الجوزهندي . (*Arab.*) Darakhte-nárgíl درخت نارگيل. (*Pers.*) Darakhte-bádinj درخت بادنج . (*Pers.*) Nariyal-ka-péŗ ناريل كا پيŗ . (*Hind.*) Nárél-ká-jháŗ ناريل كا جهاŗ (*Duk.*) Tennay-chedi தென்னஞ்செடி ; Tenna-maram தென்னமரம். (*Tam.*) Ṭenkáya-cheṭṭu టెంకాయచెట్టు. (*Tel.*) Ténna-maram തെങ്ങുമരം. (*Malyal.*) Tenginá-giḍá ತೆಂಗಿನಮರ. (*Can.*) Nári-kél-gách̲h̲ ; Náriyal-gách̲h̲. (*Beng.*) Nári-kéla-vrikshaha. (*Sans.*) Náralícha-jháḍa. (*Mah.*) Náryal-jháḍa. (*Guz.*) Pol-gahá. (*Cing.*) Oüŋ-piŋ, Oṅ-ti-piŋ *or* Oṅ-di-piñ. (*Bur.*).

208. COCOS NUCIFERA, *Linn.* (*Fruit of——Cocoanut.*)

Nárjíl نارجيل ; *Jouze-hindí* جوزهندى . (*Arab.*) Nárgíl نارگيل ; Bádinj بادنج . (*Pers.*) Náriyal ناريل . (*Hind.*) Nárél ناريل . (*Duk.*) Téngáy தேங்காய். (*Tam.*) Ṭenkáya టెంకాయ. (*Tel.*) Ténna തെങ്ങ. (*Malyal.*) Tenginá-káyi ತೆಂಗಿನಕಾಯಿ. (*Can.*) Nárikél ; Náriyal. (*Beng.*) Nárikela-phalam. (*Sans.*) Náral. (*Mah.*) Náryal. (*Guz.*) Pol. (*Cing.*) Oü-ŋ, Oṅ-ti *or* Oṅ-di. (*Bur.*).

The names of Cocoanut Oil, Dry Kernel of Cocoanut, and Cocoanut Toddy are as follows :—

Cocoanut Oil.

Dhonun-nárjíl دهن النارجيل ; *Dhonul-jouze-hindí* دهن الجوز هندي . (*Arab.*) Róghane-nárgíl روغن نارگيل . (*Pers.*) Róghane-bádinj ر وغن با دنج . Khópará-ká-tél كهو پريكا تيل ; Náriyal-ká-tél ناريل كاتيل . (*Hind. and Duk.*) Téngá-yennney தேங்காயெண்ணெய். (*Tam.*) Tenkáya-núne ‌‌‌ (*Tel.*) Ténná-enna തെങ്ങാഎണ്ണ. (*Malyal.*) Tenginá-yanne ‌‌‌ (*Can.*) Nárikél-tail ; Náriyal-tél. (*Beng.*) Nárikéla-tailam. (*Sans.*) Náralí-cha-téla ; Kóbrácha-téla. (*Mah.*) Náryal-nu-tél. (*Guz.*) Pol-tel. (*Cing.*) Ón-ṣí or Ón-ṣí. (*Bur.*).

Dry Kernel of Cocoanut.

Khóprá كهو پرا . (*Hind.*) *Khóprá* كهو پرا ; *Khópré-ki-battí* كهو پرے كي بٹي . (*Duk.*) Kobbarait-téngáy ‌‌‌ பனாத்தேங்காய். (*Tam.*) Kobbera ‌‌‌ ; Kobbera-tenkáya ‌‌‌ (*Tel.*) Kóppara ‌‌‌ (*Malyal.*) Kobari ‌‌‌ ; Kobbari ‌‌‌ (*Can.*) *Khópru*. (*Guz.*).

Cocoanut Toddy.

Táriye-nárgíl تارئي نارگيل . (*Pers.*) Náréli ناريلي . (*Hind.*) Nárél-ki-séndí ناريل كى سيندي . (*Duk.*) Téngá-kallu தேங்காகள்ளு ; Tennan-kallu தென்னங்கள்ளு. (*Tam.*) Tenkáya-kallu ‌‌‌ (*Tel.*).

The names of the Arrack and Jaggery of the above Toddy will be found under *Liquor Spirituous* and *Saccharum.*

209. COFFEA ARABICA, *Linn.* (*Seeds of——Coffee*).

Bun بن ; Qahvá قهوا . (*Arab. and Pers.*) Bun بن ; Bún بون . (*Hind.*) Bún بون ; Búnd بوند . (*Duk.*) Kápi-kottai

காபிகொட்டை. *(Tam.)*   Kápi-vittulu. కాపివిత్తులు. *(Tel.)*
Káppi-kuru കാപ്പികുരു. *(Malyal.)*   Bonda-bíjá బొండబీజా;
Kápi-bíjá కాపిబీజా. *(Can.)*   Kápi. *(Beng.)*   Cáphi. *(Guz.)*
Kópi-aṭṭa. *(Cing.)*   Káphi-si. *(Bur.)*

210. COLEUS AROMATICUS, *Benth.*
Pátér-chúr. *(Beng.)*.

211. COLOCASIA ANTIQUORUM, *Schott.* *(Root of.)*

Qulqás قلقاس. *(Arab.)*   Arví اروی; Kachú كچو.
(Hind.)   Arví اروي; Chamkúré-ká-gaḍḍah چمكورے كا گدّہ.
(Duk.)   Shámak-kizhangu சாமக்கிழங்கு. *(Tam.)*   Cháma-
gaḍḍa చామగడ్డ. *(Tel.)*   Chémpa-kizhanna ചെമ്പകിഴങ്ങ.
(Malyal.) Sháme-gaḍḍe ಶಾಮೆಗಡ್ಡೆ; Keshavaná-gaḍḍe ಕೇಶವನಾ
ಗಡ್ಡೆ. *(Can.)*   Guri-kochu. *(Beng.)*

212. COPTIS TEETA, *Wall.* *(Coptis, or Mishmi Tita.)*
Pita-karosana. *(Cing.)*

213. CORCHORUS OLITORIUS, *Linn.*
Peraṭṭi-kírai பெரட்டிகீரை. *(Tam.)*   Parinṭa పరింట;
Périnṭa-kúra పేరింటకూర. *(Tel.)*   Páṭ. *(Beng.)*

214. CORDIA LATIFOLIA, *Roxb.* *(Fruit of—— Small Sebestens.)*
Mokhátah مخاطہ; Mokhítah مخيطہ. *(Arab.)*   Sapis-
tán سپستان; Sabistán سبستان; Sagpistán سگپستان.
(Pers.)   Chhóṭá-lasórá چھوٹا لسوڑا; Chhóṭá-laslasá
چھوٹاالسلسا. *(Hind.)*   Chhóṭi-góndní چھوٹی گوندني. *(Duk.)*
Shiṛu-naṛuviḷi சிறுநறுவிளி. *(Tam.)*   Chinna-nakkera-cheṭṭu

చిన్నఁ బొటుకు ; *Chinna-boṭuku* చిన్నబొటుకు ; *Kichavirigi-chettu.* కీచవిరిగిచెట్టు. *(Tel.)* *Cheṛu-vanich-chi* ചെറുവനിച്ചി ; *Cheṛu-viri* ചെറുവിരി ; *Koṭṭá* കൊട്ടാ. *(Malyal.)* *Chhoto-bohuṛári. (Beng.)* *Nánu-gúndi. (Guz.)* Tana, Tana-ṣi *or* Ṣana-ṣi. *(Bur.).*

215. CORDIA MYXA, *Linn. (Fruit of——Large Sebestens.)*

Moḵháṭahe-kabír مخا طه كبير . *(Arab.)* Sapistáne-kalán سپستان كلان . *(Pers.)* Baṛá-lasóṛá بڑا لسوڑا . *(Hind.)* Baṛí-góndní بڑی گوندنی . *(Duk.)* Periya-naṛuviḷi പെറിയநறுவிளி. *(Tam.)* Pedda-nakkera-cheṭṭu పెద్దనక్కెరచెట్టు ; Iriki ఇరికి ; Vúra-nakkéru వూరనక్కేరు ; Pedda-boṭuku పెద్దబొటుకు ; Nak-kéru నక్కేరు ; Nakkera-cheṭṭu నక్కెరచెట్టు. *(Tel.)* Valiya-vanich-chi വലിയവന്ച്ചി ; Periya-viri പെരിയവിരി. *(Malyal.)* Baṛa-bohuṛári. *(Beng.)* Muṭṭi-gúndi. *(Guz.)* Ṣana-gi *or* Ṭana-gi ; Maiyá *or* Ṭana-maiyá. *(Bur.).*

216. CORIANDRUM SATIVUM, *Linn. (Fruits of—Coriander Fruits or Seeds.)*

Kuẓbarah كذبرہ . *(Arab.)* Kashníz كشنيز . *(Pers.)* Dhanyá. دهنيا . *(Hind.)* Dhanyáň دهنيان . *(Duk.)* Kottamalli கொத்தமல்லி. *(Tam.)* Daniyálu దనియాలు ; Kotimiri కొతిమిర. *(Tel.)* Kottam-pálari കൊത്തമ്പാലറി ; Kotta-malli കൊത്തമല്ലി. *(Malyal.)* Kottamari-bíjá ಕೊತ್ತಮರಿಬೀಜ. *(Can.)* Dhanya-á. *(Beng.)* Kustumbaru ; *Dhán-yákam. (Sans.)* Dhana. *(Mah.)* Dhána. *(Guz.)* Dhanalu ; Kottamalli-aṭṭa. *(Cing.)* Nana-zi. *(Bur.).*

Kottamalli or *Kothímír* are the names of the plant in some of the above languages, and *Dhanyá* or *Daniyálu* the names of its fruits *(seeds)*, but they are all used often indiscriminately for either or both.

217. CORNU CERVI. *(Hart's Horn).*

Qarnul-él قرن الايل . *(Arab.)* Shákhe-gavazn شاخ گوزن .
(Pers.) Bárá-singé-ki-síng باراسنگے كي سينگ . *(Hind.)*
Bárá-singí باراسنگي . *(Duk.)* Kalaimán-kombu கலைமான்
கொம்பு. *(Tam.)* Duppi-kommu దుప్పికొమ్ము. *(Tel.)* Kale-
yan-konpa കലെയൻകൊമ്പ. *(Malyal.)* Duppi-kombu ದುಪ್ಪಿ
ಕೊಮ್ಮು. *(Can.)* Gou-sor-shing. *(Beng.)* Chá-gio or Ságiyo.
(Bur.).

218. CORVINUS COITOR, *Blyth. (Indian Whiting.)*

Na-pou-tin——*smaller variety,* Nabiye. *(Bur.)*.

For the names of the *Sounds* of this fish, see *Icthyocolla.*

219. CORYDALIS GOVANIANA, *Wall.*

Bhút-kush بهو ت كش . *(Hind.)* *Bhút-kas. (Beng.).*

220. CORYPHA UMBRACULIFERA, *Linn. (Tali-pot palm.)*

Bajar-battú-ká-*jhár* بجر بتّوكاجهاز . *(Duk.)* Kottaip-
pan*ai* கொட்டைப்பனை; Tálip-pan*ai* தாளிப்பனை. *(Tam.)*
Shrítálam శ్రీతాళం. *(Tel.)* Kotap-pana കൊടപ്പന. *(Malyal.)* Shritále-mará ಶ್ರೀತಾಳೆಮರಾ. *(Can.)* Táli ; Bajar-
battulér-gá*chh. (Beng.)* Bajar-battu-nu-*jhá*da. *(Guz.)* Táli-
pat. *(Cing.)* Pé-bin. *(Bur.)*.

221. COSCINIUM FENESTRATUM, *Cobbr. (Wood of.)*

Jhár-ki-haldí جهاز كى هلد ي . *(Duk.)* Mara-manjal
மரமஞ்சள். *(Tam.)* Mánu-pasupu మానుపసుపు. *(Tel.)* Mara-
manjal മരമഞ്ഞൾ. *(Malyal.)* Marada-arishiná ಮರದ

ಆಶಿನಾ· *(Can.)* Dárú-haridrakam. *(Sans.)* Jhádi-halcdé. *(Mah.)* Venivel. *(Cing.).*

See the remarks under the species of *Berberis*, with respect to the name *Dár-hald*, which is occasionally misapplied to the wood of *C. fenestratum*.

222. COTYLEDON LACINIATA, *Linn.*

Zakhm-ḥayat-ká-pattá زخم حيات كاپتا . *(Duk.)* Ela-maruṇṇa എലമരുന്ന ; Muṟikúṭi മുറികുടി. *(Malyal.)* Tonná-haḍakana-giḍá ತೊನ್ನಾ ಹಡಕ ನ ಗಿಡಾ. *(Can.)* Kóp-pátá. *(Beng.)* Yoe-kiyá-piṇ-ba. *(Bur.).*

223. CRATÆVA RELIGIOSA, *Forst. (Leaf of.)*

Bél-patri بيل پتری ; Bél-ká-pát بيل كاپات . *(Hind.)* Vilvap-pattiri வில்வப்பத்திரி ; Bilva-ilai பில்வஇலை. *(Tam.)* Vilva-patri విల్వపత్రి ; Bilva-áku విల్వఆకు. *(Tel.)* Vilva-patram വിൽവപത്രം. *(Malyal.)* Bila-patri ಬಿಲ ಪತ್ರಿ. *(Can.)* Bilva-patram. *(Sans.).*

The meaning of all the above names is *the leaf of Bael or the fruit of Ægle marmelos*, accordingly the medicine I have obtained under these names from several places was the dry leaves of the latter plant or its cultivated variety.

224. CRETA. *(Chalk.)*

Ṭine-abyaẓ طين ا بيض . *(Arab.)* Gile-supéd گل سپيد . *(Pers.)* Khari-miṭṭi كهري منّى . *(Hind.)* Viláyati-*ch*unná ولايتي چنا . *(Duk.)* Ṣhimai-ṣhuṇṇámbu சிமைசண்ணாம்பு. *(Tam.)* Ṣhima-sunnam శిమసున్నం. *(Tel.)* Ṣhima-núra ശിമനൂര. *(Malyal.)* Ṣhima-suṇṇá ಶಿಮಸುಣ್ಣಾ. *(Can.)* Khari-máti. *(Beng.)* Dvípa-sudhá. *(Sans.)* Viláyati-*ch*uná. *(Mah.)* Chák ; Viláti-*ch*unó. *(Guz.)* Raṭa-hunu. *(Cing.)* Mie-*ph*iú or Me-biyu ; *Th*ombiyu. *(Bur.).*

See the remarks under *Clay.*

225. CRINUM ASIATICUM, *var.* TOXICARIUM, *Herbert.*

Su*kh*darsan سكهدرسن ; Bará-kanvár برا كنوار . *(Hind.)* Nágin-ká-pattá ناگن كا پتا . *(Duk.)* Visha-múṇgil விஷ மூங்கில். *(Tam.)* Visha-mungali విషముంగలి ; Lakshmi-náráyaṇa-che*ṭṭ*u లక్ష్మీనారాయణచెట్టు ; Késara-che*ṭṭ*u కేసరచెట్టు. *(Tel.)* Kántéṇṇa കാന്തെണ്ണ ; Visha-múḷa విషమూళ ; Poḷattáḷi പൊളത്താളി. *(Malyal.)* Baṛa-kanvár ; Gáer-hónár-pátá. *(Beng.)* Tolabo *or* Hín-tolabo. *(Cing.)* Kó-yánji. *(Bur.).*

The Malyalim name *Poḷattáḷi* is from the Hortus Malabaricus, which is not generally recognisable.

Kánbalu is given in some books as a Burmese name of *C. Asiaticum,* but it is the name of another plant, which is odoriferous and generally found in Siam.

226. CROCUS. *(Saffron.)*

Zaạfaráṅ زعفران . *(Arab. and Pers.)* ˙ Kumkum كمكم ; Késar كيسر . *(Hind.)* Késar-ké-*ph*úl كيسر كے پهول . *(Duk.)* Kuṇgum-pú குங்குப்பூ. *(Tam.)* Kumkuma-puvvu కుంకుమ పువ్వు ; Kumkuma-késaramu కుంకుమకేసరము. *(Tel.)* Kumkuma-puvva കുങ്കുമപ്പൂവ്. *(Malyal.)* Kumkuma-késari ಕುಂಕುಮಕೇಸರಿ ; Kumkumada-huvú ಕುಂಕುಮದಹೂವು ; Késari ಕೇಸರಿ. *(Can.)* Késur ; Jáphráṅ. *(Beng.)* Késara. *(Sans.)* Késaré. *(Mah.)* Késar. *(Guz.)* Kum-kuma-pu ; Kungama-mal. *(Cing.).*

Kurkum كركم is the Arabic name of *Turmeric (Curcuma longa,)* but applied in many Persian and other works to *Saffron;* apparently from confounding it with Kumkum كمكم . Likewise the Arabic name *Ạabír* عبير is misapplied to the same *(Saffron)*, but it is the name of a compound odoriferous powder. *Késar* is correctly the name of *Saffron* but it is misapplied to *Rottlera tinctoria* in some books.

227. CROTALARIA JUNCEA, *Linn.* *(Seeds of—Sun-hemp Seeds.)*

San-ké-bínj سن کی بیذج . (*Hind.*) Janab-ké-bínj جنب کی بیذج . (*Duk.*) Jenappa-vira*i* ஜெனப்பவிரை. (*Tam.*) Jenapa-vittulu జెనపవిత్తులు. (*Tel.*) Janapa-vera ജനപവെര; Puḷivanji-vitta പുളിവഞ്ജിവിത്ത ; Vakka-vitta വക്ക വിത്ത ; *Chaṇa-vitta* ചണവിത്ത. (*Malyal.*) Ṣhaṇa-biná-bijá ಶಣಬೀನಾಬೀಜಾ ; Puṇḍi-bijá ಪುಂಡಿಬೀಜಾ. (*Can.*) Ṣhon-bichi *or* Son-bichi. (*Beng.*) San-nu-bij. (*Guz.*) Paisán-si. (*Bur.*).

The Malyalim name assigned to this plant in the Hortus Malabaricus, (Vol. IX, Tab. 26,) viz., *Takkali-koḍi* is incorrect. The names that are generally in use are those that I have given above in the text.

228. CROTALARIA JUNCEA, *Linn.* *(Fibre of—Sun-hemp.)*

San سن . (*Hind.*) Janab جنب ; Janab-ká-nár جنب کا نار . (*Duk.*) Jenappa-nár ஜெனப்பநர். (*Tam.*) Jenapa-nára జెనపనార ; Janumu జనుము. (*Tel.*) Janapa-nára ജനപനാര ; Puḷivanji-nára പുളിവഞ്ജിനാര ; Vakkavanji വക്കവഞ്ജി ; *Chaṇam* ചണം. (*Malyal.*) Ṣhaṇabiná-náru ಶಣಬೀನಾನಾರು ; Puṇḍi-náru ಪುಂಡಿನಾರು. (*Can.*) Ṣhon *or* Ṣhon-páṭ ; Son *or* Son-páṭ. (*Beng.*) San. (*Guz.*) Paisán. (*Bur.*).

Pán or 'Pan' is the Burmese name found in some books for the above fibre, but properly it is the name of another fibre common in Thavoy, and not of the *Sun-hemp*.

229. CROTON POLYANDRUM, *Roxb.* *Syn.* C. ROXBURGHII, *Wall.*

Ḥabbussalátine-ṣaḥrái حب السلاطین صحرائی . (*Arab.*) Ḥabbussalátine-barri حب السلاطین بري . (*Pers.*) Jangli-

jamálgótá جنگلی جمال گوتا . (*Hind.*)　Janglí-jamál-*ghuttah*
جنگلی جمال غته . (*Duk.*)　Káttámanakku காட்டாமணக்கு;
Shimai-ámanakku சிமைஆமணக்கு. (*Tam.*)　Konda-ámudam
కొండఆముదం; Erra-dundiga-chettu ఎఱ్ఱదుండిగచెట్టు; Adavi-
ámudam అడవిఆముదం. (*Tel.*)　Shima-ámanakku ശീമ
ആമണക്ക; Kata-lávanakku കടലാവണക്ക. (*Malyal.*)
Káda-haralu ಕಾಡ ಹರಳು. (*Can.*)　Hákúi; Danti. (*Beng.*)
Janglí-jamálgota. (*Guz.*)　To-kanak*ho*-si *or* To-*khanakho*-
si. (*Bur.*).

The native names of *Croton polyandrum* and *Jatropha circas*
are very often confounded with each other. The reason of this
is, that in some places as well as in some languages the first plant
is considered and named as the wild variety of the *Croton-oil
plant*, and the second the wild variety of the *Castor-oil plant*;
while it is just the reverse in some other places and languages.
The names inserted under the head of each of the above plants
in this Catalogue, are those that are in use in most parts of
India.

230. CROTON·TIGLIUM, *Linn.* (*Croton-oil plant—Seeds of.*)

Habbussalátín حب السلاطين; Dand دند; Dátún داتون .
(*Arab.*)　Béd-anjíre-*khatái* بيدانجيرخطائي; Habbe-*khatái*
حب خطائي . (*Pers.*) Jépál جيپال; Jépál-gótá جيپال گوتا;
Jamál-gótá جمال گوتا . (*Hind.*)　Jamál-guttah جمال گته
; Jamál-*ghuttah* جمال غته . (*Duk.*)　Nérválam நேர்வாளம்.
(*Tam.*)　Nepála-vittulu నేపాలవిత్తులు. (*Tel.*)　Nírválam
നിർവാളം. (*Malyal.*)　Jápálada-bijá ಜಾಪಾಳದ ಬೀಜ. (*Can.*)
Jépál; Jamálgótá. (*Beng.*) Nepálácha-bi. (*Mah.*) Jamálgoto.
(*Guz.*) Jápála *or* Jaipála. (*Cing.*)　Kanak*ho*-si *or* *Khana*-
kho-si; Sa-díva *or* Tadíva. (*Bur.*).

231.   CUBEBA OFFICINALIS, *Miquel.* (*Fruit of—Cubebs.*)

Kabábah كبابه . (*Arab.*)   Kabáb-*chini* كباب چيني .
(*Pers. Hind. and Duk.*)   Válmiḷaku வால்மிளகு . (*Tam.*)
Tóka-miriyálu తోకమిరియాలు ; Çhalava-miriyálu చెలవ
మిరియాలు. (*Tel.*) Vál-muḷaka വാല്‍മുളക (*Malyal.*) Bála-
meṇasu ಬಾಲಮೆಣಸು. (*Can.*) Kábáb-chini. (*Beng.*) Kabába-
chini ; Himsi-mire. (*Mah.*) Kabáb-chini ; Taḍa-miri (*Guz.*)
Válmoḷagu *or* Vál-moḷavú. (*Cing.*).

In Southern India and other places, *Sital-chini* سيتل چيني
is the name in use for *Cubebs,* and *Kabáb-chini* كباب چيني
for the berries of *Eugenia Pimenta (Allspice);* but it is the reverse
in Calcutta and many other places, where the former (*Sital-
chini*) is applied to *Allspice,* and the latter (*Kabáb-chini*) to
Cubebs. I have adopted the latter, because it is by this name
that *Cubebs* are generally recognised in most of the Government
Hospitals and Dispensaries in India.

There is also another confusion about the name of *Kabáb-
chini* in some bazaars, particularly those at Madras, where it
is often applied to the buds of *Mesua ferrea.* This is incorrect,
for the proper name of the latter is *Nágésar* ناگيسر .

232.   CUCUMIS HARDWICKII, *Roy.* (*Fruit of.*)

Pahári-indaráyan پهاڑي اندر این . (*Hind.*) Malait-tu-
maṭṭi மலைத்துமட்டி. (*Tam.*) Konda-puçh-çha కొండపుచ్చ.
(*Tel.*) Varik-kumaṭṭi വരിക്കുമട്ടി. (*Malyal.*).

233.   CUCUMIS TRIGONUS, *Roxb. Syn.* C. PSEUDO-
COLOCYNTHIS, *Roy.* (*Fruit of.*)

Bislómbi بسلومبي ; Bislambhi بسلمبهي : Jangli-inda-
ráyan جنگلي اندراين . (*Hind.*) Káṭṭut-tumaṭṭi காட்டுத்துமட்டி.
(*Tam.*) Aḍavi-puçh-çha అడవిపుచ్చ. (*Tel.*)

234. CUCUMIS UTILISSIMUS, *Roxb.* *(Seeds of.)*

Bazrul-qiṣṣáa بزرالقثا . *(Arab.)* Tukhme-khiyáre-daráz تخم خيا رزد ; Tukhme-khiyárzah تخم خيار دراز ; Tukhme-khiyár تخم خيار . *(Pers.)* Kakrí-ké-bíj ککری کے بيج *(Hind.)* Kankri-ké-binj کنکری کے بينج . *(Duk.)* Kak-karik-káy-virai கக்கரிக்காய்விளை ; Muḷ-veḷḷirik-káy-virai முள்வெள்ளிரிக்காய்விளை. *(Tam.)* Muṭṭu-dósakáya-vittulu ముట్టుదోసకాయవిత్తులు. *(Tel.)* Kakkarikka-vitta കക്കരിക്ക വിത്ത. *(Malyal.)* Muḷḷu-savate-bíjá ಮುಳ್ಳುಸವತೆಬೀಜಾ. *(Can.)* Khírár-bíj. *(Beng.)* Ṭakhvá-ṣi. *(Bur.)*.

235. CUCURBITA MAXIMA, *Duch.* *(Fruit of.)*

Miṭhá-kaddú ميٿها کدو . *(Duk.)* Púṣhinik-káy பூஷிணிக்காய். *(Tam.)* Gummaḍi-káya గుమ్మడికాయ. *(Tel.)* Mattaṇga മത്തങ്ങ. *(Malyal.)* Kumbaḷa-káyi ಕುಂಬಳಕಾಯಿ ; Kumbaḷa-haṇṇu ಕುಂಬಳಹಣ್ಣು. *(Can).* Saphúri-komra. *(Beng.)*.

See the remarks under the next plant.

236. CUCURBITA PEPO, *Roxb.* *(Fruit of.)*

Majdabah مجدبه . *(Arab. and Pers.)* Kudímah کدیمه ; Péṭhá پيٿها ; Kóṅḍhá کونڈها *(Hind.)* Péṭhah پيٿه . *(Duk.)* Kaliyáṇa-púṣhinik-káy கலியாண பூஷிணிக்காய். *(Tam.)* Búḍide-gummaḍi బూడిదగుమ్మడి ; Pendli-gummaḍi-káya పెండ్లిగుమ్మడికాయ. *(Tel.)* Kumpaḷaṇṇá കുമ്പളങ്ങാ ; Kumpaḷam കുമ്പളം. *(Malyal.)* Búde-kumbaḷa-káyi ಬೂದ ಕುಂಬಳ ಕಾಯಿ. *(Can.)* Kumrá ; Chál-kumrá. *(Beng.)* Kúsh-pándaha. *(Sans.)*. Kohaḷa. *(Mah.)* Kóḷu ; Káṭá-bhúro-kóḷu. *(Guz.)*.

In some books the above fruit is confounded with *Miṭhú kaddú* ميٿهاکدو, which is the name o the fruit of *C. maxima.*

237. CUMINUM CYMINUM, *Linn.* *(Fruit of—Cumin Fruits or Seeds.)*

Kamún كمون . *(Arab.)* Zirá زيرا or Zirah زيره . *(Pers. and Hind.)* Jirá جيرا . *(Duk.)* Shíragam ஜீரகம். *(Tam.)* Jilakara జీలకఱ; Jiraka జీరక; Jiraṇa జీరణ. *(Tel.)* Jirakam ജീരകം. *(Malyal.)* Jirage ಜೀರಿಗೆ. *(Can.)* Jira; Zirá. *(Beng.)* Jirakaha. *(Sans.)* Jiré. *(Mah.)* Ziro. *(Guz.)* Duru; Sudu-duru. *(Cing.)* Ziyá. *(Bur.)*.

238. CUPRUM. *(Copper.)*

Noḥás نحاس . *(Arab.)* Mis مس . *(Pers.)* Táṅbah or Táṅbá تانبا . *(Hind. and Duk.)* Shembu செம்பு. *(Tam.)* Rági ತಾಮ್ರ; Túmramu తామ్రము. *(Tel.)* Shenba ചെമ്പ. *(Malyal.)* Támbra ತಾಮ್ರ. *(Can.)* Támra; Táṅba. *(Beng.)* Támram. *(Sans.)* Tambra. *(Mah.)* Trámbu. *(Guz.)* Kaiye-ni. *(Bur.)*.

239. CUPRI SUBACETAS. *(Subacetate of Copper, or Verdigris.)*

Zanjár زنجار . *(Arab.)* Zangăr زنگار . *(Pers.)* Zangár زنگار; Pitrái پترائی . *(Hind.)* Zangál زنگال . *(Duk.)* Shaṅgál-pach-ch-ai சங்காரப்பச்சை. *(Tam.)* Jengálu-pach-çha జంగాలుపచ్చ. *(Tel.)* Chengala-pach-cha ചെങ്കലപച്ച; Pach-cha-nílam പച്ചനീലം. *(Malyal.)* Jengála-pach-che ಜಂಗಾಲಪಚ್ಚೆ. *(Can.)* Támár-jhangár. *(Beng.)* Jengála-pacha. *(Sans.)* Jangár. *(Guz.)* Kihiṇ or Kihiṅ. *(Bur.)*.

240. CUPRI SULPHAS. *(Sulphate of Copper, or Blue stone.)*

Zájul-akhẓar زاج الاخضر; Záje-akhẓar زاج اخضر; Qalqand قلقند . *(Arab.)* Záke-sabz زاک سبز . *(Pers.)* Nilá-

thúthá نيلا تو تا ; Nilá-tútá نيلا تو تا . *(Hind.)*   Mór-tuttá
مور تتا ; *Mhór-tuttah* موَر تتَه . *(Duk.)*   Mayil-tuttam மயில்
தத்தம் ; Tuttam-turichi தத்தம்துரிசி. *(Tam.)*   Mayilu-
tuttam మయిలుతుత్తం. *(Tel.)*   Mayil-tutta മയില്‍തുത്ത ;
Turisha തുരിശ. *(Malyal.)* Mail-tutyá ಮೈಲ್‌ತುತ್ಯ. *(Can.)*
Tútiyá. *(Beng.)* Tuth-thánjanam. *(Sans.)* Mórtúta. *(Guz.)*
Palmánikam. *(Cing.)*   Douthá or Douthá. *(Bur.)*.

241. CURCULIGO ORCHIDIOIDES, *Gaertn.* *(Root of.)*

Káli-músli كالي موسلى ; Siyáh-músli سيا ه موسلي .
(Hind.)   Káli-músli كالي مو صلي . *(Duk.)*   Nilap-panaik-
kizhangu நிலப்பனைக்கிழங்கு. *(Tam.)*   Néla-táti-gaddalu
నేలతాటిగడ్డలు. *(Tel.)* Nelappana-kizhanna നെലപ്പനകിഴങ്ങ.
(Malyal.) Nela-táti-gadde ನೆಲತಾಟಿಗಡ್ಡೆ. *(Can.)*   Tállurá ;
Sáda-mushli; Shaphéd-mushli. *(Beng.)* Tálamúliká. *(Sans.)*
Káli-musli. *(Guz.)*.

See the remarks under *Asparagus ascendens.*

242. CURCUMA AMADA, *Roxb.* *(Root of—Mango Ginger.)*

Ám-haldi آم حلد ي . *(Hind.)*   Ám-kí-bó-kí-adrak
آم كي بو كي ادرك . *(Duk.)*   Árukamlaka-chóram ಆರುಕಂಲ
ಕಚೋರ ; Mámidi-allam కా+మిడిఅల్లం. *(Tel.)*   Phóliyá. *(Beng.)*.

Although the Malyalim name *Kúra* ಕೂರ is correctly applicable only to *Curcuma angustifolia* and *C. leucorrhiza,* it is often
used in Malabar for *C. Amada,* because the tuberous root of this
plant also yields a kind of *Arrowroot.*

243. CURCUMA ANGUSTIFOLIA, *Roxb.* *(Root of.)*

Tikhar تيكهر ; Tikhar تكهر . *(Hind.)* Viláyatí-áté-ké-
gaddé و لايتي آتے كے گڈے : Kuvé-ké-nasháraté-ké-gaddé

آر اروٹ کے گڈے ; Árárút-ké-gaḍḍé کو ے کے نشاستی کے گڈے .
(Duk.) Kúvámávu-kizhaṇgu கூவாமாவுகிழங்கு ; Ararút-
kizhaṇgu அரருட்கிழங்கு. (Tam.) Ararút-gaḍḍalu అరరూట్
గడ్డలు. (Tel.) Kúva கூவ ; Kúva-kizhaṇṇa கூவகிழங்ஞ.
(Malyal.) Árorutér-múl. (Beng.).

See the remarks under *Curcuma Amada*.

244. CURCUMA AROMATICA, *Salisb.* *Syn.* CUR-
CUMA ZEDOARIA, *Roxb.* (*Root of—Round Zedoary.*)

Áṅbé-halad آنبی هلد ; Áṅbé-haldí آنبی هلد ی ; Janglí-
haldí جنگلی هلدي . (*Hind.*) Áṅbé-haldí آنبی هلدی ; Ambé-
haldí امبی هلدي . (*Duk.*) Kastúri-maṇjal கஸ்தூரிமஞ்சள்.
(*Tam.*) Kastúri-pasupu కస్తూరిపసుపు. (*Tel.*) Káṭṭu-maṇṇal
காட்டமஞ்சம் ; Kastúri-maṇṇal കസ്തൂരിമഞ്ചം ; Ánakúva
അനക്കൂവ.(*Malyal.*) Kastúri-arishiná ಕಸ್ತೂರಿಅರಿಶಿನಾ. (*Can.*)
Jangli-haldi ; Ban-holodi ; Ámbé-holodi. (*Beng.*)   Ámbí-
haleda. (*Mah.*) Ámba-halad ; Haradal. (*Guz.*) Kiyáṣanoiṇ.
(*Bur.*).

In a great many works, (Richardson, Shakespear, Forbes'
and other Dictionaries, Materia Indica, &c.,) the Arabic name
Jadvár جدوار and its Persian and Hindustani synonymes
Mah-parvín مه پروین and *Nirbasí* نربسي are applied to *Round
Zedoary,* which is incorrect as I have already explained under
the head of '*Aconitum,*' page 31. *Round Zedoary* is undoubtedly
the *Áṅbé-haldí* of the bazaar, which is very different from
Jadvár. The cause of this error is attributable to the slight
similarity that exists between the sounds of the words *Jadvár*
or *Zadvár* and the English name *Zedoary.*

There is a root in the Indian bazaars, which bears a resemblance to the *Round Zedoary,* except the yellow color and
aromatic smell of the latter. It occurs in segments (quarters
and halves,) which show that it is originally a round tuberous
root. It is of dirty-white or pale-grey color, possesses no smell,

and has a bitter taste. It is recognised at Madras under the Sanscrit, Tamil, and Telugu names ' *Nir-visha*' and ' *Niri-visham*'; and for the reason already explained, the Hindustani name *Nirbari* is also misapplied to it. According to some Telugu practitioners it is the white variety of *Round Zedoary*, and this view is also countenanced by some works (Flora Andhrica,) in which *Tella-kastúri-pasupu* తెల్లకస్తూరిపసుపు is given as its Telugu name. How far this is correct I cannot say, because I have not as yet traced out the plant which produces the root, nor do I know any white variety of *C. aromatica* to exist.

The root under question is a strong and active medicine, and is supposed to be poisonous in large doses.

The Hindustani name *Ánbe-haldi* is used synonymously with *Dár-hald* دارهلد in some Persian works, but the latter is more correctly the name of the wood of several species of *Berberis*.

See the remarks under ' *Aconitum. Sp. of. (Root of— Jadvar.)*' and under *Berberis*.

245. CURCUMA LEUCORRHIZA, *Roxb. (Root of.)*

See the remarks under *Curcuma Amada*.

246. CURCUMA LONGA, *Linn. (Root of—Turmeric or Curcuma.)*

Kurkum كركم ; Aurúqussufr عروق الصفر ; Auruqussabbá-ghín عروق الصباغين ; Zarsúd زرسود . (*Arab.*) Zard-chóbah زردچوبه ; Zard-chób زردچوب ; Dár-zard دارزرد . (*Pers.*) Halad هلد ; Haldi هلدي . (*Hind. and Duk.*) Mañjal மஞ்சள். (*Tam.*) Pasupu పసుపు. (*Tel.*) Maññaḷ മഞ്ഞൾ ; Mariññaḷa മരിഞ്ഞള. (*Malyal.*) Arishiná ಅರಿಶಿನ. (*Can.*) Holodi. (*Beng.*) Haridrakam. (*Sans.*) Haḷede. (*Mah.*) Halad. (*Guz.*) Kahá. (*Cing.*) Sanóe or Tanún. (*Bur.*).

In many books *Kurkum* is incorrectly applied to *Saffron*, with reference to which see the remarks on *Crocus*.

The Sanscrit word *Haridra*, which is also used for *Turmeric*, is erroneously applied to the *Yellow Orpiment* in some books; the name of the latter is *Haritálakam*.

247. CURCUMA RUBESCENS, *Roxb.*

248. CURCUMA ZEDOARIA, *Roscoe. Syn.* C. ZERUM-BET, *Roxb.* (*Root of—Long Zedoary*).

Zuranbád زرنباد ; Aurúqul-káfúr عروق الكافور. (*Arab.*) Kazhúr كژور ; *Zhuranbád* ژرنباد. (*Pers.*) Kachúr كچور. (*Hind. and Duk.*) Kich-chilik-kizhangu கிச்சிலிக்கிழங்கு ; Púláŋ-kizhangu புலாங்கிழங்கு. (*Tam.*) Kich-chili-gaddalu కిచ్చిలిగడ్డలు ; Kachóram కచోరం. (*Tel*) Kach-chólam കച്ചോലം ; Kach-chúri-kizhanna കച്ചുരികിഴങ്ങ ; Pulá-kizhanna പുലാകിഴങ്ങ. (*Malyal.*) Kachórá ಕಚೋರಾ. (*Can.*) Kochúr ; Shorí. (*Beng.*) Kachhúraha. (*Suns*) Kachóra. (*Mah.*) Káchúr. (*Guz.*).

In some Arabic, Persian and other medical works, *Aarqul-káfúr* عرق الكافور is the Arabic name assigned to the above root, which means *the Spirit or Liquor of Camphor*. It should be *Aurúqul-káfúr* عروق الكافور (*the root of Camphor*), and the *Long Zedoary* is so named in allusion to its aromatic smell.

249. CYBIUM COMMERSONII, *Cuv. et Val.* (*Sier Fish—Oil of*).

See the names under *Oleum Piscis.*

250. CYCAS CIRCINALIS, *Linn.*

Jangli-madan-mast-ká-*jhár* جنگلي مدن مست كا جهاڑ ; Paháṛi-madan-mast-ká-*jhár* پہاڑي مدن مست كا جهاڑ. (*Duk.*) Úrai ஊரை ; Káma-maram காமமரம் (*Tam.*) Varaguna వరగుణ ; Raṇaguvva రణగువ్వ. (*Tel.*) Úránbú ഉറാമ്പു. (*Malyal.*) Múdaiñ or Múdang. (*Bur*).

251. CYCAS CIRCINALIS, *Linn. (Cone of the male variety of).*

Jangli-madan-mast-ká-*phúl* جنگلی مدن مستکا پھول ; Pahári-madan-mast-ká-*phúl* پہاڑي مدن مستکا پھول *(Duk.)* Madana-kámé*sh*urap-pú மதனகாமேசுரப்பூ ; Madana-kámam-pú மதனகாமப்பூ ; Kamappú காமப்பூ. *(Tam.)* Madana-mastu మదనమస్తు ; Madana-kámák*sh*i మదనకామాక్షి. *(Tel.)* Rinbadam റിമ്പദം. *(Malyal.)*.

The scales of the above cone is one of the most useful narcotic medicines in India, and are commonly sold in the bazaars of Southern India. I showed this cone to Dr. Bidie some time ago, and he kindly examined and identified it to be the produce of the male variety of *C. circinalis.* We have subsequently found it produced by a male plant of that species in the Agri-horticultural Society's garden at Madras.

I believe that the male variety of another species *(C. revoluta?)* of the genus *Cycas* also produces a similar cone, which possesses the same medicinal properties.

252. CYPERUS ROTUNDUS, *Linn. (Root of).*

Móthá موتھا ; Bará-nágar-mó*th*á بڑا ناگرموتھا *(Hind.)* Kóré-ki-jar جڑ کي کورے. *(Duk.)* Kórai கோரை. *(Tam.)* Bhadra-tunga-muste భద్రతుంగముస్తె ; Bhadramuste భద్రముస్తె ; Tunga-muste తుంగముస్తె ; Mustakamu ముస్తకము ; *Sh*ákha-tunga-véru శాఖతుంగవేరు ; Kaivartaka-muste కైవర్తకముస్తె. *(Tel.)* Mó*th*á. *(Beng.)*.

253. CYPERUS PERTENUIS, *Roxb. (Root of).*

So*a*de-kú*ss* سعد کوفي ; So*a*d سعد. *(Arab.)* Mushke-zamín مشک زمين. *(Pers.)* Nágar-mó*th*á ناگرموتھا. *(Hind.)* Nágar-mótah ناگرموته. *(Duk.)* Kóraik-kizhangu கோரைக்கிழங்கு ; Mutta-kách முத்தகாசு. *(Tam.)* Tungagaḍḍala-véru కుందగడ్డలవేరు; Kólatunga-muste కోలతుంగముస్తె. (Tel.) Kóra-kizhaṇṇa കോരകിഴണ്ണ. (Malyal.) Konnári-gaḍḍe కున్నారిగడ్డె. (Can.) Nágor-móthá. (Beng.) Mustá. (Sans.) Nágar-mótá. (Mah.) Jaṭamakuṭu. (Cing.) Vomou-ŋiu or Vo-mou-ng-ie. (Bur.).

See the remarks under *Nardastachys Jatamansi.*

D.

254. DÆMIA EXTENSA, *R. Br.*

Utran اترن ; Utran-ki-bél اترن کی بیل . (Hind.) Utran انرن ; Juṭuk جٹك ; Juṭup جنٹپ . (Duk.) Vélip-parutti வேலிப்பருத்தி ; Uttámaṇi உத்தாமணி. (Tam.) Jiṭṭupáku జిట్టుపాకు ; Dushṭupu-cheṭṭu దుష్టుపుచెట్టు ; Guruṭi-cheṭṭu గురుటి చెట్టు. (Tel.) Vélip-paritti വെലിപ്പരിത്തി. (Malyal.) Hála-kóratíge ಹಾಲಕೊರ ತೀಗೆ. (Can.) Chhágul-báti. (Beng.).

255. DALBERGIA SISSOO. *(Wood of.)*

Sásam ساسم or Sásim ساسم . (Arab.) *Shisham* شیشم ; Sisam سیسم ; Sísu سیسو . (Hind.) *Shisham-ki-lakṛi* شیشم کی لکڑی ; *Shisham* شیشم . (Duk.) Núkku-kaṭṭai நூக்குகட்டை. (Tam.) Sissú-karra సిస్సూకర్ర. (Tel.) Ṣhiṣhu-káṭ. (Beng.) Sísam. (Guz.).

In Dukhni, the word *Shisham* is used for any wood which is black or reddish black and heavy, whatever tree may produce it. Ṣhiṣhu-káṭ is the Bengali name for the above wood, not *Shiṣhu* or ' Sissoo' by itself, which means a young boy.

256. DATURA ALBA, *Linn.* (*White flowered Dhatura.*)

Jouz-másal جوز ماثل ; Jouz-másale-abyaẓ جوز ماثل ابيض ; Jouz-másame-abyaẓ جوزماثم ابيض. (*Arab.*) Kouz-másale-supéd كوزماثل سپيد ; Tátúrahe-supéd تا تورهٔ سپيد ; Kouz-kunáe-supéd كوزكناٴ سپيد. (*Pers.*) Suféd-*dhatúrá* سفيد دهتورا ; Sádah-*dhatúrá* سادهدهتورا. (*Duk.*) ساد دد هتورا. (*Hind.*) Ujlá-*dhatúrah* اجلادهتوره. Úmattai உம்மத்தை. (*Tam.*) Ummetta ఉమ్మెత్త ; Duttúramu దత్తూరము. (*Tel.*) Ummatta ഉമ്മത്ത ; Ummam ഉമ്മം. (*Malyal.*) Ummatte-gidá ಉಮ್ಮತ್ತಿಗಿಡಾ. (*Can.*) *Dhútúrá* ; Sádá-*dhútúrá*. (*Beng.*) Ummatta-vriksha. (*Sans.*) *Dhatúro*. (*Guz.*) Attana ; Sudu-attana. (*Cing.*) Padáyiṅ-phiṅ. (*Bur.*).

See the remarks in the following No.

257. DATURA FASTUOSA, *Willd.* (*Purple flower-ed Dhatura.*)

Jouz-mágale-asvad جوز ماثل اسود ; Jouz-másame-asvad جوزماثماسود. (*Arab.*) Kouz-másale-siyáh كوزماثل سياه ; Tátúrahe-siyáh تا تورهٔ سياه ; Kouz-kunáe-siyah كوزكناٴى سياه. (*Pers.*) Kálá-*dhatúrá* كالادهتورا ; Kálá-*dhatúrah* كالادهتوره ; Udah-*dhatúrá* اود دد هتورا. (*Hind. and Duk.*) Karu-vúmattai கருவுமத்தை. (*Tam.*) Nalla-ummetta నల్లఉమ్మెత్త. (*Tel.*) Karu-ummatta കറുഉമ്മത്ത. (*Malyal.*) Kare-vummatte ಕರೆವುಮ್ಮತ್ತೆ. (*Can.*) Kálá-*dhútúrá*. (*Beng.*) Kúla-bémiká ; Krishṇa-datúra. (*Sans.*) Kálo-*dhatúro*. (*Guz.*) Kalu-attana. (*Cing.*) Padáyiṅ-khatta. (*Bur.*).

The imperfect flowers or buds of both the above species of Datura *(D. alba and D. fastuosa,)* are sold in the bazaars of Madras under the following names :—

Ghar-bhúli كهربهولي . *(Duk.)* Úmattai-pú உமத்தைப்பூ. *(Tam.)* Umetla-puvvu ఉమెత్తపువ్వు. *(Tel.).*

Forgetfulness of house is the meaning of Gharbhúli, which is one of the results of the intoxication of the drug, and this name is occasionally applied to the plants themselves.

The buds of *Datura* appear to be sold in some bazaars of South India, under the name of *Maráti-moggu,* with reference to which see the remarks under *Eriodendron anfractuosum.*

The Burmese names ' pa-daing-phoo', ' pa-daing-khate' and ' pa-daing-ame' are used synonymously and applied to either of the above species in some books, but according to their meaning, the first should be confined to *D. alba,* and the two last to *D. fastuosa.*

258. DAUCUS CAROTA, *Linn. (Root of—Carrot.)*

Jazar جزر . *(Arab.)* Gazar گزر ; Zardak زردک *(Pers.)* Gájar گاجر . *(Hind. and Duk.)* Maŋjaḷ-muḷḷángi மஞ்சள்முள்ளாங்கி ; Kárttu-kizhaŋgu கார்ட்டுகிழங்கு. *(Tam.)* Paçh-çha-mullangi పచ్చమల్లంగి ; Píta-kanda పీతకంద; Shikhá-múlamu శిఖామూలము. *(Tel.)* Gajjari ಗಜ್ಜರಿ. *(Can.)* Gájar. *(Beng.)* Garjaram ; Shikhá-múlam. *(Sans.)* Gázara. *(Mah.)* Gájar. *(Guz.)*

The Sanscrit name *Garjaram* is confounded in some books with ' *Grijjanam.*'

259. DAUCUS CAROTA, *Linn. (Seeds of.)*

Bazrul-jazar بزرالجزر . *(Arab.)* Tukhme-gazar تخم گذر ; Tukhme-zardak تخم زردک . *(Pers.)* Gájar-ké-bínj گاجر کے بیج . *(Hind. and Duk.)* Kárttu-kizhaŋgu-virai கார்ட்டுகிழங்குவிரை. *(Tam.)* Gajjara-gaddala-vittulu

గజరగడ్డలవిత్తులు. *(Tel.)* Kempu-mullangi-bíjá కెంపుముల్లంగి
బీజ. *(Can.)* Gájar-bíchi. *(Beng.)* Garjara-bíjam ; Shikhá-
múla-bíjam. *(Sans.)* Gázarácha-bi. *(Mah.)*. Gajar-nu-bíj.
(Guz.).

260. DIOSPYROS EMBRYOPTERIS, *Pers. Syn.* E. GLUTINIFERA, *Roxb.*

Ábnúse-hindí آ بنو س هندي . *(Arab. and Pers.)*
Téndú تیند و ; Gáb گاب . *(Hind.)* Téndú تیند و . *(Duk.)*
Tumbilik-káy தும்பிளிக்காய். *(Tam.)* Tumiki తుమికి ; Tinduki
తింఉకి; Tubiki తుబికి. *(Tel.)* Panich-chi പണിച്ചി; Vananchik-
ká-maram വനഞ്ചിക്കാമരം. *(Malyal.)* Gáb. *(Beng.)* Tin-
duka*ha.* *(Sans.)* Timbiri. *(Cing.).*

Ábnús is the name of *D. Ebinaster (Ebony),* but often
applied in books to *D. embryopteris.* *Ábnúse-hindí* would be a
proper name for the latter.

261. DIPTEROCARPUS LÆVIS, *Ham. (Exudation of—Wood Oil or Gurjun Balsam.)*

Garjan-ká-tél گرجن کا تیل . *(Hind.)*   Gorjon-tail.
(Beng.) Hora-tel. *(Cing.)* Kaḷiṇ-si *or* Kaṅyeṇ-si. *(Bur.)*.

262. DRACOCEPHALUM ROYLEANUM, *Wall.* (Seeds of.)

Bálanko با لنکو *or* Bazrul-bálanko بزر ا لبا لنکو . *(Arab.)*
Bálango با لنگو *or* Tukhme-bálango تخم با لنگو . *(Pers.)*
Bálango با لنگو . *(Hind.)* Balanká بالنکا . *(Duk.).*

E.

263. ECHIUM. *Sp. of.*

Lasánussour لسان‌الثور . (*Arab.*)   Gáv-zabán گاو زبان .
(*Pers. Hind. and Duk.*).

As I have remarked under *Cacalia kleinia,* the ' *Gow-zaban*' of bazaar is neither the produce of that plant, nor of any other species of *Compositæ.* On examining the dry leaves sold under that name in many Indian bazaars, together with the seeds or nuts often found in them, I considered them to be the produce of one of the species of *Boraginacœ,* and to make myself certain on this point, I raised a few plants from the seeds, and sent one of them to Dr. Waring at London. It had been submitted by him to Drs. Wight and Hooker, and pronounced by them to belong to one of the genera of the same Natural Order, viz., *Echium.* The species was not determined by them from want of flowers.

Some of the plants I raised were more than ⁓ years old, but did not flower, nor did they appear to thrive well in this country.

The medicine sold in many Indian bazaars under the Persian name of *Gule-gáv-zabán* گل گاو زبان are dry flowers of a pink color, and the meaning of the name is *flowers of Gáv-zabán* or *Echium.* I cannot say, however, whether they are the flowers of *Gáv-zabán* or not, because I have never found them with it when it is newly brought in large quantities to Madras, though I have found every other part of the plant.*

264. ECLIPTA PROSTATA, *Linn.*

Bharangráj بهرنگراح : *Bhangrá* بهنگرا . (*Hind.*)
Bhangrá بهنگرا . (*Duk.*) Karisha-lánganni கரிசலாங்கண்ணி ;

---

* Since making the above remarks I have found ' Gaw-zaban' mentioned under the name of ' Onosma bracteatum' in Royles' 'Illustrations of the Botany of the Himalayan Mountains,' page 301.

Kaíkéshi கைகேசி ; Kaivíshi-ilai கைவீஷியிலை. (Tam.)
Gunṭa-galijéru గుంటగలిజేరు ; Galagara-cheṭṭu గలగరచెట్టు ;
Gunṭa-kalagara గుంటకలగర. (Tel.) Karishánganṇi കരിശാ
ങ്കണ്ണി ; Mukuṭri മുകുറി ; Kalenṇiyam കലെലഞ്ഞിയം ;
Kaṇṇunṇi കണ്ണുണ്ണി. (Malyal.) Garagada-sappu గరగడ
సప్పు ; Bara-garagada-giḍá బరగరగడగిడా ; Káḍigga-garagá
కాడిగ్గగరగా. (Can.).

265. EHRETIA BUXIFOLIA, *Roxb.* (*Root of.*)

266. ELEODENDRON ROXBURGHII, *W. et A.*

Cheluppai-maram செலுப்பைமரம். (*Tam.*) Nirija నీరిజ ;
Bíra బీర ; Nerasi నేరసి. (*Tel.*).

267. ELETTARIA CARDAMOMUM, *Maton.* (*Capsules of—Officinal or Malabar Cardamoms.*)

See the names and remarks under *Cardamomum*, and also
the remarks under *Amomum.*

268. EMBELIA RIBES, *Burn.* (*Berries of.*)

Biranje-kábali برنج كابلى . (*Arab. and Pers.*) Bába-
rang با برنگ . (*Hind.*) Bái-barang بائی برنگ . (*Duk.*)
Váyu-viḷangam வாயுவிளங்கம். (*Tam.*) Váyu-viḷangam-
cheṭṭu వాయువిళంగంచెట్టు. (*Tel.*) Váyi-vaḷanṇam വായി
വിളങ്ങം. (*Malyal.*) Váyi-vuḷanga ವಾಯಿವುಳಂಗ. (*Can.*)
Bábrang. (*Beng.*) Bávaḍanga. (*Mah.*) Váyi-vaḷang. (*Guz.*).

These berries are supposed to be used in some places for
adulteration with *Black Pepper*. If so, they can be easily distinguished from the following characters:—

The berries of *E. ribes* are much smaller than *Black-pepper*;
very smooth; almost always have a thin peduncle or stalk
attached to them with a persistent calyx; and possess a very

slight pungent taste, which is different from that of *Black-pepper*.
With regard to their color, there are 2 varieties of them sold
in the bazaar; one is grey or reddish-grey, and the other dull-
brown.

269. ERIODENDRON ANFRACTUOSUM, *D. C.*

Suféd-sémal سفيد سيمل ; Suféd-señbal سفيد سينبل ;
Túlá-pér تو لا پيز . (*Hind.*) K̲hatyán ختيان ; K̲hatyán-ká-
jhár كا جهاز ختيان . (*Duk.*) Ilava-maram இலவமரம்.
(*Tam.*) Búraga-cheṭṭu బూరగచెట్టు. (*Tel.*) Paṇṇi-maram
വെണ്ണിമരം ; Muḷḷillá-púḷa മുള്ളിലാപൂള. (*Malyal.*) Búra-
maṛá ಬೂರಮರ. (*Can.*) Túlá-gáchh ; Shémal-gáchh.
(*Beng.*) Shalmaní-vrikshaha. (*Sans.*) Imbul. (*Cing.*)
Ṭimbo-le-biṇ. (*Bur.*).

There is much confusion about the Tamil and Telugu
name *Maráṭi-moggu* மராடிமொாக்கு, in the bazaars of Southern
India. What is sold in Madras under that name, are very
young fruits of *Eriodendron anfractuosum*. They are about 1 or
1¼ inches in length, and about 2 lines in thickness; attached
to a portion of the peduncle with the brim of the calyx; and
of brown color. If the young fruits of this plant, when about
1½ or 2 inches long, are dried in the sun, and a portion
of the calyx removed, they assume the appearance I have
just described. When not old, they are demulcent and
astringent, and are used as such in Diarrhœa and Dysentery.
In some other places, however, the buds of *Datura alba* and
D. fastuosa appear to be sold under the same name; and in a
few others, again, the buds of *Artabotrys odoratissima*, which
is a narcotic medicine used occasionally by the natives in
the manner described in the Materia Indica, Vol. II, page 185,
under the article 'Maratia Mooghoo'. The fact is, that the
drug to which that name was originally applied, or ought
to be applied now, is not known, and therefore it is unsafe
to buy any medicine under that name. Any medicine which
is really intended by that name, can be obtained by other
and more sure names. The confusion about the name is still
great, when we know that other names used synonymously with

Marúṭi-moggu in the above work *(Jangli-lóng* جنگلي لونگ *, &c.),*
are the names of drugs which are totally different from one
another. If the dry buds of *Datura* are sold under the above
name, they can be distinguished by the following characters :—
They are conical, of greenish brown color, and consists of
two envelopes and one bundle. The first or outer envelope is
the *calyx;* when this is torn, the second or inner one *(corolla)*
will be exposed, which is oblong in form and encloses the bundle
of 5 *stamens* and 1 *style.* See the remarks under *Gossypium.*

270. ERYTHRINA INDICA, *Linn.*

Pángrá پانگرا . *(Hind. and Duk.)* Kaliyáṇa-murukku
கலியாணமுருங்கு. *(Tam.)*   Báḍidapu-*cheṭṭu* బాడిదపుచెట్టు;
Báḍchipa-cheṭṭu బాడ్చిపచెట్టు. *(Tel.)* Karu-murukkin-maram
കരുമുരുക്കിൻമരം ; Murukka മുരുക്ക ; Kalyáṇa-murukku-
maram കല്യാണമുരുക്കമരം. *(Malyal.)*   Páravál̤ada-mará
ಪಾರವಾಳದಮರಾ. *(Can.)* Pányaá-mandár ; Pálitá-mandár.
(Beng.) Erabadu-gahá. *(Cing.)* Kaṣi. *(Bur.).*

Mahámeda occurs as one of the Telugu names of this plant
in some Dictionaries and other works, but it is properly the
name of another plant.

271. EUGENIA ACRIS, *Wight. (Berries of——Indian Allspice.)*

Sital-*chíni* سيتل چيني . *(Hind. and Duk.).*

Allspice is known in Southern India and some other places
as *Kabáb-chíni* كباب چيني, with reference to which and some
other points connected with that name, see the remarks under
Cubeba officinalis.

272. EUPATORIUM AYAPANA, *Vent.*

Ayappana*i* அயப்பணை. *(Tam.).*

273. EUPHORBIA ANTIQUORUM, *Linn.*

Zaqqúme-hindí زقوم هندي . *(Arab.)*   Zaqúniyáe
hindí زقونياے هندي . *(Pers.)* Tidhárá تدهارا : Tidhárá-

séhnḍ سينڈ ا ر ها تد ; Tidhárá-séhńṛ اسينهڗ تدهار . *(Hind.)*
Tidhári-sénḍ تدهاری سينڈ ; Tín-dhári-sénḍ تين دهاری سينڈ ·
(Duk.) Shadurak-kaḷḷi சதுரக்கள்ளி ; Tirikkaḷḷi திரிக்கள்ளி.
(Tam.) Bonta-jemuḍu బొంతజెముడు ; Bomma-jemuḍu బొమ్మ
జెముడు ; Múḍu-múla-jemuḍu మూడుమూలజెముడు. *(Tel.)*
Kaṭak-kaḷḷi കടക്കള്ളി ; Chatirak-kaḷḷi ചതിരക്കള്ളി. *(Mal-*
yal.) Tékáṭá-ṣhij ; Láriyá-dáonú. *(Beng.)* Vajra-kanṭaká.
(Sans.) Tandhári-sénḍ. *(Guz.)* Dalúk. *(Cing.)* Sházávngi
or Shazáñv-ji. *(Bur.)*.

274. EUPHORBIA CATTIMANDO. *W. Elliot.*
Katti-mandu కత్తిమండు. *(Tel.)*.

275. EUPHORBIA NIVULIA, *Ham.*
Ṣhij. *(Beng.)*.

276. EUPHORBIA NERIFOLIA, *Linn.* Syn. E.
LIGULARIA, *Roxb.*

Síj سيج ; Pattón-kí-sénḍ پتون كي سينڈ ; Thóhar
تهوهر . *(Hind.)* Kutté-kí-jibh-kí-sénḍ كتے كي جيبه كي سينڈ
Kutté-kí-jíbh-ká-pattá كتے كي جيبه كا پتا. *(Duk.)* Ilaik-
kaḷḷi இலைக்கள்ளி. *(Tam.)* Áku-jemuḍu ఆకుజెముడు. *(Tel.)*
Elakkaḷḷi എലക്കള്ളി. *(Malyal.)* Yalekaḷḷi ಯಲೆಕಳ್ಳಿ.
(Can.) Pátá-ṣhij ; Munsa-ṣhij ; Hij-dáoná. *(Beng.)*
Shazávn-mina. *(Bur.)*.

277. EUPHORBIA TIRUCALLI, *Linn.* *(Milk-*
hedge plant.)
Zaqqume-hindí زقوم هندي. *(Arab.)* Zaquní-
yáe-hindí زقونيائي هندي. *(Pers.)* Séhńṛ سيهنڗ ; Séhnḍ
سيهنڈ ; Kónpal-séhnḍ كونپل سينڈ. *(Hind.)* Sénḍ سينڈ ;

Kári-ki-sénd كاري كي سينڈ ; Báṛ-ki-sénd باڑ كي سينڈ . *(Duk.)*
Kaḷḷi கள்ளி; Kaḷḷi-kombu கள்ளிகொம்பு. *(Tam.)* Jemuḍu
జెముడు ; Jemuḍu-káḍılu జెముడుకాడెలు ; Káḍa-jemuḍu కాడ
జెముడు. *(Tel.)* Kól-kaḷḷi കൊൽകള്ളി ; Tiruk-kaḷḷi
തിരുക്കള്ളി ; Kaḷḷi കള്ളി. *(Malyal.)* Bonta-kaḷḷi ಬೊಂತಕಳ್ಳಿ.
(Can.) Látá-dáoná ; Lanká-shíj. *(Beng.)* Vajraduhú.
(Mah.) Thóvar ; Navahandí. *(Jing.)*

278. EURYCOMA LONGIFOLIA, *Jack.*

Penvar-pét. *(Malay)*.

279. EXACUM BICOLOR, *Roxb.* *(Country Kariyat.)*

Baṛá-charáyatah بڑا چرايته ; Ḥabshí-charáyatah
حبشي چرايته . *(Hind.)*.

280. EXACUM PEDUNCULATUM, *Linn.*

281. EXACUM TETRAGONUM, *Roxb.* *(Purple Chiretta.)*

Údah-charáyatah اودہ چرايته . *(Hind. and Duk.)*
Kúchoṛi. *(Beng.)*.

F.

282. FAGRÆA FRAGRANS, *Roxb.*

283. FEL BOVINUM. *(Ox Gall or Ox Bile.)*

Ṣafrául-baqar صفرا البقر . *(Arab.)* Zahrahe-gáv
زہرگا و . *(Pers.)* Baíl-ká-ṣafrá بیل كاصفرا . *(Hind.)* Baíl-
ká-pit بیل كا پت . *(Duk.)*.

284. FERONIA ELEPHANTUM, *Corr. (Fruit of—Wood-apple.)*

Kabit كبيب. *(Arab. and Pers.)*   Kaṭbél كت بيل.
(Hind.) Kavíṭ كويت. *(Duk.)* Viḷám-pazham விளாம்பழம்.
(Tam.) Velaga-panḍu వెలగపండు ; Kapi*dh*-dhamu కపిత్థము.
(Tel.) Viḷám-pazham വിളാമ്പഴം. *(Malyal.)* Byálada-
haṇṇa ಬ್ಯಾಲದಹಣ್ಣು. *(Can.)*   Ko*th*-bél; Káṭ-bél. *(Beng.)*
Kapid*tha*-phalam. *(Sans.)* Kaviṭa. *(Mah.)*   Kavíṭ; Kóṭhu.
(Guz.) Divúl. *(Cing.)* Ṣi-ṣi *or* Ti-di. *(Bur.)*.

Máhę or 'Hman' is the name of a fruit only found in
Burmah, which bears some resemblance to *Wood-apple*, but it is
incorrectly applied to the latter itself in some works, including
Mason's Natural Productions of Burmah.

From its great abundance and cheapness, the *Wood-apple*
is occasionally substituted for the *Bael-fruit (Ægle marmelos)*,
when the latter is sold in large quantities, but they can be easily
distinguished from each other by the following characters :—

Bael-fruit.	*Wood-apple.*
1. Generally round and slightly obovate, and often oblong.	1. Almost always round or spherical.
2. Generally about the size of an orange, and often as big as a pomegranate or larger.	2. Generally about the size of an orange, and some times as large as a pomegranate.
3. Greenish-yellow in color, smooth, and slightly shining.	3. Dull white or greenish white in color, and not smooth.
4. Rind very hard and woody.	4. Rind hard and woody, but more easily broken.
5. In the centre of the pulp, there are from 5 to 18 cells, each of which contains from 1 to 12 or more seeds* and mucus.	5. No cells at all, and the seeds are embedded in the pulp.

---

* In small *Bael-fruits*, the seeds are often absent in the cells.

Bael-fruit.

6. The seeds are oblong, flat or compressed, woolly, and about the size of a lime-seed.

7. The mucus is thick, very tenacious, transparent, and terbinthinate in smell and taste.

8. When the fruit is quite ripe, the pulp is of brownish red color, with a strong balsamic odour and taste.

9. When very ripe or dry, the pulp is very adherent to the rind.

Wood-apple.

5. The seeds are small, round, and smooth.

7. Contains no mucus.

8. In the same condition, the pulp is of reddish grey color, with a very sweet and agreeable taste and smell.

9. In the same condition, the pulp and seeds are more or less loose from the rind.

See the remarks under the next plant and also under *Gummi Acaciæ.*

285. FERONIA ELEPHANTUM, *Corr.* (*The small variety of.*)

Bhuiñ-kat-bél بهُنِين كت بيل . (*Hind.*) *Bhúiñ-kaviṭ* بِهرُ ئن كويت . (*Duk.*) Kutti-viḷám குட்டிவிளாம் ; Nila-viḷám நிலவிளாம். (*Tam.*) Néla-velaga నేలవెలగ. (*Tel.*) *Bhú-kapidtha-phalam.* (*Sans*).

From the very small size of this plant, which is often not more than a foot, it is some times considered to be a different species from *F. Elephantum* (*Wood-apple tree*). The difference in size, however, is only enough to constitute a variety, and as the plant does not differ in any other respect, it may be considered to be the same species.

286. FERRI OXIDUM MAGNETICUM. (*Magnetic Oxide of Iron, Magnet, or Load-stone.*)

Miqnátis مقْنا طيس ; Mighnátis مغنا طيس ; Hajrul-mighnátis حجر المغنا طيس . (*Arab.*) Sange-áhanrubá سنگ آهن ربا ; Sangé-chamak سنگ چمک . (*Pers.*) Chamak-ká-patthar چمک كاپتَر ; Chamak چمک . (*Hind.*) Chamak-patthar چمک پتَر . (*Duk.*)

287. FERRI PEROXIDUM. (*Rust or Impure Red Oxide of Iron.*)

Khabṣul-ḥadíd خبث الحديد ; Zaafaránul-ḥadíd زعفران الحديد (*Arab.*) ; Zanjárul-ḥadíd زنجار الحديد ; Zange-áhan زنگ آهن ; Chirke-áhan چرک آهن ; Rime-áhan ریم آهن Zangáre-áhan زنگار آهن (*Pers.*). Lóhéká-zang لوهیکا زنگ ; Lóhé-ká-gú لوهیکا گو ; Mandór مندور . (*Hind. and Duk.*) Ayach-chendúram அயச்செந்தூரம் ; Irumbu-chiṭṭam இரும்புசிட்டம். (*Tam.*) Inapa-chiṭṭam ఇనప చిట్టం ; Aya-shindúramu అయశిందూరము. (*Tel.*) Irumbuk-kiṭam ഇരുമ്പുക്കിടം. (*Malyal.*) Khabbaṇada-kiṭṭá ಖಬ್ಬಣದಕಿಟ್ಟ. (*Can.*) Lohár-gú ; Lohár-*jhangár.* (*Beng.*) Mandúram. (*Sans.*) Lokhan-dhácha-kaṭai. (*Mah.*) Lohá-nu-zang. (*Guz.*) Yakkaḍa-kiṭṭam ; Mallokoḍá. (*Cing.*) Ṣánpiyá or Ṭámbiyá ; Ṣánkhí or Ṭánkhí. (*Bur.*).

288. FERRI SULPHAS. (*Sulphate of Iron or Green Vitriol.*)

Zálje-aṣfar زاج اصفر . (*Arab.*) Záke-zard زاک زرد (*Pers.*) Kasís کسیس ; Hirá-kasís هیرا کسیس . (*Hind.*) Kashísh کشیش ; Hirá-kashísh هیرا کشیش . (*Duk.*) Anna-bédi அன்னபேதி. (*Tam.*) Anna-bhédi అన్న భేది. (*Tel.*) Anna-bhédi അന്നഭേദി. (*Malyal.*) Anná-bhédi ಅನ್ನಭೇದಿ (*Can.*) Hirá-kos or Hirá-kosís. (*Beng.*) Hira-kasis. (*Guz.*).

289. FERRUM. (*Iron.*)

Ḥadíd حدید . (*Arab.*) Áhan آهن . (*Pers.*) Lohá لوہا or Lohah لوہ . (*Hind. and Duk.*) Irumbu இரும்பு. (*Tam.*) Inumu ఇనుము. (*Tel.*) Irumba ഇരുമ്പ. (*Malyal.*) Kabbiṇa ಕಬ್ಬಿಣ. (*Can.*) Lohá or Láhá. (*Beng.*) Ayam ; Lóham. (*Sans.*) Lokhanda. (*Mah.*) Lévu. (*Guz.*) Dán. (*Bur.*).

290. FICUS BENGALENSIS, *Linn. Syn.* F. INDICA, *Roxb. (Banyan-tree——Milk of.)*

Baṛ-ká-dúdh بڑ کا دودھ. *(Hind. and Duk.)* Álam-pál ஆலம்பால் *(Tam.)* Marri-pálu మర్రిపాలు. *(Tel.)* Férá-lin-pála പേരാലിൻപാല. *(Malyal.)* Álada-hálu ಆಲದ ಹಾಲು. *(Can.)* Baṭer-khir. *(Beng.)* Vaṭa-kshíram. *(Sans.)* Vaḍecha-dúda. *(Mah.)* Nuga-kiri. *(Cing.)* Náṇ-kí-ḍáv or Niyáv-ki-ḍáv. *(Bur.)*.

Nugu or *Nugu-gaha* is the Cingalese name of *F. Indica*, but in some books *Kiri-palla* is given. It means *milk-plant*, and may therefore be applied to several plants which abound in milk, without any particular distinction.

291. FICUS CARICA, *Linn. (Fruit of——Fig.)*

Tin تين *(Arab.)* Anjír انجير *(Pers. Hind. and Duk.)* Shímai-atti சீமையத்தி; Tén-atti தேன்அத்தி. *(Tam.)* Shí-ma-atti ಶೀಮಅತ್ತಿ; Téne-atti తేనెఅత్తి; Anjúru అంజూరు. *(Tel.)* Shíma-atti ശീമഅത്തി. *(Malyal.)* Shíme-atti ಶೀಮೆಅತ್ತಿ. *(Can.)* Dumur. *(Beng.)* Anjír. *(Guz.)* Raṭa-atti-ká. *(Cing.)* Ṣa-phán-ṣí; Ṭimbo-thán-di or Ṣimbo-Ṣaphán-ṣí. *(Bur.)*.

292. FICUS ELASTICA, *Roxb. (Indian Caout-chouc-tree.)*

Viláyatí-baṛ-ká-jháṛ ولايتي بڑ کا جهاز. *(Duk.)* Shímai-álai-maram சீமையாலைமரம். *(Tam.)* Shíma-marri-cheṭṭu ಶೀಮಮರ್ರಿಚೆಟ್ಟು. *(Tel.)* Shíme-álada-mará ಶೀಮೆಆಲದಮರಾ. *(Can.)* Viláyatí-vaḍécha-jháḍa. *(Mah.)*.

293. FICUS GLOMERATA, *Roxb. (Fruit of.)*

Jammaiz جميز; Tínul-aḥmaq تين الاحمق. *(Arab.)* Ṣamare-pash-shah ثمر پشه; Anjíre-aḥmaq انجير احمق. *(Pers.)* Gúlar گولر. *(Hind.)* Gullar گلر; Gullér گلير.

(*Duk.*) Atti-pazham அத்திபழம். (*Tam.*) Atti-pandu అత్తిపండు ; Médi-pandu మేడిపండు ; Bóda-mámidi బోడమామిడి ; Bramha-médi బ్రమ్మమేడి ; Bodda-pandu బొడ్డపండు ; Paidi-pandu పైడిపండు. (*Tel.*) Atti-yálum അത്തിയാലും. (*Malyal.*) Atti-hannu ಅತ್ತಿಹಣ್ಣು. (*Can.*) Jogiaá-dumur; Gullér. (*Beng.*) Udumbara-*phalam.* (*Sans.*) Umdécha-phal. (*Mah.*) Gullar. (*Guz.*) Atti-ká. (*Cing.*) Ṣáphán-si or Ṣaphán-ti. (*Bur.*).

294. FICUS OPPOSITIFOLIA, *Roxb.* (*Fruit of.*)

Tine-barri تين برى . (*Arab.*) Anjíre-dashtí انجير دشتي . (*Pers.*) Jangli-anjír جنگلي انجير ; Jangli-gullér جنگلي گلير . (*Duk.*) Pé-attip-pazham பேஅத்திப்பழம். (*Tam.*) Verri-atti-pandlu వెఱ్ఱి అత్తిపండ్లు. (*Tel.*) Pé-yatti ചെയത്തി ; Páraka-pazham പാറകപഴം. (*Malyal*) Adavi-atti ಅಡವಿ ಅತ್ತಿ. (*Can.*) Káku-dumur. (*Beng.*) Ummattó-dumbara-*phalam.* (*Sans.*) Jangli-anjír. (*Guz.*) Véda-umdécha-*;háda.* (*Mah.*).

295. FICUS POLYCARPA, *Roxb.* (*Fruit of.*)

Chhótá-jangli-anjír چھوٹا جنگلي انجير ; *Chhótá*-jangli-gullér چھوٹا جنگلي گلير . (*Duk.*) Chiṛiya-pé-atti சிறியபே அத்தி. (*Tam.*) Chinna-verri-atti-pandu చిన్నవెఱ్ఱి అత్తిపండు. (*Tel.*) Cheṛiya-kát-tatti ചെറിയകാട്ടത്തി ; *Cheṛu*-páraka-pazham ചെറുപാറകപഴം. (*Malyal.*).

296. FLACOURTIA CATAPHRACTA, *Roxb.*
(*Leaves of.*)

Zarnab زرنب . (*Arab.*) Tálispatar تا ليسپتر ; Tális-patrí تا ليسپتري ; Barahmí بر همي . (*Hind.*) Taj-pát تج پات ; Barmí برمي . (*Duk.*) Táḷisha-pattiri தாளிசபத்திரி. (*Tam.*) Tálisa-patri తాళీసపత్రి. (*Tel.*) Tálisa-patri

ತಾಲೀಸಪತ್ರಿ. (*Can.*) Tálishpatri ; Pániála. (*Beng.*) Tálisha. (*Sans.*) Talis-patari. (*Mah.*) Talis-patturu. (*Cing.*).

The vernacular names of the above plant, and of *Cinnamomum eucalyptoides* and *C. Tamala,* are generally the same. See the remarks under the latter plants.

297. FLUGGEA LEUCOPYRUS, *Willd.*

Suféd-madh-ká-péṛ سفيد مدھ کا پيڑ. (*Hind.*) Suféd-madh-ká-jháṛ سفيد مدھ کا جھاڑ. (*Duk.*) Veḷḷai-pilláṇji வெள்ளைபில்லாஞ்சி. (*Tam.*) Tella-puruguḍu తెల్లపురుగుడు. (*Tel.*).

The names of this plant in Tamil, Hindustani, and some other languages inserted in several books (Materia Indica, Shakespears' and other Dictionaries, &c.,) are incorrect.

The Syrup prepared from the fruits of this plant is considered to be equal to honey (*vegetable honey*), hence the name *Suféd-madh* سفيد مدھ (*white honey*). The word *white* distinguishes the plant from *Kálá-madh* کالا مدھ (*black honey*), a name given to *Phyllanthus multiflorus,* for a similar reason.

298. FŒNICULUM DULCE, *D. C. (Fruit of——Sweet Fennel.)*

Sweet fennel is not to be found in India, at least, I was not able to procure it from any bazaar. It has no native name, but the names generally applied to it in books (Materia Indica, &c.,) are those belong to *Aniseeds.* See the remarks under *Pimpinella anisum.*

299. FŒNICULUM PANMORIUM, *D. C. (Fruits of).*

Pánmohúri. (*Beng.*).

The names of *Aniseeds* are often confounded with those of the above fruits. See the remarks under *Pimpinella anisum.*

G.

300. GALBANUM.

Qinnah قنه . *(Arab.)*   Bárazd بارزد ; Bárazhd بارزد ;
Bérazd بیرزد . *(Pers.)*   Barijá بریجا ; Barijá-gónd
بریجاگوند . *(Hind. and Duk.).*

301. GALLA. *(Galls or Oak Galls.)*

Áafs عفص . *(Arab.)*   Mázú ماز و . *(Pers.)* Mázú-phal
ماجوپهل ; Máphal مايهل . *(Hind.)*   Májú-phal ما ز و پهل ;
Mái-phal مانی پهل . *(Duk.)* Máshik-káy மாஷிக்காய். *(Tam.)*
Máshi-káya ఈారిశికాయ. *(Tel.)*   Máshik-káya മാശിക്കായ.
(Malyal.)   Máchi-káyi ಮಾಚಿಕಾಯಿ. *(Can.)*   Máju-phal.
(Beng.)   Máyuhu. *(Sans.)*   Mái-phala ; Máshi-ká. *(Mah.)*
Máyi-phal. *(Guz.)*   Mása-ká. *(Cing.)*   Pinzakání-si or
Pinz-gáni-di. *(Bur.).*

302. GARCINIA MANGOSTANA, *Linn. (Fruit of.)*

Mangústán منگوستان . *(Hind.)*   Mangustán. *(Beng.)*
Mango-si or Mengo-ti. *(Bur.).*

303. GARCINIA MORELLA, *Desv. var.* G. PEDI-CELLATA. *(Gum Resin of—Gamboge.)*

See the names and remarks under *Cambogia.*

304. GARCINIA PICTORIA, *Roxb.*

Múkki-maram முக்கிமரம். *(Tam.)*   Kochi-goraka.
(Cing.)   Sanoto-pin, Tanato-bin or Sanatho-bin. *(Bur.).*

305. GARCINIA PICTORIA, *Roxb.* *(Gum Resin of—Gamboge.)*

See the names and remarks under *Cambogia*.

306. GARCINIA PURPUREA, *Roxb.* *(Concrete Oil of—Kokum-butter.)*

Kokam-ká-tél كو كم كا تيل . *(Hind.)*.

307. GARDENIA CAMPANULATA, *Roxb.*

308. GARDENIA LUCIDA, *Roxb.*
309. GARDENIA GUMMIFERA, *Linn.* } Resin of.

Ḍikmali نَ كملي . *(Hind.)* Ḍikámalí نَ كاملي . *(Duk.)* Kumbai கும்பை ; Ḍiká-malli டிகாமல்லி. *(Tam.)* Tella-manga తెల్లమoౝ ; *Chinaká-ringuva* చినకారింగువ.   *(Tel.)* Ḍikke-malli ಡಿಕ್ಕಮಲ್ಲ. *(Can.)* Kola-lákaḍa. *(Cing.)*.

310. GENIOSPORUM PROSTRATUM, *Benth.*

311. GENTIANA KURROO, *Roy.* *Syn.* PNEUMA-NANTHE KURROO, *Don.*

312. GENTIANÆ RADIX. *(Gentian Root.)*

Jintiyáná جنطيا نا . *(Arab.)*   Kou-shád كو شاد . *(Pers.)* Pakhán-béd پكهان بيد . *(Hind.)* Juntiyánah جنطيا نه . *(Duk.)*.

See the remarks under *Clay* with regard to the above Hindustani name, *Pakhánbéd*, being applied to a *mineral Clay*, with a slight alteration, viz., *Pakún-béd* پكا ن بيد .

313. GISEKIA PHARNACIOIDES, *Linn.*

Bálú-ká-ság با لوكا ساگ ; Bálú-kí-bhájí بالوكا بهاجي . *(Duk.)* Maṇal-kírai மணல்கீரை. *(Tam.)* Isaka-dásari-kúra ఇసకదాసరికూర. *(Tel.)* Attirilla-púla. *(Cing.)*.

314. GLORIOSA SUPERBA, *Linn. (Root of.)*

Nát-ká-bachhnág ناٹ کابحھناگ . *(Duk.)* Kalaippaik-
kizhaṅgu கலப்பைக்கிழங்கு; Kárttikaik-kizhaṅgu கார்த்திகைக்
கிழங்கு. *(Tam.)* Aḍavi-nábhi అడవినాభి; Potti-dumpa పొత்தి
దుంప; Agni-ṣhikha అగ్నిశిఖ; Kalappa-gaḍḍa కలప்பగడ్డ.
(Tel.) Ventóni വെൻതോണി. *(Malyal.)* Oloṭ-chandal.
(Beng.) Ṣíma-dou *or* Símmi-dáv. *(Bur.)*.

The above root is considered by the native practitioners
and druggists in Southern India to possess nearly the same
medicinal properties as the root of *Aconitum ferox;* hence its
names *Nát-ká-bachhnág (Country Aconite), Aḍavi-nábhi (Wild
Aconite),* &c. For the same reason, it is some times wilfully
substituted for, or adulterated with, the *true Aconite-root,* though
there is a great difference between their physical characters.

The root of *Gloriosa Superba* is tuberous, cylindrical, bent
at a right angle near one end, knotty at the angle, and
occasionally much pointed at both ends; varies in length from
3 to 5 or more inches; generally about the size of a finger or
thumb, and some times much larger when the plant grows in the
sandy and wet soil. The knot bears a mark of the stem on the
upper surface, and gives an attachment to many thin rootlets by
the lower. The root is covered with a thin, loose, and wrinkled,
epidermis, which is of brownish-grey or pale-brown color, and
the surface underneath the latter is brown or dark-brown if it is
a well dried root. The substance internally is of white color.
Its taste is faintly bitter, not acrid, and it is *farinaceous* in
structure. It is not poisonous in 12 grain doses, which I have
taken myself and then given to others; but on the contrary, it
is an alterative-tonic and antiperiodic. It might be poisonous
in a much larger quantity, but as far as I was able to examine,
it contains no *Aconitia.**

---

* The roots I have used internally were dug out by myself to avoid all doubts with
regard to their genuineness. I first took 1 grain of the root, and then increased its dose
gradually to 12 grains three times a day. Being thus assured of its possessing no
deleterious effects, I have used it in some cases among my patients.

This root does not dry well for months in its entire state, and it should therefore be
sliced before exposed to the sun.

315. GLYCYRRHIZÆ RADIX. *(Liquorice Root or Liquorice.)*

Aslussús اصل السوس. *(Arab.)* Bíkhe-mahak بیخ مهک. *(Pers.)* Jéthí-madh جیٹھی مدھ ; Jathí-madh جٹھی مدھ ; Mulatthí ملٹھی. *(Hind.)* Mitthí-lakrí ملٹھی لکڑي. *(Duk.)* Ati-maduram அதிமதுரம். *(Tam.)* Yashti-madhukam యష్టిమధుకం; Ati-madhuramu అతిమధురము. *(Tel.)* Yashti-madhukam ಯಷ್ಟಿಮಧುಕಂ; Ati-madhuram ആതിമധുരം; Iratti-madhuram ഇരട്ടിമധുരം. *(Malyal.)* Yashti-madhuká ಯಷ್ಟಿಮಧುಕಾ; Ati-madhurá ಅತಿಮಧುರಾ. *(Can.)* Jai-shtomodhu. *(Beng.)* Madhu-yashtikam; Yashti-madhukam. *(Sans.)* Jéshtá-madha. *(Mah.)* Jethí-madh. *(Guz.)* Ati-maduram; Velmí. *(Cing.)* Noe-khiyu; Noe-khiyu-ami; No-e-giyu *or* Simbo-noegiyu. *(Bur.)*

See the remarks under *Abrus precatorius* with reference to the above names being misapplied to the root of this plant, &c.

316. GLYCYRRHIZA. *(Extract of——Extract of Liquorice.)*

Rubbussús رب السوس. *(Arab.)* Ausárahe-mahak عصارهٔ مهک ; Jathímadh-ká-ras جٹھی مدھ کا رس. *(Pers.)* Mulatthi-ká-ras ملٹھی کا رس. *(Hind.)* Mitthí-lakrí-ká-ras ملٹھی لکڑي کا رس. *(Duk.)* Ati-maduram-pál அதிமதுரம் பால். *(Tam.)* Yashti-madhuram-pálu యష్టిమధురంపాలు; Ati-madhuram-pálu అతిమధురంపాలు. *(Tel.)* Iratti-madhuram-pál ഇരട്ടിമധുരംപാല്. *(Malyal.)*

317. GMELINA ASIATICA, *Linn.*

318. GMELINA PARVIFOLIA, *Roxb.*

Nilak-kumizh நிலக்குமிழ். *(Tam.)* Challa-gummudu చల్లగుమ్ముడు; Kavva-gummudu కవ్వగుమ్ముడు. *(Tel.)* Nilak-kumazh നിലക്കുമഴ്. *(Malyal.)*

319.   GOSSYPIUM HERBACEUM, *Linn.*

320.   GOSSYPIUM ARBOREUM, *Linn.* ⎫ *Cotton-*
                                                 ⎬ *plant.*
321.   GOSSYPIUM BARBADENSE, *Linn.* ⎭

Nabátul-quṭn نبات القطن ; *Shajratul-quṭn* شجر ةالقطن . (*Arab.*) Daraḵhte-punbah درخت پنبه . (*Pers.*) Kapás-ká-péṛ کپاس کا پیڑ ; Kapás کپاس . (*Hind.*) Kapás-ká-jháṛ کپاس کا جهاڑ . (*Duk.*) Parutti-cheḍi பருத்திசெடி. (*Tam.*) Patti-cheṭṭu பத்திசெட்டு ; Kárpásamu కార్పాసము. (*Tel.*) Parittich-cheṭi പരിത്തിച്ചെടി. (*Malyal.*) Hatti-giḍá ಹತ್ತಿಗಿಡ. (*Can.*) Karpásh-gachh ; Shútér-gáchh. (*Beng.*) Kárpása-vrikshaha. (*Sans.*) Kápúsá-cha-jháḍa. (*Mah.*) Rú-nu-jháḍa ; Kapás-nu-jháḍa. (*Guz.*) Kapu-gahá. (*Cing.*) Wá-biṇ. (*Bur.*).

The following are the names of *Cotton-seeds*, which are frequently used in medicine by the Hakeems:—

Ḥabbul-quṭn حب القطن . (*Arab.*) *Punbah-dánah* پنبه دانه (*Pers.*) *Banólá* بنولا or *Banólah* بنوله . (*Hind. and Duk.*) *Parutti-virai* பருத்திவிதை. (*Tam.*) *Patti-vittulu* పత్తివిత్తులు ; *Kárpása-vittulu* కార్పాసవిత్తులు. (*Tel.*) *Paritti-vitta* പരിത്തി വിത്ത. (*Malyal.*) *Hatti-bíjá* ಹತ್ತಿಬೀಜ. (*Can.*) *Karpásh-bíj* ; *Karpásh-bíchi.* (*Beng.*) *Kárpúsa-bíjam.* (*Sans.*) *Kápúsú-cha-bí.* (*Mah.*) *Rú-nu-bíj* ; *Kapás-nu-bíj.* (*Guz.*) *Kapu-aṭṭa.* (*Cing.*) *Wá-si.* (*Bur.*).

322.   GOSSYPIUM. (*Cotton.*)

Quṭn قطن or Quṭun قطن . (*Arab.*) Punbah پنبه . (*Pers.*) Rúí رونی . (*Hind. and Duk.*) Parutti பருத்தி. (*Tam.*) Patti பத்தி ; Pratti ப்ரத்தி. (*Tel.*) Parutti പരുത്തി. (*Malyal.*) Hatti ಹತ್ತಿ. (*Can.*) Ruí ; Phútá ; Karpásh or Kapás. (*Beng.*) Kárpásaha. (*Sans.*) Kápús. (*Mah.*) Rú. (*Guz.*) Kapu. (*Cing.*) Gúṅ or Goṅ ; Wá. (*Bur.*).

In some Bengali and Sanscrict Dictionaries, *Kapás* or *Kár-pása* and *Túlá* or *Túla,* are used synonymously, but the former is the name of the *common Cotton* and the latter of that produced by *Eriodendron anfractuosum.*

323. GRACILARIA LICHENOIDES, *Greville.*
324. GRACILARIS CONFERVOIDES, *do.*   } *Ceylon Moss.*

Daryá-ki-páchí د ر یا کي پا چي ; Mós مو س . *(Duk.)* Kaḍal-pách-chi கடல்பாச்சி. *(Tam.)* Samudrapu-páchi సముద్రపుపాచి. *(Tel.)* Kiyáv-poé. *(Bur.).*

The above Burmese name is also often applied to *Permelia perlata* and *P. perforata.*

325. GUMMI ACACIÆ. *(Gum Arabic.)*

Ṣamaghe-aarabbí صمغ عربي . *(Arab. and Pers.)* Babúl-ki-gónd ببول کي گوند . *(Hind.)* Kikar-ká-gond کيکر کا گوند . *(Duk.)* Vélam-piṣhin வேலம்பிஷின் ; Karu-vélam-piṣhin கருவேலம்பிஷின். *(Tam.)* Nalla-tumma-banka నల్లతుమ్మబంక ; Tumma-banka తుమ్మబంక. *(Tel.)* Vélakam-paṣha വേലകംപശ ; Karu-vélakam-paṣha കരുവേലകംപശ. *(Malyal.)* Gobbaḷi-góndu ಗೊಬ್ಬಳಿಗೊಂಡ ; Karé-gobbaḷi-góndu ಕರೆಗೊಬ್ಬಳಿಗೊಂಡ. *(Can.)* Bábúlér-gun. *(Beng.)* Kála-barbúra-niriyasam. *(Sans.)* Kála-bábḷi-cha-gónda. *(Mah.)* Kálo-bával-nu-gúndar. *(Guz.).*

Though in many works, the Arabic name *Ṣamaghe-garabbí* as well as its English synonyms *Gum Arabic* or *Indian Gum Arabic* are applied to the gum of *F. ronia Elephantum,* they are not correctly applicable to any other gum but that of *Acacia Arabica* and other species of *Acacia.* It is the latter which is most abundantly produced in India and found in every bazaar, and although there are several other gums, including that of *F. Elephantum,* which resemble the *true Gum Arabic,* they are comparatively very scarce. *Samaghe-garabbi* is more properly the name of the *true Gum Arabic (Acacia vera, &c.)*, but as the latter is quite identical with the gum of *A. Arabica*, the same name is applied to both gums in India.

The names in the text are those properly belong to the gum of *A. Arabica*, and those of the gum of *F. Elephantum* are as follows :—

Ṣamaghe-kabit صمغ كبيت . *(Arab. and Pers.)* Kaṭbél-ki-gónd كت بيل كي گو ند . *(Hind.)* Kaviṭ-ká-gónd كت بيل كي گو ند *(Duk.)* · Viḷúm-piṣhin விளாம்பிசின். *(Tam.)* Velaga-banka వెలగబంక . *(Tel.)* Viḷúm-pasha വിളാമ്പശ. *(Malyal.)* Byúlada-góndú ಬ್ಯೂಲದ ಗೊಂದು. *(Can.)* Koth-bél-gun ; Káṭ-bél-gun *(Beng.)* Kapidtha-niryúsam. *(Sans.)* Kariṭa-gónda *(Mah.)* Kaviṭ-gón. *(Guz.)* Divul-melliyam. *(Cing.)* Ti-si. *(Bur.)*.

It will be seen from the above names that the Tamil synonyme for the gum of *Acacia A. alɩea*, *Vélam-piṣhin*, sounds very much like the synonyme in the same language for the gum of *Feronia Elephantum*, *Viḷam-piṣhin*, and it is not improbable, therefore, that this was originally the cause of confounding those gums with each other.

326. GYMNEMA SYLVESTRE, *R. Br.*

Parpatrah پڑ پتر . *(Duk.)* Ṣhiru-kuruṇjá சிறுகுறுஞ்சா *(Tam.)* Chhóta-dúdhí-lata. *(Beng.)* Binnúg. *(Cing.)*

327. GYNANDROPSIS PENTAPHYLLA, D. C.

Hurhur هردر ; Hurhur-ká-pér هردركا پیڑ . *(Hind.)* Hulhul هلهل ; Hulhul-ká-jhár هلهل كا جهاڑ . *(Duk.)* Véḷai வேளை. *(Tam.)* Váminta వామింత. *(Tel.)* Tai-véḷá തൈവേള; Kara-véḷá കരവേള; Véḷá വേള. *(Malyal.)* Hurhuriyá ; Kánúlá. *(Beng.)*.

328. GYNOCARDIA ODORATA, *R. Br. Syn.*
HYDNOCARPPUS ODORATUS, *Lindly. (Seeds of)*.

Chál-mógré-ké-binj چال موگرے کے بینج or Chnál-mógré-ké-bínj چهال موگرے کے بینج . *(Hind.)*.

H.

329. HELIANTHUS ANNUUS, *Linn.* *(Seeds of).*

Aẕaryún آذريون . (*Arab.*) Vartáj ورتاج , Tukhme-gule-áftáb-parast تخم گل آفتاب پرست ; Tukhme-áftáb-parast تخم آفتاب پرست . (*Pers.*) Súrij-makkhí سورج‌مکهی or Súrij-mukkhí سورج مکهی . (*Hind.*) Súrij-ké-jhár-ké-bínj سورج کے جهاڑ کے بینج . (*Duk.*) Ṣhúriya-kánti-virai. சூரியகாந்திவிளை (*Tam.*) Súrya-kánti-vittulu సూర్యకాంతి విత్తులు; Súryá-vartamu సూర్యావర్తము; Poddu-tiruguḍu-vittulu పొద్దుతిరుగుడువిత్తులు. (*Tel.*) Súryya-kántam-vitta സൂര്യകാന്തം വിത്ത. (*Malyal.*) Súrya-kánti-bijá సూర్యకాంతిబీజ. (*Can.*) Súrya-kánti-bí. (*Mah.*) Negiya-si *or* Négiyá-si. (*Bur.*).

See the remarks under *Acacia speciosa.*

330. HEMIDESMUS INDICUS, *R. Br.* *(Hemi-desmus or Country Sarsaparilla .*

Zaiyán غيان Ạushbatunnár عشبت النار . (*Arab.*) Ạushbahe-hindí عشبهٔ هندی ; Yásamíne-barrí ياسمين بري (*Pers.*) Janglí-chaṅbélí جنگلی چنبیلی ; Hindí-sálsá هندي سالسا . (*Hind.*) Sugandí-pá'á سگندي پالا ; Nannárí نناری ; Náṭ-ká ạushbah ناٹ کا عشبه (*Duk.*) Nannári நன்னறி. (*Tam.*) Sugandhi-pála సుగంధిపాల ; Pála-sugandhi పాలసుగంధి; Pála-chukkam-déru పాలచుక్కందేరు; Gaḍi-sugandhi గడిసుగంధి. (*Tel.*) Nannári-kizhanna നന്നാരികിഴങ്ങ; Naru-ninṭi നറുനിണ്ടി. (*Malyal.*) Sugandha-pálada-gidá

రిఃనఁంಔ. (*Can.*) Ananto-múl ; Ananto. (*Beng.*) Sugand͟hi ; Gópi-múlam. (*Sans.*) Irimusu. (*Cing.*).

From the close resemblance of the sound of the Bengali names *Ananto-múl* and *Antomul,* they are some times confounded with each other. The former is the name of the *Country Sarsaparilla,* and the latter of the *Country Ipecacuanha (Tylophora asthmatica).*

In some Persian works, there is a much confusion about the above names in the text, and they are misapplied to more than one plant ; and in a few others, again, the Hindustani name *Makó* مكو or *Makóé* مكوئي is given to *H. Indica,* while it is correctly a synonyme of *Solanum nigrum* of Blume and *S. rubrum.* See the remarks under *Sarsæ Radix.*

331. HERMODACTYLUS. (*Hermodactyl.*)

Loabate-barbarí لعبت بر برى ; Súrinján سورنجان ; Aaknah عكنه . (*Arab.*)   Súrinján سورنجان . (*Pers. Hind. and Duk.*)   Shuriljján கரிஞ்சான். (*Tam.*) Shurinján ꮶ౦ಜ౯౬౯. (*Tel.*).

The *Súrinján* is of two kinds, named according to its taste as *Súrinjáne-shírín* سور نجان شيرين (*sweet Súrinján*), and *Súrinjáne-talk͟h* سور نجان تلخ (*bitter Súrinján*).

332. HERPESTIS MONNIERA, *H. B. et K.*

Suféd-chamni سفيدچمني . (*Hind.*) Nír-brami நீர்பிரமி. (*Tam.*)   Sámbráni-áku సాంబ్రాణిఆకు ; Sámbráni-cheṭṭu సాంబ్రాణిచెట్టు. (*Tel.*)   Dhóp-chamni ; Adha-birni. (*Beng.*) Jala-primmi. (*Sans.*) Sunu-vila. (*Cing.*).

333. HIBISCUS ROSA-SINENSIS, *Linn.* (*Flowers of.*)

Ang͟haráe-hindí انغرا' هندى . (*Arab. and Pers.*) Jásún جاسون ; Javá جوا . (*Hind.*) Jásút جاسوت ;

Guḍhél هيل گَدّ ; Kuḍhal هل كَدّ . (*Duk.*)   Ṣhappáttup-pú
சப்பாத்துப்பூ. (*Tam.*)   Dásáni-puvvu దాసానిపువ్వు ; Japá-
pushpam జపాపుష్పం ; Java-pushpamu జవపుష్పము. (*Tel.*)
Chemparattip-púva ചെമ്പരത്തിപ്പൂവ ; Ayim-paratti
ആയിമ്പരത്തി. (*Malyal.*) Dásváḷada-huvu దాసవాళదహువు.
(*Can.*)   Ór-phúl ; Jobá-phúl. (*Beng.*)   Japá-pushpam.
(*Sans.*)   Dásindá-cha-phúla. (*Mah.*)   Jásút-nu-phúl.
(*Guz.*)   Kh-ounyan. (*Bur.*).

334. HIBISCUS SABDARIFFA, *Linn.* (*Roselle or Red Sorrel.*)

Lál-anbári لال انباري . (*Hind.*) Lál-anbárá لال انبارا .
(*Duk.*)   Ṣhivappu-káṣhuruk-kírai சிவப்புகாசுருக்கிரை ;
Ṣhímai-káṣhuruk-kírai சிமைகாசுருக்கிரை. (*Tam.*)   Erra-
gómgúra ఎఱ్ఱగోంగూర ; Shíma-gómgúra శిమగోంగూర. (*Tel.*)
Lál-mishṭá. (*Beng.*)   Ṭénbo-khénbouṅ. (*Bur.*).

335. HIPTAGE MADABLOTA, *Gœrtn.*

Kurindai குரிந்தை ; Ṣhiru-kuriṇjá சிறுகுறிஞ்சா. (*Tam.*)
Mádhaví-tíge మాధవీతీగ ; Vaḍla-yárála వడ్లయారాల ; Pótu-
vaḍla పోతువడ్ల. (*Tel.*)   Mádhúbi ; Mádhúbi-latá ; Bos-antí.
(*Beng.*).

336. HIRUDO. (*Leech.*)

Ạalaq علق ; Zaló زلو . (*Arab.*)   Zaló زلو ; Zalók
زلوك . (*Pers.*)   Jók جوك . (*Hind.*)   Jónk جونك .
(*Duk.*)   Aṭṭai அட்டை. (*Tam.*)   Jelagalu జెలగలు ; Aṭṭalu
అట్టలు. (*Tel.*)   Aṭṭa അട്ട. (*Malyal.*)   Jigaṇi జిగణి. (*Can.*)
Joṅk. (*Beng.*)   Jaḷúkaha. (*Sans.*)   Jaḷa. (*Guz.*)   Kudallu-
Púṇḍal. (*Cing.*)   Miyoṅ or Miṅyoṅ. (*Bur.*).

337. HIRUDO GRANULOSA, *Sav.. (Indian Leech.)*

See the names under *Hirudo.*

338. HOLARRHENA ANTIDYSENTERI-CA, R. Br.

339. HOLARRHENA PUBESCENS, *Wall.*

} *Seeds of.*

Lasánul-aaṣáfírul-murr لسان العصافير المر . (*Arab.*) Indar-jave-talḵh ا ندرجو تلخ ; Zabáne-kunjaṣhke-talḵh زبان كنجشك تلخ ; Tuḵhme-ahare-talḵh تخم اهرتلخ . (*Pers.*) Karvá-indarjou كڙو ا ا ندرجو . (*Hind. and Duk.*) Kaṣhappu-veṭpá-lariṣhi கசப்புவெட்பாலரிஷி ; Kuḷap-páḷai-virai குளப்பாளைவிரை. (*Tam.*) Chédu-kodiṣha-vittulu శేడుకోడిషవిత్తులు ; Amkuḍu-vittulu అంకుడువిత్తులు. (*Tel.,* Kaipa-koṭakap-pála-vitta കൈപകൊടകപ്പാലവിത്ത. (*Malyal.*) Títá-indarjou. (*Beng.*) Kaḍú-indra-jou. (*Mah.*) Kaḍvo-indarjou. (*Guz.*).

See the remarks under *Wrightia tinctoria* with regard to the sweet and bitter varieties of *Indarjou* ا ندرجو , &c.

340. HOPEA ODERATA, *Roxb.*

341. HORDEI SEMINA. *(Barley.)*

Shaaír شعير . (*Arab.*) Jou جو . (*Pers. Hind. and Duk.*) Bárali-ariṣhi பாரலிஅரிஷி. (*Tam.*) Bárali-biyyam బారలిబియ్యం. (*Tel.*) Jóo. (*Beng.*) Jav. (*Guz.*) Múyo (*Bur.*).

342. HOYA VIRIDIFLORA, *R. B*

Nak-chhikní نک چهکني . (*Hind.*).

343. HYDNOCARPUS INEBRIANS, *Vahl.* *(Nut of.)*

Jangli-bádám جنگلی با د ا م . *(Hind. and Duk.)* Niraḍi-muttu நீரடிமுத்து. *(Tam.)* Níraḍi-vittulu నీరడివిత్తులు. *(Tel.)* Raṭa-kekuna. *(Cing.)*.

344. HYDRARGYRI BISULPHURETUM. *(Impure Bisulphuret of Mercury, or Cinnabar.)*

Shanjarf شنجرف ; Zanjafr زنجفر . *(Arab.)* Shangarf شنگرف ; Hingól هنگول . *(Pers. and Hind.)* Shangraf شنگرف . *(Duk.)* Liṇgam லிங்கம்; Jádi-liṇgam சாதிலிங்கம். *(Tam.)* Ingili-gamu ఇంగిలికము. *(Tel.)* Cháyilyam ചായില്യം ; Cháliyam ചാലിയം ; Játi-lingam ജാതിലിംഗം. *(Malyal.)* Ingaḷiká ಇಂಗಳಿಕ. *(Can.)* Hingól ; *Shangraf.* *(Beng.)* Inghúlam *(Sans.)* Sangraf. *(Guz.)* Lingam ; Játi-lingam. *(Cing.)*.

Zanjarf زنجرف , *Dardúr* دردار , *Sarúre-aḥmar* سرور احمر , and some other names are found applied to *Cinnabar* in some Persian and other works ; but they are neither restricted to it, nor in use at present, and I have, therefore, omitted them from the text.

345. HYDRARGYRI PERCHLORIDUM. *Syn.* Hydrargyri corrosivum sublimatum. *(Corrosive Sublimate, or Perchloride of Mercury.)*

Shavíram شویرم ; Shavir شویر . *(Duk.)* Víram வீரம்; Ṣhav-víram சவ்வீரம். *(Tam.)* Ṣhaviramu శవీరము ; Víramu వీరము. *(Tel.)* Ṣhavíram. *(Cing.)*.

The medicine sold in the bazaars of Southern India under the above names is *Perchloride of Mercury (Corrosive Sublimate)*, and responds to all the chemical tests of that salt. It is less crystalline and more dull and opaque in appearance than the salt in use in Hospitals, and occasionally contains a small quantity of *Subchloride of Mercury (Calomel).* As far as I was able to examine this salt, I found it to contain no other impurity. It is quite fit for use both externally and internally as a substitute for the *Corrosive Sublimate* imported from Europe.

In some books, the Arabic name *Sulaimáni* سليماني is considered to be applicable to *Corrosive Sublimate;* but this is incorrect, because the *Sulaimani* contains *Arsenic* in its combination.

246. HYDRARGYRI SUBCHLORIDUM. *(Impure Subchloride of Mercury, Calomel, or Calomelas.)*

Ras-kapúr رسكپور . *(Hind. and Duk.)* Raṣha-karuppúram சசகருப்பூரம்; Púram பூரம். *(Tam.)* Rasa-karpúramu రసకర్పూరము ; Púramu పూరము. *(Tel.)* Rasa-karppúram രസകപൂരം. *(Malyal.)* Rasa-karpúram. *(Cing.).*

The medicine obtained by these names in the Indian bazaars, is, according to chemical tests, an impure *Subchloride of Mercury (Calomel)*, though it differs much in some of the physical characters of that salt supplied to Hospitals. It does not occur in powder, but in heavy crystalline masses, and bears some resemblance to *Camphor;* hence the names *Ras-kapúr, Rasa-karpúram*, &c., which mean *Mercurial-camphor.* When powdered in a mortar, it is rendered yellowish-white, and this powder generally corresponds with the *common Calomel.* Its chief impurity is *Perchloride of Mercury*, which it occasionally contains in a minute quantity; and it is not, therefore, a safe medicine to be used internally. Used in the form of *Ointment* or *Lotion*, it is more sure and effectual medicine than *Calomel,* probably from its containing a small quantity of *Perchloride of Mercury.*

The native practitioners, particularly the Vaiddiyans, resort to this medicine both for external and internal use, more frequently than any other preparation of Mercury, and they consider it poisonous in more than a few grain doses.

In some medical and other works, *Ras-kapúr* is applied to *Corrosive Sublimate,* while in a few others, *Dég-bar-dég* دیگ بردیگ

is considered to be its Persian synonyme. Both these asser-
tions are incorrect, because the former is applicable only to
the Medicine I have just described; and the latter is generally
in use for a preparation of Arsenic. *Déy-bar-déy* is, moreover,
a very uncertain name, and could be applied to all the medicines
prepared by sublimation. It means *a kettle on a kettle*, in
reference to the manner in which some solid volatile medicines
are prepared by sublimation by keeping one vessel upon another.

347. HYDRARGYRUM. *(Mercury.)*

Zibaq زيبق . *(Arab.)* Símáb سيماب ; Jívah جيوه .
(Pers.) Para پارا . *(Hind. and Duk.)* Irasham இரசம்.
(Tam.) Rasam ರಸಂ ; Páda-rasam పాదరసం. *(Tel.)* Rassam
രസ്സം. *(Malyal.)* Páda-rasá ಪಾದರಸಾ. *(Can.)*   Párá.
(Beng.) Páradaha ; Rasam. *(Sans.)* Pára. *(Mah.)* Páro.
(Guz.) Rasadiyá. *(Cing.)* Padá or Padá. *(Bur.)*.

348. HYDROCOTYLE ASIATICA, *Linn.* *(Indian Hydrocotyle or Penny-wort.)*

Artáníyáe-hindí ارتانيائے هندي . *(Arab.)* Vallári
ولاري ; Vallári-ká-pattá ولاري كا پتا . *(Duk.)* Vallárai
வல்லாணை. *(Tam.)* Mandúka-bramha-kúráku మండూకబ్రమ్హ
కూరాకు ; Pinna-élaki-chettu పిన్నఏలకిచెట్టు ; Bokkudu-chettu
బొక్కుడుచెట్టు. *(Tel.)* Kutakan കുടകന്. *(Malyal.)* Von-de-
lagá ವೊಂದೆಲಗಾ. *(Can.)* Thol-kuri. *(Beng.)* Hingotu-kola.
(Cing.) Minkhuá-bin. *(Bur.)*.

The Tamil names *Vallárai* and *Vilári* are some times confounded with each other on account of the resemblance of their
pronunciation. The latter is the name of *Hymenodictyon excelsum.*

349. HYMENODICTYON EXCELSUM, *Wall.* Syn. CINCHONA EXCELSA, *Roxb.*

Bandárú بندارو : Bandarú بندرو . *(Hind.)* Bandári
بندارني ; Jangli-anár-ká-*jhár* جنگلي انار كا جهاڙ . *(Duk.)*

Vilári அலரி. *(Tam.)*   Bandára-*chettu* బండారచెట్టు; Búrija బూరిజ; Búrja బూర్జ; *Chétippa* చేటిప్ప. *(Tel.)*   Vallári വല്ലാരി. *(Malyal.)*.

The Hindustani name *Kálá-bachhnáy* كالا بچهناگ is very erroneously applied to this plant in many books, with reference to which see the remarks under *Aconitum ferox*. See also the remarks on *Hydrocotyle Asiatica*. The meaning of *Jangli-anár-ká-jhár* is *the wild Pomegranate plant*, and this is applied to *H. Excelsum* in S. India on account of the resemblance of its leaves to those of the former.

350. HYOSCYAMUS INSANUS, *Stocks.*

Kóhi-bang كو ﻫﻲ بنگ . *(Hind.)*.

351. HYOSCYAMUS NIGRUM, *Linn. (Seeds of—Henbane-seeds.)*

Bazrul-banj بزرا لبنج . *(Arab.)*   Khurásáni-ajváyan خراساني اجوان . *(Hind.)*   Khurásáni-ajván خرساني اجو این . *(Duk.)*   Kúrásháni-yómam கூராசானியோமம். *(Tam.)*   Kúrásáni-vámam కూరాసానివామం; Kurinji-vámam కురింజ వామం. *(Tel.)*   Khurásáni-vómá ಖುರಾಸಾನಿವೋಮಾ; *Khurásáni-vádakki* ಖುರಾಸಾನಿವಾಡಕ್ಕಿ. *(Can.)*   *Khórásáni-vóvá.* *(Mah.)*   *Khorásáni-ájmo*; *Khorásáni-ajván.* *(Guz.)*.

Kurásáni-vámam is a correct Telugu name of the above seeds, but it is improperly applied to the seeds of *Cnidium diffusum* and considered to be synonymous with *Kuranji-vámam* in Flora Andhrica.

352. HYSSOPUS OFFICINALIS, *Linn. (Husk of the seeds of.)*

Zúfáé-yábis زوفائے یا بس . *(Arab. and Pers.)*.

I.

353. ICTHYOCOLLA. *(Isinglass.)*

G ḥirriyus-samak غري السمك ; *G ḥarriyus-samak*
غر السمك . *(Arab.)* Siréshame-máhí سريشم ماهي *(Pers.)*
Mach-chhí-ká-sirish مجهي كا سريش . *(Hind.)* Mach-chhí-
kí-sirish مجهي كي سرش *(Duk.)* Mín-vajjaram மீன்
வச்சரம் *(Tam.)* Chépa-vajramu చేపవజ్రము. *(Tel.)*.

354. IGNATIA AMARA, *Linn.* *(Seeds of—St.
Ignatius' Bean.)*

Papítah پپيته . *(Hind. and Duk.)* Kayappaṇ-koṭṭai
கயப்பங்கொட்டை. *(Tam.)*.

355. ILLICIUM ANISATUM, *Linn. (Fruit of—
Star Anise.)*

Bádiyáne-ḳhaṭái باد يان خطا ني ; Ráziyánaje-ḳhaṭái
رازيانه خطائي . *(Arab.)* Ráziyánahe-ḳhaṭái رازيانج خطائي
Bádiyáne-ḳhaṭái باد يا ن خطا ني . *(Pers.)* Anás-phal
ا نا س پهل . *(Hind.)* Anas-phal نس پهل *(Duk.)*
Aṇṇáshup-pu அணணசுப்பு. *(Tam.)* Anása-puvvu అనాస
పువ్వు. *(Tel.)* Nanat-poén. *(Bur.)*.

From the resemblance of the above fruit to a flower, it is
incorrectly named in some books as *Anas-phúl* instead of *Anas-
phal*. In addition to this, the word *Anas* is confounded in some
Persian works with *Anánás*, and the *Star-anise* is accordingly
and. erroneously named *Gule-anánás* گل ا نا نا س ,which
means the flower of *Ananas sativus*.

356. INDIGOFERA TINCTORIA, *Linn.*

Nabátun-nílaj نبات النيلج . (*Arab.*) Darakhte-níl درخت نيل . (*Pers.*) Níl-ká-pér نيل کا پير . (*Hind.*) Níl-ká-jhár نيل کا جها ڙ . (*Duk.*) Aviri அவிரி ; Nili-maram நீலிமரம். (*Tam.*) Níli-chettu నీళ్ళచెట్టు ; Aviri అవిరి. (*Tel.*) Amari അമരി. (*Malyal.*) Nili-gidá ನೀಲಿಗಿಡ. (*Can.*) Níl-gáchh. (*Beng.*) Níla-vrikshaha. (*Sans.*) Nílicha-jháda. (*Mah.*) Avari ; Nil-gahá. (*Cing.*) Mé-biṉ. (*Bur.*).

See the remarks under *Cassia lanceolata, C. Obovata,* and *Pharbitis Nil.*

357. INDIGOFERA TINCTORIA, *Linn* (*Express-ed juice of—Indigo.*)

Nilaj نيلج . (*Arab.*) Nílah نيله ; Auṣárahe-níl عصار‍ة نيل ; Níl نيل . (*Pers.*) Níl نيل . (*Hind. and Duk.*) Nílam நீலம். (*Tam.*) Níli-mandu నీలిమండు. (*Tel.*) Nílam നീലം. (*Malyal.*) Nili ನೀಲಿ. (*Can.*) Nil. (*Beng.*) Nílam. (*Sans.*) Nílh. (*Mah.*) Níl ; Gali. (*Guz.*) Nila or Níla. (*Cing.*) Mé or Mai ; Maine or Méné ; Ṣham-me. (*Bur.*).

See the remarks under *Cassia lanceolata, C. obovata,* and *Pharbitis Nil.*

358. IPOMŒA CYMOSA, *Röm. et Schu-letes.*

359. IPOMŒA SEPARIA, *Kön.*

} *Seeds of.*

Lál-dánah لا لـ دانه ? (*Hind.*).

360. IPOMŒA TURPETHUM, *R. Br.* (*Root of—Turbith root.*)

Turbud تربد . (*Arab.*) Nisút نسوت . Nákpatar نا ک پتر ; Pitóhri پتوهري . (*Hind.*) Tikṛá تکڙا . (*Duk.*)

Shivadai சிவதை; Shivadai-vér சிவதைவேர். (Tam.) Tegaḍa
తెగడ ; Tegaḍa-véru తెగడవేరు. (Tel.)   Chiváka-véra ചിവാക
വെര. (Malyal.)   Turbut ; Tribrit ; Téurí. (Beng.) Tri-
puṭa. (Sans.) Trista-válu-múl. (Cing.).

J.

361.   JALAPA. (Jalap.)

Sháṭil شاطل . (Arab.) Róshanak روشنك ; Biḵhe-
jallabah بيخ جلا به . (Pers.)   Béḵhe-jullabah بيخ جلا به ;
Béḵhe-jallabah بيخ جلابه ; Jálap-kí-jaṛ جا لپ كي جڑ ; Jálap
جا لپ . (Duk)   Bédik-kizhaṇgu பேதிக்கிழங்கு. (Tam.)
Bédi-gaḍḍa బేదిగడ్డ. (Tel.).

362.   JASMINUM SAMBAC, Aiton. (Flowers of.)

Suman سمن or Saman سمن ; Yásaman ياسمن ; Varde-
abyaẓ ورد ابيض. (Arab.) Gule-supéd گل سپيد . (Pers.)
Mógrá موگرا ; Mógré-ké-phúl موگرے كے پهول . (Hind.
and Duk.) Malligaip-pú மல்லிகைப்பூ ; Mallip-pú மல்லிப்பூ.
(Tam.)   Malle-puvvulu మల్లెపువ్వులు ; Mallelu మల్లెలు. (Tel.)
Mullách-cha-pú മുല്ലാച്ചപൂ ; Mullappú മുല്ലപ്പൂ. (Malyal.)
Mallige-huvvu ಮಲ್ಲಿಗೆಹುವ್ವು. (Can.) Mogra ; Mogra-phúl.
(Beng.) Mográ-cha-phúla. (Mah.) Mogra-nu-phúl. (Guz.)
Pich-chi-mal. (Cing.).

The following are the names of the double-flowered variety
of the above plant :—

Baṭ-mógrá بٹ موگرا . (Hind. and Duk.) Kuḍa-malli
கு—மல்லி. (Tam.) Gundu-malle గుండుమల్లె. (Tel.) Baṭ-mogra.
(Beng. and Guz.).

363. JATROPHA CURCAS, *Linn.* (*Nut of—English Physic Nut.*)

Dande-nahrí دند نهري ; Dande-barrí د ند بري . (*Arab. and Pers.*) Jangli-arandi جنگلي ا رندى . (*Hind.*) Jangli-yarandí جنگلى يرندي . (*Duk.*) Káṭṭámaṇakku சாட்டா மணக்கு. (*Tam.*) Pépálam పేపాలం. (*Tel.*) Káṭṭá-vanakka കാട്ടാവണക്ക. (*Malyal.*) Beṭṭada-haraḷu ಬೆಟ್ಟದ ಹರಳು. (*Can.*) Bon-*bhéranḍá* ; Erandá-*gáchh.* (*Beng.*) Parvata-yeranḍa. (*Sans.*) Ráṇa-yerandí. (*Mah.*) Jangli-arandí. (*Guz.*) Val-endaru ; Erandu. (*Cing.*) Késu-gi ; Ṣimbo-kesu *or* Ṭimbo-kesu. (*Bur.*).

The Bengali name ' *Bagh-bheranḍa*' which occurs in some books, ought to be *Ban-bheranḍa.* See the remarks under *Croton polyandrum* and *Ricinus communis.*

364. JATROPHA GLANDULIFERA, *Roxb.*

Úḍaḷai உடலை. (*Tam.*) Néla-ámudamu నేలఆముదము. (*Tel.*).

In some books *Aabab* عبب is assigned as the Arabic name of the above plant, but it is the name of a species of Solanaceæ.

365. JATROPHA MULTIFIDA, *Linn.* (*Nut of—French Physic Nut.*)

366. JUGLANS. (*Walnut.*)

Jouz جوز . (*Arab.*) Girdagán گرد گان ; *Chár-maghz* چار مغز ; *Chahár-maghz* چهار مغز . (*Pers.*) Aḳhróṭ اخروٹ ; Akróṭ اکروٹ . (*Hind. and Duk.*) Akróṭṭu அக்ரோட்டு. (*Tam.*) Akróṭu అక్రోటు. (*Tel.*) Akróḍu ಅಕ್ರೋಡು. (*Can.*) Aḳhróṭ. (*Beng.*) Akróḍa. (*Mah.*) Ṣis-khyá-si *or* Ṭikyá-zi. (*Bur.*).

See the remarks under *Aleurites triloba.*

367. JUNIPERI FRUCTUS. *(Juniper Berries.)*

Abhal ابهل ا ; Ḥabbul-aaraar حب العرعر ; Ṣamratul-
aaraar ثمرة العرعر. *(Arab.)* Aaraar-ká-*phal* عرعركا پهل.
(Hind.) Abhal ابهل ا. *(Duk.)*.

368. JUSTICIA GENDARUSSA, *Linn. Syn.* GENDA-

RUSSA VULGARIS, *Nees.*

Aslaqe-asvad اثلق ا سود. *(Arab.)*   Banj-angashte-
siyáh بجنگشتاسيا ه. *(Pers.)* Údi-san*bhálú* اودىسنبها لو ;
Nílí-nirgandí نيلي نرگندب. *(Hind.)*   Kálí-*shanbáli*
كالي شنبالي. *(Duk.)* Karu-no*ch*-*chi* கருநொச்சி ; Karuppu-
no*ch*-*chi* கருப்புநொச்சி. *(Tam.)*   Nalla-vávili నల్లావావిలి ;
Nalla-no*ch*-*chili* నల్లనొచ్చిలి ; Néla-vávili నేలవావిలి. *(Tel.)*
Karun-no*ch*-*chi* കരുനൊച്ചി ; Vátak-koṭi വാതക്കൊടി ;
Vátan-golli വാതകൊള്ളി. *(Malyal.)*   Karelakkí-giḍá ಕರೆ
ಲಕ್ಕಿಗಿಡಾ. *(Can.)* Jogmodon. *(Beng.)*   Níla-nirgundí ;
Kri*sh*ṭṇa-surasa. *(Sans.)* Kalu-varaniá. *(Cing.)* Bavanet.
(Bur.).

The meaning of the Telugu and Bengali synonymes *Gandha-
rasamu* and *Gandros* is *a smelling or fragrant juice,* and they are
therefore, applied in some books either to some fragrant drugs,
as *Myrrh,* &c., or to some odoriferous plants. They are also
applied in some books (Flora Andhrica, Hortus Suburbanus
Calcuttensis, &c.,) to *Justicia Gendarussa;* but this plant possesses
no particular smell, unless it is mistaken for a variety of *Vitex
negundo* or *V. trifolia,* which is often indicated or intended by
the native names applied to the former.

K.

369. KÆMPFERIA GALANGA, *Linn. (Root of.)*

*Ch*andra-múla ; Humúla ; *Ch*andú-múlá. *(Beng.)*
Pánvu ; *Khamou or* Gamou ; Pán-vu-kamún. *(Bur.)*.

The Malyalim and Mahratti names given to this plant in the Hortus Malabaricus, (Vol. XI., Tab. 41) are those properly belong to *Curcuma zerumbet*.

370. KÆMPFERIA ROTUNDA, *Linn.*

Bhú-*ch*ampá. *(Beng.)*.

371. KINO *(the drug)*.

Dammul-a*kh*vain دم ا لا خو ين ; Dammus-saabán دم التعبان ; Dammut-tanín دم التنين ; Qáterud-dam قا طر ا لد م . *(Arab.)* *Kh*úne-siyávashán خون سيا وشا ن (Pers.) Dammul-a*kh*vain دم ا لا خوين . *(Hind. and Duk.)* S*h*ímai-kándá-miruga-mirattam சீமைகாண்டாமிருக மிரத்தம். *(Tam.)* - S*h*íma-gándá-mrugam-netturu శీమాగాండా ముగోనెత్తురు. *(Tel.)* S*h*íma-vénnap-pas*h*a ശീമവെണ്ണപ്പശ. *(Malyal.)*.

The above are properly the names of the *Kino* which was known formerly as *Dragon's Blood*, and which was imported into India chiefly from Africa. It is not to be found now in the bazaar.

Of the two varieties of *Kino* commonly met with in the Indian markets at present, one is the produce of *Pterocarpus marsupium*, and the other of *Butea frondosa* and *B. superba*. The above names are also used for the *Kino* of *P. marsupium*, but they are correctly applicable to it only in the manner I have marked them under the head of that plant. The names of *Butea Kino* are quite different from those of other varieties of *Kino*, and are already given under its proper head.

L.

372.　LAC. (Milk.)

Labn لبن. (Arab.) Shír شیر. (Pers.) Dúdh دودھ. (Hind. and Duk.) Pál பால். (Tam.) Pálu పాలు. (Tel.) Pál പാൽ; Kshíram ക്ഷീരം. (Malyal.) Hálu ಹಾಲು. (Can.) Dúdh. (Beng.) Kshíram. (Sans.) Dúda. (Mah.) Dúdh. (Guz.) Kiri. (Cing.) No. (Bur.).

The milk which is most frequently used for the sick as a diet in this country is that of *Cow* and *Goat*; and the milk of *Ass* is a valuable medicine in *Phthisis*. The names of these milks are as follows :—

a. Cow's milk—*Labnul bajar* لبن البقر. (*Arab.*) *Shíre-gáv* شیر گاو. (Pers.) *Gái-ká-dúdh* گائی کا دودھ. (Hind. and Duk.) *Pashum-pál* பசும்பால். (Tam.) *Áru-pálu* ఆవుపాలు. (Tel.) *Pashuvin-pál* പശുവിൻപാൽ. (Malyal.) *Ákalu-hálu* ಆಕಳಹಾಲು. (Can.) *Gáicha-dúda* (Mah.) *Gai-nu-dúdh.* (Guz.) *Mi-kiri.* (Cing.).

b. Goat's milk—*Labnul-magz* لبن المعز. (Arab.) *Shíre-buz* شیر بز; *Shíre-tis* شیر تیس. (Pers.) *Bakri-ká-dúdh* بکری کا دودھ. (Hind.) *Chhéli-ká-dúdh* چھیلی کا دودھ. (Duk.) *Velláttup-pál* வெள்ளாட்டுப்பால். (Tam.) *Kanchi-méka-pálu* కంచిమేకపాలు. (Tel.) *Velláttup-pál* വെള്ളാട്ടുപ്പാൽ. (Malyal.) *Bakri-cha-dúda.* (Mah.) *Bakri-nu-dúdh.* (Guz.) *Yelu-kiri.* (Cing.).

c. Ass' milk—*Labnul-atán* لبن الاتان. (Arab.) *Shíre-khar* شیر خر. (Pers.) *Gadhi-ká-dúdh* گدھی کا دودھ. (Hind.) *Gaidhé-ká-dúdh* گدھے کا دودھ. (Duk.) *Kazhudaip-pál* கழுதைப்பால். (Tam.) *Gúdide-pálu* గాడిదపాలు. (Tel.) *Kazhutap-pál* കഴുതപ്പാൽ. (Malyal.) *Katte-hálu* ಕತ್ತೆಹಾಲು. (Can.) *Gádhara-cha-dúda.* (Mah.) *Gadha-nu-dúdh.* (Guz.) *Buro-kiri.* (Cing.).

373. LACTUCA SATIVA, *Linn.* *(Seeds of.)*

Bazrul-*khas* بزرالخس. *(Arab.)* Tukhme-káhú تخم كاهو.
(Pers.) Káhú-ké-bínj کاہو کے بیذج. *(Hind. and Duk.)*
Shalláttu-virai சல்லாத்துவிரை. *(Tam.)* Kávu-vittulu కావు
విత్తులు. *(Tel.)*.

374. LAVANDULA. *Sp. of.*

Ustokhúdús اسطو خودوس. *(Arab. Pers. and Duk.)*.

375. LAWSONIA ALBA, *Lam.* *(Henna plant.)*

Hinná حنا; Yoranná يرنا. *(Arab.)* Hiná حنا. *(Pers.)*
Mhindi مهندي. *(Hind.)* Mhéndi مهيندي; Ménhdi.
ميهندي. *(Duk.)* Marutónri மருதோன்றி; Aivanam
ஐவணம். *(Tam.)* Góranta గోరంట. *(Tel.)* Mayilánchi
മയിലാഞ്ചി; Marutónni മരുതൊന്നി. *(Malyal.)* Góranțe
గోరంటె. *(Can.)* Méhédi. *(Beng.)* Kuravaka. *(Sans.)*
Méndhí. *(Mah.)* Méndi. *(Guz.)* Mariṭoṇḍi. *(Cing.)* Dán-
biṇ. *(Bur.)*.

The Persian names *Isband* اسبند or *Ispand* اسپند are
applied to the seeds of *L. alba* in Southern India, while the
same are in use for the seeds of *Pajanum harmala* in Hyderabad,
Calcutta, Patna, Benares, and Northern India. The latter is
correct.

376. LEDEBOURIA HYACINTHOIDES, *Roth.*
(Bulb of.)

Chhóṭí-janglí-píyáz چهوتی جنگلی پیاز. *(Duk.)* Shiṛu-
nari-veṇgáyam சிறுநரிவெங்காயம்; Shiṛu-káṭṭu-veṇgáyam
சிறுகாட்டுவெங்காயம். *(Tam.)* Chiru-aḍavi-vulli-gaḍḍa ఛిరు
అడవివుల్లిగడ్డ. *(Tel.)* Náni-jangli-kándo. *(Guz.)*.

See the remarks under *Urginea Indica* with reference to
the bulbs of *L. hyacinthoides* being confounded with those of
the former, &c.

377. LEPIDIUM SATIVUM, *Linn.* *(Seeds of.)*[1]

Ḥabbur-rashád حب الرشاد ; Ḥurf حرف . *(Arab.)*
Tukhme-turrah-tézak تخم تره تیزک . *(Pers.)* Hálim هالم ;
Chansar چنسر . *(Hind.)*   Halim هلیم . *(Duk.)* Áḷi-virai
அளிவிளை . *(Tam.)*   Áḍéli అడేలి ; Áḍiyúlu అడియూలు . *(Tel.)*
Hálim. *(Beng. Mah. and Guz.)* Samah-ni. *(Bur.).*

378. LINUM USITATISSIMUM, *Linn.* *(Seeds of—*
Linseed.)

Bazrul-kattán بزرا الکتان . *(Arab.)*   Tukhme-zaghír
تخم زعیر ; Tukhme-katán نخم کتان . *(Pers.)* Alsí السی ;
Tísí تیسی . *(Hind.)*   Alsí-ké-bínj السی کے بیذج . *(Duk.)*
Alishi-virai அலிஷிவிளை . *(Tam.)*   Atasí అతసి ; Madana-
ginjalu మదనగింజలు . *(Tel.)*   Cheru-chánattinté-vitta చెరు
ചാണത്തിൻതെവിത്ത . *(Malyal.)* Alaṣhi అలఫ . *(Can.)*
Tísɩ ; Mosíná. *(Beng.)*   Atasí. *(Sans.).*

By some mistake, 'Atees' is applied in some books to *Lin-
seeds,* which is correctly the name of the root of *Aconitum
heterophyllum.*   The above names *Alsí, Alishi* or *Alaṣhí,* and *Tísí
Atasí* or *Tɩsi,* are confounded occasionally with *Avisi* or *Agaṣhi,*
and *Agatti* or *Agti.* The latter are the names of *Agati-grandiflora.*

379. LINUM USITATISSIMUM, *Linn.* *(Oil of—*
Linseed oil.)

Dhonul-kattán دهن الکتان . *(Arab.)* Roghane-zaghír
روغن زغیر , Roghane-katán روغن کتان . *(Pers.)* Alsí-
ká-tél السی کا تیل ; Tísí-ká-tél تیسی کا تیل . *(Hind.)* Alsí-
ká-tél السی کا تیل . *(Duk.)* Alishi-virai-yenney அளிஷிவிளை
யெண்ணெய் . *(Tam.)* Madana-ginjala-núne మదనగింజలనూనె ;
Atasi-núne అతసినూనె . *(Tel.)* Cheruchána-vittinté-eṇṇá
ചെറുചാണവിത്തിൻതെഎണ്ണാ . *(Malyal.)* Alaṣhi-yaṇṇe
అలఫయణ్ణ . *(Can.)* Tísí-tail. *(Beng.).*

380. LIQUIDAMBER ALTINGIA, *Blume.* (*Resin of—Liquid Storax.*)

Méaahe-sáyelah ميعة سا يله . (*Arab*) Asle-lubní عسل لبني . (*Pers.*) Siláras سلارس . (*Hind.*) Neri-ariṣhip-pál தெரிஅரிஷிப்பால். (*Tam.*) Ṣhilá-rasam జిలారసం. (*Tel.*) Seláras. (*Guz.*) Nantayu. (*Bur.*).

See the remarks under *Ophelia Elegans* and *O. multiflora*.

381. LOBELIA NICOTIANÆFOLIA, *Heyné.*
Déva-nal ; Bók-nal ; Davul. (*Mah.*).

382. LODOICEA SECHELLARUM. *Labill.* (*Nut of.*)

Nárjíle-baḥrí نارجيل بحري . (*Arab.*) Nárgíle-baḥrí نارگیل بحري . (*Pers.*) Daryá-ká-náríyal دریاکا ناریل . (*Hind.*) Daryá-ká-nárél دریاکا ناریل . (*Duk.*) Kadaṭ-rengáy கடற்றெங்காய். (*Tam.*) Samudrapu-ṭenkáya సముద్రపు టెంకాయ. (*Tel.*) Kaṭal-ténná കടൽതെങ്ങാ . (*Malyal.*) Daryá-nu-naríyal (*Guz.*) Múdú-pol. (*Cing.*) Penle-on-ṣí. (*Bur.*).

See the remarks under *Xylocarpus granatum* with regard to the above Burmese name.

383. LUFFA AMARA. *Roxb* (*Fruit of.*)

Karví-turí كرزوي ترائي . (*Hind.*) Karví-turái كرزوي ترئي . (*Duk*) Pé-pírkkam பேப்பீர்க்கம். (*Tam.*) Chédu-bíra చేదు బీర ; Verri-bíra వెర్రిబీర. (*Tel.*) Títo-jhiṅgá ; Ṭito-torai ; Tito-dhuṅdul. (*Beng.*).

Karólá or ' Kerula' is the Hindustani name assigned to the above plant in some books, but it is correctly the name of *Momordica charantia* in that language as well as in Bengali.

384. LUFFA ECHINATA, *Roxb.*

M.

385. MALVA MAURITIANA,

Vilâyati-kangai-ká-pér ولايتي كنگئي كا پيڙ . *(Hind.)*
Vilâyati-kangói-ká-*jhár* ولايتي كنگوئي كا جهاڙ . *(Duk.)*.

See the remarks under *Abutilon Indicum* with reference to the names of that plant being incorrectly applied to *M. Mauritiana.*

386. MALLOTUS PHILLIPIENSIS, *Müll. Syn.* Rottlera tinctoria, *Roxb. (Pubescence of the Capsules—Kamala.)*

Qinbil قنبيل *(Arab.)* Kanbélá كنبيلا . *(Pers.)* Kamélá كيلا : Kamúd كود . *(Hind.)* Kamélá-mávu கெமேலா மாவு. *(Tam.)* Kápila-poḍi కాపిలపొడి. *(Tel.)* Kaméla. *(Beng.)* Kapila *(Sans.)* Kaméla. *(Guz.)* Hampirilla-geḍivella-buvá. *(Cing.)*.

Vars ورس is the Arabic name of a medicine which resembles *Saffron* when not powdered, and *Kamélá* when powdered, and therefore often confounded with these drugs. It is neither the produce of *Crocus Sativus* nor of *Mallotus Phillippiensis (Rottlera tinctoria)*; and is found only in Arabia.

The Arabic word *Qinbil* is applied to more than one drug in some Arabic and Persian works, but according to the present usage of the language in India, it is restricted to *Kamélá.*

Késar and *Kunkuma-puvvu* are the correct Hindustani and Telugu names of *Saffron*, but are confounded in some books with those of *R. tinctoria, Nyctanthes arbor tristis,* and *Mesua ferrea,* &c. See the remarks under *Crocus.*

387. MANGIFERA INDICA, *Linn.* *(Mango-tree.)*

Shajratul-anbaj شجرة الانبج . *(Arab.)* Darakhte-anbah درخت انبه ; Darakhte-naghzak درخت نغزک . *(Pers.)* Ánb-ká-péṛ آنب کا پیڑ ; Ám-ká-péṛ آم کا پیڑ . *(Hind.)* Ám-ká-jhár آم کا جھاڑ . *(Duk.)* Mángá-maram மாங்காமரம் ; Má-maram மாமரம். *(Tam.)* Mámiḍi-chettu మామిడిచెట్టు ; Mákandamu మాకందము ; Mávi మావి. *(Tel.)* Mávva మావ్వ ; Múch-chi-maram മൂച്ചിമരം. *(Malyal.)* Máviná-mará మావినామరా. *(Can.)* Ám-gáchh. *(Beng.)* Ámra-vrikshaha. *(Sans.)* Ambá-cha-jháḍa. *(Mah.)* Kairi-nu-jháḍa ; Ambá nu-jháḍa. *(Guz.)* Amba-gahá. *(Cing.)* Ṣiya-piṇ or Ṭiye-piṇ. *(Bur.)*.

388. MANIHOT UTILISSIMA, *Phol.* *(Root of.)*

Pinḍálú پنڈالو ; Pinḍalam پنڈلم *(Duk.)* Mara-vallik-kizhaṇgu மரவள்ளிக்கிழங்கு ; Ál-vallik-kizhaṇgu ஆல்வள்ளிக்கிழங்கு. *(Tam.)* Mánu-penḍalam మానుపెండలం; Karra-penḍalam కఱ్ఱపెండలం. *(Tel.)* Mara-kizhaṇṇa മരകിഴങ്ങ ; Mara-valli-kizhaṇṇa മരവള്ളികിഴങ്ങ ; Maram-chíni-kizhaṇṇa മരംചീനികിഴങ്ങ. *(Malyal.)* Pálopinaṅ-ú ; Pálo-pínaṅ-mi. *(Bur.)*.

389. MANNA.

Mann من ; Shir-khisht شیرخشت . *(Arab.)* Shir-khisht شیرخشت . *(Pers. Hind. and Duk.)* Méná மேனை. *(Tam.)* Méná మేనా. *(Tel.)* Manná മന്ന. *(Malyal.)*.

The above are the general names of *Manna* from whatever source it may be, but at present they are generally meant for the *Ash-manna* imported from Europe. The names of each of the varieties of *Manna* supposed to be found in India, are given under their respective heads, viz., *Alhagi maurorum, Calotropis procera,* and *Tamarix gallica.*

390. MASTICHE. *(Mastich or Mastic.)*

Maṣṭakí مصطكي ; Maṣṭakié-rúmí مصطكي رومي ; Aalake-rúmi علك رومي . *(Arab.)* Kundure-rúmi *(Pers.)* Rúmí-maṣṭaki كند رومي ; Maṣṭaki مصطكي . *(Hind.)* Irúmi-malait-taki இரூமிமலைத்தகி ; Púnaik-kaṇ-kuṇgiḷikam பூனைக்கண்குங்கிளிகம். *(Tam.)* Rúmardhakamu రూమర్ధకము ; Pilli-kaṇḍla-guggilam పిల్లికండ్లగుగ్గిలం. *(Tel.)* Rúmi-mostoki. *(Beng.)* Rumí-mastaki. *(Mah.)* Rúmi-mastaki. *(Guz.).*

391. MEL. *(Honey.)*

Aasl عسل ; Aaslun-naḥal عسل النحل . *(Arab.)* Shahad شهد ; Angabín انگبين . *(Pers.)* Shahad شهد ; Madh مده . *(Hind.)* Shahad شهد . *(Duk.)* Tén தேன். *(Tam.)* Téne తేనె. *(Tel.)* Tén തേൻ. *(Malyal.)* Jénu ಜೇನು. *(Can.)* Modhu. *(Beng.)* Madhu. *(Sans.)* Mada. *(Mah.)* Madh. *(Guz.)* Páni. *(Cing.)* Piyá-ye. *(Bur.)*

A preparation of *Honey* and *Vinegar* is sold in many Indian markets, which corresponds to *Oxymel.* It has the following names :—

Sikanjabín سكنجبين . *(Arab.)* Sirkangabín سركنگبين . *(Pers.)* Sikanjabín سكنجبين . *(Hind.)* Shikajabín شكنجبين . *(Duk.).*

392. MELANORRHÆA USITATISSIMA, *Wall.*
(Resinous juice of—Black Varnish.)

Ṭisi or Ṣissi. *(Bur.).*

393. MELIA AZEDARACH, *Linn.*

Bakáyan ; Mahá-nínb مها نينب . *(Hind.)* Gouri-nim ; Gouli-nim گولي نيم . *(Duk.)* Malai-

vémbu மலைவேம்பு ; Malai-véppam மலைவேப்பம். *(Tam.)*
Konda-vépa కొండవేప ; Turaka-vépa తురకవేప. *(Tel.)*
Bettadá-bévina ಬೆಟ್ಟದಾಬೇವಿನ. *(Can.)* Mahá-nim. *(Beng.)*
Parvata-nimba-vri*kshaha*. *(Sans.)* Dóngrá-*cha*-limbá*cha*-
*j*há*d*a. *(Mah.)* Mahá-nimba. *(Cing.)* Simbo-tamá-bi ;
Simbo-*tha*mákhá *or* Simbo-*tha*mágá ; Simbo-*kha*mákha *or*
Simbo-kamákhá. *(Bur.)*.

Whether *Melia azedarach* and *M. Sempervirens* are distinct
species or mere varieties of the same species, the native names of
both are generally the same.

See the remarks under *Moringa pterygosperma*.

394. **MENTHA SATIVA**, *Linn.* *(Indian Pepper-
mint.)*

Naanaaul-hind نعناع الهند ; Naanáae-hindí نعناع هندي ;
Habaqul-hind حبق الهند ; Fódanaje-hindí فودنج هندي ;
Fótanaje-hindí فوتنج هندي . *(Arab.)* Púdinah پودنه .
(Pers.) Púdínah پودينه . *(Hind. and Duk.)* Pudíná
புதீனை ; Í-ech-chak-kírai ஈச்சக்கீரை. *(Tam.)* Pudíná
పుదీనా ; Íga-engili-kúra ఈగఎంగిలికూర. *(Tel.)* Putiyina
പുതിയിന. *(Malyal.)* Chetni-maragu ಚೆಟ್ನಿಮರಗು. *(Can.)*
Pódina. *(Beng.)* Pudíná. *(Mah.)* Pudina. *(Guz.)* Bhúdina.
(Bur.).

395. **MERIANDRA BENGALENSIS,**
Benth.

396. **MERIANDRA STROBILIFERA,**
Benth.

Leaves of.

Káfúr-ká-pát كافور كا پات . *(Hind.)* Káfúr-ká-pattá
كافور كا پتا . *(Duk.)* Shima-karpúram-áku శిమకర్పూరంఆకు.
(Tel.).

The meaning of all the above names is *the leaf of camphor
plant*, and they are applied to the leaves of *M. Bengalensis* and
M. Strobilifera, simply because they smell of camphor.

397. MESUA FERREA, *Linn.*

Nágésar ناگيسر ; Nág-késar ناگ كيسر . (*Hind.*) Shiṟu-nágap-pu சிறுநாகப்பூ ; Nágasháp-pú நாகசாப்பூ. (*Tam.*) Nága-késaram నాగకేసరం ; Geja-pushpam గెజపుష్పం. (*Tel.*) Veḷutta-chenpakam വെള്ളച്ചെമ്പകം. (*Malyal.*) Nága-késaram. (*Sans.*).

The meaning of the Malyalim name *Veḷutta-chenpakam* is the white *Michelia champaca,* and is applied to *Mesua ferrea* on account of the resemblance of its flowers to those of the former, particularly with regard to their smell.

See the remarks under *Cubeba officinalis* in reference to the buds of *M ferrea* being called *Kabáb-chíní* at Madras.

398. MESUA FERREA, *Linn.* (*Oil of.*)

Nágésar-ká-aiṭr ناگيسر كا عطر ;   Nág-késar-ká-aiṭr ناگ كيسر كا عطر . (*Hind.*)   Nágésar-ká-aaṭar ناگ كيسر كا عطر (*Duk.*).

399. MEZEREI RADIX. (*Mezereon.*)

Mázariyún مازريون . (*Arab.*)

400. MICHELIA CHAMPACA, *Linn.* (*Flowers of.*)

Champá جمپا ; *Champé-ké-phúl* جمپے كے پهول . (*Hind. and Duk.*) Shampaṇgi-pushpam சம்பங்கிபுஷ்பம். (*Tam.*) Sampangi-puvvu సంపంగిపువ్వు ; *Champakamu* చంపకము ; Kánchanamu కాంచనము ; *Champéyamu* చాంపేయము ; Gandha-phalí గంధఫలి ; Hémángamu హేమాంగము ; Héma-pushpakamu హేమపుష్పకము. (*Tel.*) Chempakap-pú ചെമ്പകപ്പൂ. (*Malyal.*) Sampage-huvvu ಸಂಪಗೆಹುವ್ವು.(*Can.*) *Chámpá.* (*Beng.*) Champaka-pushpam. (*Sans.*) *Chámpécha-phúla.* (*Mah.*) Sappu. (*Cing.*)

Sapenga is considered as synonymous with *Manóranjitam* in some Telugu works, which is incorrect, the former with a slight alteration *(Sampangi)* being the name of *Michelia champaca,* and the latter of *Artabotrys odoratissima.*

Sagá-pán occurs in some books as the Burmese name of *M. champacu,* but it is the name of the flower of another plant, which is also fragrant and bears some resemblance to the flower of the former.

401. MIMUSOPS ELENGI, *Linn.*

Mólsarí مولسري . *(Hind.)* Ghólsari كهولسري; Bhólsari بهولسري . *(Duk.)* Mogaḍam மொகடம். *(Tam.)* Pogaḍa-mánu పొగడమాను. *(Tel.)* Elangi എലങ്കി *(Malyal.)* Bakal. *(Beng.).*

402. MIRABILIS JALAPA, *Linn.*

Gule-aabbás گل عباس . *(Pers. and Hind.)* Gulá-básh گلا باش . *(Duk.)* Pattaṛáṣhu பத்தராசு. *(Tam.)* Bhadrákshi భద్రాక్షి; Chandra-malli చంద్రమల్లి; Chandra-kánta చంద్ర కాంత. *(Tel.)* Anti-mantáram ആന്തിമന്താരം; Anti-malari ആന്തിമലരി. *(Malyal.)* Chandra-mallige ಚಂದ್ರಮಲ್ಲಿಗೆ; Gulamáji ಗುಲಮಾಜ; Sanja-mallige ಸಂಜಮಲ್ಲಿಗೆ. *(Can.)* Krishno-kéli; Gulá-bás. *(Beng.)* Sindrika-gahá. *(Cing.)* Mizu-biṇ. *(Bur.).*

403. MOMORDICA BALSAMINA, *Linn.*

404. MOMORDICA CHARANTIA, *Linn.*

Qiṣául-barrí قثا البري . *(Arab.)* Simá-hang سيماهنگ . *(Pers.)* Karólá کرولا . *(Hind.)* Karélá کريلا . *(Duk.)* Pávakká-cheḍi பாவக்காசெடி. *(Tam.)* Kákara-cheṭṭu కాకరచెట్టు. *(Tel.)* Kaippa-valli കൈപ്പവള്ളി;

Pávakká-*cheṭi* പാവക്കാചെടി ; Pánṭi-pávél പാണ്ടിപാ
വെത ; Kappakka കപ്പക്ക. *(Malyal.)*   Hágala-káyi-giḍá
ಹಾಗಲಕಾಯಿಗಿಡಾ. *(Can.)*   Korolá. *(Beng.)*   Kára-valli-latá.
(Sans.)   Kárli. *(Mah.)*   Karélo. *(Guz.)*   Ke-hiṇ-gá-biṇ.
(Bur.)l

The Malyalim name *Púnṭipávél* is from the Hortus Malabaricus, (Vol. VIII, Tab. 9), and it is a rather doubtful one.
See the remarks under *Luffa amara.*

405.   MOLLUGO CERVIANA, *Ser.*

Hazár-dánah هزاردانه . *(Duk.)*   Porpáṭakam பொற்
பாடகம் ; Parpáṭakam பர்பாடகம். *(Tam.)*   Parpáṭakamu
చర్పాటకము. *(Tel.)*   Parpáshṭaká ರರ್ಪಾಷ್ಟಕಾ. *(Can.).*

406.   MORINGA PTERYGOSPERMA, *Gærtn.*

(Horse-radish tree.)

Shajnah سهجنه or Shajná سهجنا ; Ségvá سیگوا . *(Hind.)*
Mungé-ká-*jhár* منگے کا جهاڑ . *(Duk.)*   Muruṇgai முருங்கை.
(Tam.) Munaga మునగ. *(Tel.)*   Muriṇṇa മുരിങ്ങ. *(Malyal.)*
Nugge-giḍá. ನುಗ್ಗೆಗಿಡಾ. *(Can.)*   Sojná. *(Beng.)*   Ṣhóbhán-
jana-vri*ksha*ha. *(Sans.)*   Munagác*ha-jhá*ḍa ;   Baḍadí-
ṣhingác*ha-jhá*ḍa. *(Mah.)*   Murungá. *(Cing.)*   Dándalon-
biṇ. *(Bur.).*

The Arabic or Persian name *Bán* بان is generally considered to be applicable to the above plant, but it is the name
of a quite different one, probably not to be found in India. In
some books, (Shakespear, Forbes, and Richardson's Dictionaries,
&c.,) it is confounded with no less than five or six plants, viz.,
Melia sempervirens, Hyperanthera moringa (Moringa pterygosperma),
Tamarisk tree, Myrobalan tree, and *Béd-mushk (Salix Babylonica*
or S. Ægyptica).   There is almost the same confusion about
the nut, *Ḥabbul-bán* حب البان , which is often substituted by
some other seeds, particularly those of *Melia sempervirens,* and

Moringa pterygosperma under the name of *Ben-nut*. The true Ḥabbul-bán bears a great resemblance to *Pistachio-nut* and it is not *Ben-nut*. The cause of confounding Ḥabbul-bán with *Ben-nut* is apparently the resemblance of the sound of *bán* and *ben*.

Munaga is the Telugu name of *Moringa pterygosperma*, but *Aḍavi-munaga* is found applied to it in some books (Flora Andhrica, &c.). The meaning of the latter is *the wild munaga*, and it is therefore applicable to the wild variety of that plant (*M. pterygosperma*) if it exists at all.

407. MORUS INDICA, *Linn.* (*Indian Mulberry plant*).

Tút توت (*Arab. Pers. and Hind.*) Sháh-tút شاه توت (*Duk.*) Kambili-púch-chi-cheḍi கம்பிளிப்புச்சிசெடி; Múshu kaṭṭai-cheḍi மூசுகட்டைசெடி. (*Tam.*) Kambaḷi-cheṭṭu కంబళిచెట్టు; Kambaḷi-búchi-cheṭṭu కంబళిబూచిచెట్టు. (*Tel.*) Hippal-neraḷi-giḍá ಹಿಪ್ಪಲ್ನೆರಳಿಗಿಡ (*Can.*) Tút. (*Beng.*) Shálmali-vrikshaha. (*Sans.*) Shátú-tácha-jháḍa. (*Mah.*).

408. MOSCHUS. (*Musk*).

Misk مسك; Mishk مشك; Mushk مشك. (*Arab.*) Mushk مشك. (*Pers.*) Kastúrí كستوري; Mushk مشك (*Hind. and Duk.*) Kastúri கஸ்தூரி. (*Tam.*) Kastúri కస్తూరి. (*Tel.*) Kastúri കസ്തൂരി. *Malyal.*) Kastúri ಕಸ್ತೂರಿ. (*Can.*) Kashtúri *or* Kastúri. (*Beng.*) Kastúri. (*Sans.*) Kasturí. (*Mah.*) Kastúri; Mushk. (*Guz.*) Kastúri. (*Cing.*) Kaḍo. (*Bur.*).

409. MUCUNA PRURIENS, *D. C.* (*Hairs covering the Legume of—Cowhage or Cow-itch*).

Kivánchh كوانچھ; Kiváchh كواچھ. (*Hind.*) Kách-kúri كاچكوري; Kánch-kúri كانچكوري. (*Duk.*) Púnaik-káli புனைக்காலி. (*Tam.*) Pilli-aḍugu పిల్లిఅడుగు; Dúla-gonḍi దూలగొండి; Pedda-dúlagonḍi పెద్దదూలగొండి. (*Tel.*)

Náyik-koraṇa നായിക്കൊരണ. *(Malyal.)* Nasaguni-giḍá ನಸಗುನಿಗಿಡಾ; Turachi-giḍá ತುರಚಿಗಿಡಾ. *(Can.)* Ákolṣhi; Kámách; Bichhoti. *(Beng.)* Kavacha. *(Mah.)* Kivánch. *(Guz.)* Ácháriyapalbe. *(Cing.* Khwele *or* Khu-e-le. *(Bur.).*

Utangan اتنگن, *Anjarah* انجره, *Kaznah* کزنہ, &c., are often found misapplied to the above plant in several Persian and other works. They are the names of another plant, possessing nearly the same medicinal properties.

410. MURRAYA (BERGERA) KONIGII, *Linn.*

Karé-pák کری پاک; Karyá-pák کریا پاک; Karyá-pát کریاپات. *(Duk.)* Karu-véppilai கருவேப்பிலை; Karu-vémbu கருவேம்பு. *(Tam.)* Kari-vépa-cheṭṭu కరివేపచెట్టు. *(Tel.)* Karu-véppa കറുവെപ്പ. *(Malyal.)* Kari-béviná-giḍá ಕರಿಬೇವಿನಗಿಡಾ. *(Can.)* Barsungá. *(Beng.)* Surabhi-nimba-vrikshaha. *(Sans.)* Karépákácha-jháda. *(Mah.)* Karri-pincha. *(Cing.)* Pido-ṣin *or* Pindo-ṣiṅ *(Bur.).*

411. MUSA SAPIENTUM, *Linn.*

Shajratul-talḥ شجرة الطلح: *Shajratul-mouz* شجرة الموز. *(Arab.)* Darakhte-mouz درخت موز *(Pers.)* Kélé-ká-péṛ کیلے کا پیڑ. *(Hind.)* Mouz-ká-jháṛ موز کا جهاڑ. *(Duk.)* Vázh-ai-ch-cheḍi வாழைச்செடி; Kadali கதலி. *(Tam.)* Araṭi-cheṭṭu అరటిచెట్టు; Anaṭi-cheṭṭu అనటిచెట్టు; *Antḥ*-cheṭṭu అంటచెట్టు; Kadali కదళి. *(Tel.)* Vázha-maram വാഴമരം. *(Malyal.)* Baḷe-giḍa ಬಾಳೆಗಿಡಾ. *(Can.)* Kéla-gáchh *(Beng.)* Kadali-vrikshaha. *(Sans.)* Kéḷa-jháḍa; Kéḷicha-jháḍa. *(Mah.)* Kéla-nu-jháḍa. *(Guz.)* Kehal-gahá. *(Cing.)* Napiyá-biṅ. *(Bur.).*

412. MUSA SAPIENTUM, *Linn. (Fruit of——*
Plantain or Banana.)

Talḥ طلح ; Mouz موز . *(Arab. and Pers.)* Kélá كيلا or
Kélah كيله . *(Hind.)* Mouz موز . *(Duk.)* Vázhaip-pazham
வாழைப்பழம் ; Kadali கதலி. *(Tam.)* Araṭi-panḍu అరటి
పండు; Anaṭi-panḍu అనటిపండు; Amṭipanḍu అంటిపండు; Kadaḷi
కదళి. *(Tel.)* Vázhap-pazham വാഴപ്പഴം. *(Malyal.)* Bále-
haṇṇu ಬಾಳೆಹಣ್ಣು. *(Can.)* Kélá. *(Beng.)* Kadaḷi-*phalam.*
(Sans.) Kéḷa or Pikli-kéḷi. *(Mah.)* Kéla. *(Guz.)* Kehal
or Kessel. *(Cing.)* Naṇivá-ṣi. *(Bur.).*

413. MYLABRIS CICHORII, *Fabr.*

414. MYLABRIS INDICA, *Fussl.*

415. MYLABRIS PUSTULATA, ——.

416. MYLABRIS PUNCTUM, ——.

} *Telini
Fly.*

Zaráriḥul-hind ذراريح الهند ; Zaráriḥe-hindí
ذراريح هندى . *(Arab.)* Dabáne-hindí دبان هندي
(Pers.) Télní تيلني ; Télní-mak*khi* تيلني مكهي . *(Hind.)*
Bad-bó-ki-zirangí بدبوكى زيرنگي ; Zirangí زيرنگي . *(Duk.)*
Pinsṭṭariṇ-í பிணற்படரிங்கீ. *(Tam.)* Blish*ṭ*ering-ígelu బ్లిష్
టెరింగ్ ఈగలు. *(Tel.).*

Although the Dukhni name *Zirangí* زيرنگي is not a correct
one either for *Mylabris cichorii* or *Cantharis vesicatoria,* yet their
preparations, such as the *Blistering-ointment,* &c., are commonly
known by that name in Southern India.

417. MYRICA SAPIDA, *Wall. (Bark of.)*

Azúri ازوزي ; Áúdul-barq عود البرق ; Qandól قندول .
(Arab.) Dárshishaạáñ دارششعان . *(Pers.)* Káíphal
كائي پهل . *(Hind. and Duk.)* Marudam-paṭṭai மருதம்

படை. (*Tam.*) Kaiḍaryamu ఙెడర్యము. (*Tel.*) Marutam-
toli മരുതംതൊലി. (*Malyal.*) Kái-*phal.* (*Beng.*) Káya-
phala. (*Mah.*).

418. MYRISTICA MALABARICA, *Lam.* (*Nut of—Malabar Nutmeg ?*)

419. MYRISTICA OFFICINALIS, *Linn.* (*Nut of—Nutmeg.*)

Jouzbuvá جوز بوا ; Jouzuṭṭib جوز الطيب . (*Arab.*)
Jouzbóyah جوز بويه . (*Pers.*)   Jáé-*phal* جانے پهل (*Hind.*)
Jáphal جا پهل . (*Duk.*)   Jádikkáy ஜாதிக்காய். (*Tam.*)   Jáji-
káya జాజికాయ ; Játí-*phalamu* జాతీఫలము. (*Tel.*)   Játikká
ജാതിക്കാ. (*Malyal.*)   Jájikáyi ಜಾಜಕಾಯಿ. (*Can.*)   Jáe-*phal.*
(*Beng.*)   Jáji-*phalam.* (*Sans.*)   Jáiphala. (*Mah.*)   Jáye-
phal. (*Guz.*)   Jádi-ká ; Sádika. (*Cing.*)   Zádiphu. (*Bur*).

The Telugu name *Lavangam* is generally considered to be
synonymous with *Lavangálu* and *Lavangapú,* which are the
names of *Cloves;* but it is misapplied in some books (Flora
Andhrica, &c.,) to Nutmeg or its plant, *Myristica officinalis.* *Játi-
phalamu* or *Jáji-káya* is the proper name of the latter.

420. MYRISTICA OFFICINALIS, *Linn.* (*Arillus of the Nut—Mace.*)

Basbásah بسبا سه ; Basbás بسبا س . (*Arab.*)   Bazbáz
بزباز . (*Pers.*)   Jávatrí جا و تری ; Javattari جو تري ;
Jápatrí جا پتري . (*Hind.*)   Joutrí جو تری . (*Duk.*)   Jádi-
pattiri ஜாதிபத்திரி. (*Tam.*)   Jápatri జాపత్రి. (*Tel.*)   Játi-
pattiri ജാതിപത്തിരി. (*Malyal.*)   Jápatri ಜಾಪತ್ರಿ. (*Can.*)
Jótri. (*Beng.*)   Jájipatri. (*Sans.*)   Jáyapatri. (*Mah.*)
Jávantari ; Jápatri. (*Guz.*)   Vasávasi ; Vaduvághu. (*Cing.*)
Zádiphu-apóén. (*Bur.*)

421. MYRRHA. *(Myrrh.)*

Mur مر or Murr مرّ . *(Arab.)* Ból بول . *(Pers. Hind. and Duk.)* Vellaip-pólam வெள்ளைப்போளம். *(Tam.)* Bálimṭra-pólam బాలింట్రపోళ్లో. *(Tel.)* Bóla బోళ. *(Can.)* Ból. *(Beng.)* Gandha-rasaha ; Rasa-gandhaha. *(Sans.)* Bálata-bóla. *(Mah.)* Ból. *(Guz.)* Gandarassa ; Bólam. *(Cing.)*.

Kalane-ṣói is occasionally confounded with *Myrrh*, but it is the Burmese name for a kind of *Mummy*, which is supposed ' to be the dried flesh and bones of a human body embalmed with *Myrrh* and *Spice*.' See the remarks under *Justicia Gendarussa*.

N.

422. NARDOSTACHYS JATAMANSI, *D. C.*
(Indian Spikenard—Root of.)

Sunbuluttibe-hindí سنبل الطيب هندي ; Sunbulul-aaṣáfíre-hindí سنبل العصافير هندي . *(Arab.)* Sunbuluttibe-hindí سنبل الطيب هندي . *(Pers.)* Jaṭámásí جتّا ما سي ; Jhaṭá-mánsí جهتّا ما نسي . *(Hind.)* Bál-chhaṛ بال چهڑ . *(Duk.)* Jaṭámáshi ஜடாமாஷ. *(Tam.)* Jaṭámámshi జటామాంషి. *(Tel.)* Jeṭá-mánchi ജടാമാഞ്ഞി. *(Malyal.)* Jeṭá-mávaṣhí ಜಟಾಮಾವಷಿ. *(Can.)* Jaṭámámsí. *(Beng. and Sans.)* Jeṭá-mávasi. *(Mah.)* Jaṭamámsi *or* Jaṛamánsi. *(Cing.)*.

Billi-lóṭan بلي لوٹن is another Dukhni name of *N. jatamansi*, but it is also often applied to *Acalypha Indica*. The cat is supposed to be very fond of these plants, hence the meaning of the name *cat's struggle*. The Cingalese name *Jaṭamakuṭu* is applied to *N. Jatamansi* in some books, but it is correctly the name of the root of *Cyperus pertenuis*.

423. NAUCLEA OVALIFOLIA, *Roxb.*
Shál. *(?)*.

424. NERIUM ODORUM, *Aiton. (Sweet-scented Oleander.)*

Diflí د فلي . *(Arab.)* Ḳhar-zahrah خرزهر . *(Pers.)* Kanér كنير ; Kanél كذيل ; Karbér كربير . *(Hind.)* Ganér گنير . *(Duk.)* Alari அலரி. *(Tam.)* Gannéru గన్నేరు. *(Tel.)* Alari അലരി. *(Malyal.)* Kaṇagale ಕಣಗಲೆ. *(Can.)* Kanér ; Karabí. *(Beng.).*

There are several varieties of this plant, the whole of which are distinguished and named according to the color of their flowers, as *red, white,* &c.

See the remark under *Tamarix Gallica.*

425. NICOTIANA TABACUM, *Linn. (Leaves of— Tobacco.)*

Tanbák تنباك . *(Arab.)* Tanbákú تنباكو . *(Pers. and Hind.)* Tamákú تماكو ; Tamáqú تماقو . *(Duk.)* Pugai-ilai புகையிலை *(Tam.)* Pogáku పొగాకు ; *Dhúmra-patramu* ధూమ్రపత్రము. *(Tel.)* Puka-yilá പുകയില ; Pokala പൊകല. *(Malyal.)* Hógesappu ಹೊಗೆಸಪ್ಪು. *(Can.)* Támák ; Támáku. *(Beng.)* *Dhúma-patram.* *(Sans.)* Tambákúcha-pálá. *(Mah.)* Tamáku. *(Guz.)* Dungazha ; Dimkola ; Dungkola. *(Cing.)* Ṣé. *(Bur.).*

The names of the principal varieties of Tobacco sold in the bazaars of Southern India are—

a.—Bandar-ká-tambákú بندركاتمباكو . *(Hind. and Duk.)* *Bandar-pugai-ilai* பந்தர்புகையிலை. *(Tam.)* *Bandaru-pogáku* బందరుపొగాకు. *(Tel.).*

b.—Séndúr-ká-tambákú سيندوركا تمبا كو . *(Hind. and Duk.)*

c.—Kórvai-pugai-ilai கோர்வைபுகையிலை. *(Tam.)* *Kórva-pogáku* కోర్వపొగాకు. *(Tel.).*

d.—Kámbu-pugai-ilai காம்புபுகையிலை. *(Tam.)* *Kúḍa-pogáku* కడపొగాకు. *(Tel.).*

426. NIGELLA SATIVA, *Linn. Syn.* N. Indica, *D. C. (Seeds of.)*

Sh-ouníz شونيز ; Kamúne-asvad كمون اسود ; Ḥabba-tussoudá حبة السودا . *(Arab.)* Siyáh-dánah سياد دانه ; Siyah-biranj سياه برنج . *(Pers.)* Kalónjí كلونجي ; Kálá-zírá كالزيرا . *(Hind. and Duk.)* Karuṇ-ṣhíragam கருஞ்சீரகம். *(Tam.)* Nalla-jilakara నల్లజీలకఱ. *(Tel.)* Karun-chírakam കരുഞ്ജീരകം. *(Malyal.)* Karé-jírage ಕರೆಜೀರಗೆ. *(Can.)* Kálá-jírá *or* Kál-zírá. *(Beng.)* Káraví ; Sushaví. *(Sans.)* Káḷajire. *(Mah.)* Kaluduru. *(Cing.)* Samou-né. *(Bur.).*

The only difference between the Hindustani and Dukhni names *Kálá-zírá* كالزيرا and *Káli-zírí* كالى زيري is, the one is in masculine and the other in feminine gender, yet according to the present usage the former is applied to the seeds of *N. sativa*, and the latter to those of *Vernonia anthelmintica.* The literal meaning of the Arabic and Persian names *Ḥabba-tussoudá* حبّ السودا and *Siyáh-dánoʰ* سياه دانه in Hindustani is *Kálá-dánah (black seeds)* which is the name in the latter language for the seeds of *Pharbitis Nil.* From this similarity in the meaning, the seeds of *N. sativa* and *P. Nil* are often confounded with each other. See the remarks on *Alpinia galanga* with reference to the names *Kalónjí* and *Kulanjan.*

427. NIMA (BRUCEA) QUASSIOIDES, *Ham.*

Bharangi بهرنگى . *(Hind.).*

428. NOTONIA CORYMBOSA, *Linn.*

429. NYMPHÆA EDULIS, *D. C.*

Nílú-far نيلوفر . *(Arab. and Pers.)* Kaṅval كنول ; Chhóṭá-kaṅval چهوٹا كنول . *(Hind.)* Chhóṭá-kaṅval چهوٹا كنول ; Aali-phúl علي پهول ; Alli-phúl الي پهول

(*Duk.*) Alli அல்லி ; Alli-támara*i* அல்லிதாமரை ; Ámbal
ஆம்பல். (*Tam.*) Alli-támar*ə* అల్లితామర. (*Tel.*) Allit-támara
അള്ളിത്താമര ; Ánpala ആമ്പല. (*Malyal.*) Nyadale-huvu
ನ್ಯದಲೆಹುವು. (*Can.*) Kanval. (*Beng.*) Kamala. (*Sans.*)
Kamula. (*Mah.*) Kanval. (*Guz.*) Nalun *or* Nelun. (*Cing.*)
Kiyá-nu. (*Bur.*).

See the remarks under *Pharbitis Nil.*

O.

430. OCIMUM ALBUM, *Linn.*

Bádrúje-abya*z* بادروج ابيض . (*Arab.*) Raiháne-
kóhi ريحان كوهي . (*Pers.*) Saféd-tulsí سفيد تلسى ; Janglí-
tulsí ا اجلي تلسي . (*Hind.*) Ujlí-tulsí جنگلي تلسي
Kukká-tulsí ككاتلسى . (*Duk.*) Kanján-kórai கஞ்சாங்கோரை ;
Náy-tolashi நாய்தொளளி. (*Tam.*) Tella-tulasi తెల్లతులసి ;
Kukka-tulasi కుక్కతులసి. (*Tel.*) Vella-tolasi വെള്ള
തൊളസി ; Nákkanni നാക്കഞ്ഞി. (*Malyal.*) Sádá-tulshi.
(*Beng.*) Saphéd-tulsi. (*Guz.*).

431. OCIMUM BASILICUM, *Linn.*

*Sh*áhasfaram شاهسفرم ; Raiháñ ريحان . (*Arab.*)
*Sh*áhasparam شاهسپرم ; Názbó نازبو ; Dabáñ-*sh*áb
دبان شاب . (*Pers.*) Sabzah سبزه . (*Hind. and Duk.*)
Tiruní*t*ru-pac*h*-c*h*-ai இருநீற்றுபச்சை ; Tiruní*t*rup-pattiri
இருநீற்றுபத்திரி. (*Tam.*) Vibúdi-patri విభూదిపత్రి ; Rudra-
jeḍa రుద్రజెడ ; Vépuḍu-pac*h*-c̣ha వేపుడుపచ్చ. (*Tel.*) Tiruní*t*ru-pac*h*-c*h*á തിരുനീറുപച്ച ; Pac*h*-c*h*a-pushpam പച്ച

ഹിപ്പം. (*Malyal.*) Kám kastúri ಕಂಗಸ್ತೂರಿ. (*Can.*)
Sabja ; Náshbó ; Násbón ; Bábú-tulshi. (*Beng.*) Vishva-
tulasi. (*Sans.*) Sabjá ; Tukamirái. (*Mah.*) Sabza. (*Guz.*)
Kalá-pinzain ; Pinzain *or* Pinzin. (*Bur.*).

432. OCIMUM GRATISSIMUM, *Linn.*

Faranjmishk فرنجمشک . (*Arab.*) Palangmishk
پلنگمشک ; Raiháne-qaranfuli ريحان قرنفلي —— *seeds of,*
Bálankúe-khurd با لنكوے خرد . (*Pers.*) Rám-tulsi
رام تلسي . (*Hind. and Duk.*) Elumich-cham-tolashi
எலுமிச்சம்தொளஷி. (*Tam.*) Nimma-tulasi నిమ్మతుళసి.; Ráma-
tulasi రామతుళసి. (*Tel.*) Káttu-tuttuvá കാട്ടുതുത്തുവാ. (*Malyal.*) Ráma-tulashi ರಾಮತುಳಶಿ. (*Can.*) Rám-tulshi.
(*Beng.*) Ráma-tulasi. (*Sans.*).

433. OCIMUM SANCTUM, *Linn.*

Barandá برندا ; Varandá ورندا ; Tulsi تلسي . (*Hind.*)
Tulsí تلسي . (*Duk.*) Tulashi துளஷி. (*Tam.*) Tulasi
తుళసి ; Krushna-tulasi కృష్ణతుళసి ; Gaggera-chettu గగ్గెరచెట్టు.
(*Tel.*) Tulasi തുളസി ; Nalla-tirttá നല്ലതിത്താ ; Nalla-
tuttuvá നല്ലതുത്തുവാ. (*Malyal.*) Tulashi-gidá ತುಳಶಿಗಿಡಾ.
(*Can.*) Tulshi. (*Beng.*) Tulashi-vrikshaha. (*Sans.*)
Tulasicha-jhádạ. (*Mah.*) Tulsi. (*Guz.*) Maduru-talla.
(*Cing.*) Lún. (*Bur.*).

434. ODINA WODIER, *Roxb.*

Jingam جنگم ; Kashmalá كشملا . (*Hind.*) Bésharam-
ká-jhár بے شرم كاجهار . (*Duk.*) Odiya-maram ஒடியமரம்.
(*Tam.*) Oddi-manu ఒడ్డిమాను. (*Tel.*) Udi-maram ഉടിമരം.
(*Malyal.*) Jival. (*Beng.*).

435. ODINA WODIER, *Roxb.* *(Gum of.)*

Jingan-ki-gónd کنجگی گوند ; Kinné-ki-gónd جنگن کی گوند *(Hind.)*.

The Gum known as *Kinné-ki-gónd* in Upper India is different from *Kinyí-gónd* کنیا گوند of Southern India, and also from *Qinnah* قنه *(Galbanum)*.

436. OLDENLANDIA UMBELLATA, *Linn.* *(Root or Wood of.)*

Chirval چرول or *Chirval-ki-lakṛi* چرول کی لکڑی . *(Hind. and Duk.)* Imburá-vér இம்புராவேர் ; Shiṛu-vér சிறுவேர் ; Imbúṛal இம்பூறல். *(Tam.)* Chiru-véru చిరువేరు. *(Tel.)*.

Chirval is misapplied to *Rubia cordifolia* in some books.

437. OLEUM NIGRUM. *(Black Oil.)*

Málkangní-ká-jantar مال کنگی کا جنتر . *(Duk.)* Válu-luvai-tailam வாலுளுவைத்தைலம். *(Tam.)* Málkangini-tailamu మాల్‌కంగిని తైలము. *(Tel.)*.

The above black, thick, and oily liquid, which is obtained by destructive distillation of the seeds of *Celastrus paniculata*, is quite different from the oil of the same seeds extracted in the usual way by expression. The latter is yellow, of rather thin consistence, and sold in many bazaars under its proper name, *Málkangní-ká-tél* مال کنگی کا تیل . This name, however, is more in use for *Black Oil* than the other in some parts of Northern Circars.

438. OLEUM OLIVÆ. *(Olive Oil.)*

Zait زیت . *(Arab.)* Róghane-zaitún روغن زیتون . *(Pers.)* Zaitún-ká-tél زیتون کا تیل . *(Hind. and Duk.)* Jaitú-neṇṇey ஜைதூநெண்ணெய். *(Tam.)* Jaitún-núne జైతూన్‌నూనె. *(Tel.)* Zaitún-tél. *(Beng.)*.

439. OLEUM PISCIS. *(Fish oil.)*

Dhonus-samak دهن السمك . *(Arab.)* Roghane-máhí روغن ماهي . *(Pers.)* Mach-chhi-ká-tél مجهي كاتيل . *(Hind. and Duk.)* Mın-yenney மீன்யெண்ணெய். *(Tam.)* Chépa-núne చేపనూనె. *(Tel.)* Maleyam-nai മത്സ്യംനൈ ; Mín-nai മീൻനൈ. *(Malyal.)* Mininá-yanne ಮೀನಿನಾಯೆಣ್ಣೆ. *(Can.)* Machár-tail. *(Beng.)* Machhya-tailam. *(Sans.)* Mósólicha-téla. *(Mah.)* Min-tel ; Mál-tel. *(Cing.).*

440. OLEUM RICINI. *(Castor oil.)*

Dhónul-khirvaa دهن الخروع . *(Arab.)* Róghane-bédanjír روغن بيدانجير ; *(Pers.)* Arand-ká-tél ارنڈكاتيل . *(Hind.)* Yarandi-ká-tél ارندي كا تيل . *(Duk.)* Ámanak-kenney ஆமணக்கெண்ணெய். *(Tam.)* Ámudam ఆముదం. *(Tel.)* Kottenna കൊട്ടെണ്ണ. *(Malyal.)* Haralenne ಹರಳೆಣ್ಣೆ. *(Can.)* Bhérandá-tail. *(Beng.)* Vátyálaka-tailam. *(Sans.)* Eran-déla. *(Mah.)* Diváá · Yerandi-nu-tél ; Yerandium. *(Guz.)* Endaru-tel. *(Cing.)* Kegu-si. *(Bur.).*

The above are the general names for *Castor Oil*, whether obtained from the seeds of the *Large-seeded* variety, or from the *Small-seeded.* But there is a great difference between these two articles as found in the bazaars of Southern India ; so much so, the one is used by natives only for Lamp, and the other for medicinal purposes. The latter is viscid, nearly colorless or of pale-yellow color, and has a peculiar bland oily taste with a slight nauseous smell. The former is much thicker, more or less of brown color, and has an acrid and very disagreeable nauseous taste and odour. Its action as a purgative is much stronger, and generally accompanied with much griping. It is often used in Hospital practice with Purgative Enemata, for which purpose it is more suited, in my opinion, than the other article.* These oils are distinguished in the bazaar by the following names :—

Castor Oil, or the oil obtained from the seeds of the Small-seeded Castor Oil plant.—

Dhonul-khirvaạạus-ṣaghír دهن الخروع الصغير . (*Arab.*) *Róghane-bédanjíre-khurd* روغن بيد انجير خرد . (*Pers.*) *Chhóṭí-araṇḍ-ká-tél* چهوٹي ارنڈ كا تيل ; *Chhóṭí-araṇḍí-ká-tél* چهوٹي ارنڈي كا تيل . (*Hind.*) *Chiṭlí-yaraṇḍi-ká-tél* جھوٹى يرنڈي كاتيل ; *Chhóṭı-yaraṇḍi-ká-tél* چهوٹي يرنڈي كاتيل . (*Duk.*) Chiṭṭámaṇak-keṇṇey சிட்டாமணக்கெண்ணெய். (*Tam.*) Chiṭṭámudam-núne చిట్టాముదంనూనె. (*Tel.*) Cheṛu-koṭṭennấ ചെറുകൊട്ടെണ്ണ ; Chiṭrávaṇakka-eṇṇá ചിററവണക്കെണ്ണ. (*Malyal.*) Chiṭṭa-baraleṇue ಚಿಟ್ಟಬರಲೆಣ್ಣೆ. (*Can.*) Chhóṭa-bhérandá-taīl. (*Beng.*) Lahana-earaṇḍéla. (*Mah.*) Náni-yeraṇḍi-nu-tél. (*Guz.*) Punji-endaru-tel ; Sudu-endaru-tel. (*Cing.*) Angéṅ-keṣu-ṣí. (*Bur.*).

Lamp Oil, or the oil obtained from the seeds of the Large-seeded Castor Oil plant.—

Dhonul-khirvaạạul-kabír دهن الخروع الكبير . (*Arab.*) *Róghane-bédanjíre-kalán* روغن بيد انجير كلان . (*Pers.*) Baṛí-araṇḍ-ká-tél بڑي ارنڈ كا تيل ; Baṛí-araṇḍí-ká-tél بڑي ارنڈي كا تيل . (*Hind.*) Charágh-ká-tél چراغ كا تيل ;

---

* The above remarks are applicable only to the varieties of Castor Oil sold in the bazaar; but I believe that there is no difference between the Oils of small and large seeds, if they be prepared in a proper manner, or by cold-drawn process. Dr. Bidie has kindly furnished the following note on the subject, when the proof of this form was submitted to his examination :—

‘I have prepared oil from both varieties of the seeds by cold-drawn process, and there was not the least difference as regards quality or action between them. Several dozen bottles of each were prepared, so there could be no chance of error.’

Baṛí-yarandí-ká-tél بَڑي يرنّدي كا تيل . *(Duk.)* Viḷak-kenney மிளக்கெண்ணெய். *(Tam.)* Ámudam ఆముదం; Dípamu-samuru �దీపముసముఱు. *(Tel.)* Dípa-yaṇṇe ೞಿೆಠಯೆಣ್ಣೆ. *(Can.)* Baṛá-bhéraṇḍá-tail. *(Beng.)* Thóra-eraṇḍéla. *(Mah.)* Móḷu-yerandi-nu-tél. *(Guz.)* Lokka-endaru-tel. *(Cing.)* Agi-kegu-ṣí *(Bur.)*.

By some mistake, *Castor oil* is called ' *Tilácha-tel*' in some Mahratti works. It is the name of the oil of *Sesamam Indicum*.

441. OPHELIA CHIRATA, *D. C.* }
442. OPHELIA ANGUSTIFOLIA, *D. Don.*
443. OPHELIA DENSIFOLIA, *Gris.*   Chiretta
444. OPHELIA ELEGANS, *Wight.*
445. OPHELIA MULTIFLORA, *Dalz.*

Qaṣabuzzarírah قصب الزرير ه . *(Arab. and Pers.)* Charáyatah چرايته . *(Hind. and Duk.)* Shiraṭ-kuch-chi சிரட்சச்சி; Nila-vémbu நிலவேம்பு. *(Tam.)* Néla-vému నేలవేము. *(Tel.)* Nila-véppa നീലവെപ്പ. *(Malyal.)* Nela-bévu ನೆಲಬೇವು. *(Can.)* Cherota. *(Beng.)* Bhú-nimbaha. *(Sans.)* Chiráyitá. *(Mah.)* Chíráyata. *(Guz.)* Bin-cohamba. *(Cing.)* Ṣekhági. *(Bur.)*.

The names of all the varieties of *Chiretta* or *Chiretta-yield-ing plants* as well as *Andrographis paniculata* are nearly the same in India. In some places, however, a few of these plants have different names, which are confined to those localities. For example, *O. elegans* and *O. multiflora* are well known by the following names in Northern Circars:—

Siláras سلار س ; *Salájit* سلاجت . *(Duk.)* *Saláras* ౩ౌరాస; Ṣhílájatu ೖౌಜಜు. *(Tel.)*.

But these names, all over India, are applied to quite different substances, viz., *Siláras* to *Storax*, and *Salájit* or *Salájit* to a *mineral-clay (Alum Earth of Nepaul)*.

446. OPHIORHIZA MUNGHOS, *Linn.*

Kiri-puraṇḍán ஓரிபுரண்டான். *(Tam.)* Sarpákshi-chettu సర్పాక్షిచెట్టు. *(Tel.)* Datkattiya. *(Cing.)*.

447. OPHIOXYLON SERPENTINUM, *Linn.*

Pátala-gandhi పాతలగంధి. *(Tel.)* Chuvanna-avilpori ചുവന്നഅവിൽപൊരി. *(Malyal.)* Chandrá; Chhoṭo-chárd. *(Beng.)*.

448. OPIUM.

Afyún افیون; Labnul-ḳhash-ḳhásh لبن الخشخاش. *(Arab.)* Mahánul مهانل; Tiryák تریاک. *(Pers.)* Afyún افیون. *(Hind.)* Afím افیم. *(Duk.)* Gaṣha-gaṣhá-pál கசகசாபால்; Abini அபினி. *(Tam.)* Gasa-gasála-pálu గసగసాలపాలు; Abhini అభిని. *(Tel.)* Kaṣha-kaṣha-karappa കശകശകരപ്പ; Kaṣha-kaṣhap-paṣhá കശകശപ്പശാ. *(Mal-yal.)* Aphímu అఫీము. *(Can.)* Aphim or Aphin. *(Beng.)* Aphim; Aphinam. *(Sans.)* Aphin. *(Mah.)* Aphim. *(Guz.)* Abin. *(Cing.)* Bhain or Bhín. *(Bur.)*.

The following are the most common varieties of Opium found in Southern India :—

a. Malwa Opium——*Málví-afyún* مالوی افیون. *(Hind.)* *Málví-afím* مالوي افیم. *(Duk.)* *Málví-abini* மாளவிஅபினி. *(Tam.)* *Málva-mandu* మాళ్వమండు. *(Tel.)* *Málví-aphim.* *(Beng. Mah. and Guz.)*.

b. Dúdhí Opium.——*Dúdhí-afím* دودهي افیم. *(Duk.)* Pál-abini பால்அபினி. *(Tam.)* Pál-mandu పాల్మండు. *(Tel.)*.

The first variety is the same what is described in many books under the title of *Malwa Opium.* The second variety is very soft, darker in color, and contains a large quantity of milky juice, whence the meaning of its names *milky-opium.* 1½ grains of this Opium is equal to 1 of the former in strength.

449. OPUNTIA DILLENII, *Haw.* *Syn.* Cactus Indicus, *Roxb.*

Nág-phaná ناگ پهنا . (*Hind.*) Chappal-sénḍ چپل سینڈ . (*Duk.*) Nága-dáḷi நாகதாளி. (*Tam.*) Nága-dáli నాగదాలి. (*Tel.*) Nága-muḷḷa നാഗമുള്ള. (*Malyal.*) Nág-phana. (*Beng.*) Koḍu-gaha. (*Cing.*).

450. ORYZA SATIVA. *Linn.* (*Seeds or Grains without husk—Rice.*)

Urz ارز ; Arruz ا ورز . (*Arab.*) Biranj برنج . (*Pers.*) Chával چاول . (*Hind.*) Chánval چانول . (*Duk.*) Ariṣhi அரிசி. (*Tam.*) Biyyam బియ్యం. (*Tel.*, Ari അരി. (*Malyal.*) Akkí ಅಕ್ಕಿ. (*Can.*) Chál ; Chánvol. (*Beng.*) Taṇḍulam. (*Sans.*) Tándúla. (*Mah.*) Chókha. (*Guz.*) Hál. (*Cing.*) Sán ; Ṣan *or* Chán. (*Bur.*).

The rice with and without husk, and *straw* have generally distinct names in many of the languages in this country, but much confusion is caused in some books by using them indiscriminately when the *rice without husk* is only intended. The above names in the text are those properly and only belong to the latter.

451. OSSA. (*Bones.*)

Aaẓm عظم . (*Arab.*) Ustaḵhán استخوان . (*Pers.*) Haḍḍí هڈی ; Hár هاڙ . (*Hind.*) Haḍ هڈ . (*Duk.*) Elumbugaḷ எலும்புகள். (*Tam.*) Emikalu ఎమికలు. (*Tel.*) Asti അസ്ഥി ; Ella എല്ല. (*Malyal.*) Eluvu ಎಲುವು ; Múle ಮೂಲೆ. (*Can.*) Asti ; Haḍḍí. (*Beng.*) Asti. (*Sans.*) Haḍa. (*Mah.*) Ayu. (*Bur.*).

452. OVUM. (*Egg.*)

Baiz بیض ; Baizah بیضه . (*Arab.*) Tuḵhme-murgh تخم مرغ . (*Pers.*) Anḍá انڈا . (*Hind. and Duk.*)

Muṭṭai وطـَّــــ. *(Tam.)* Guḍḍu గుడ్డు. *(Tel.)* Muṭṭa ముట్ట.
(Malyal.) Moṭṭe ಮೊಟ್ಟೆ. *(Can.)* Andaha. *(Sans.)* Ándé.
(Mah.) Andá; Indu. *(Guz.)* Bíju. *(Cing.)* Aú or Ú.
(Bur.).

453. OXALIS CORNICULATA, *Linn.*

Anbótí سه پتی; Seh-pattí ا نبوتي . *(Hind.)* Anbóti-
ki-bháji ا نسوتی کي بها جي . *(Duk.)* Puḷi-yárai புளியாரை.
(Tam.) Puli-chintáku పులిచింతాకు. *(Tel.)* Puḷiyárala
പുളിയാരല. *(Malyal.)* Puḷḷam-purachí-sappu ಹುಳ್ಳಂ
ಪುರಚಿಸಪ್ಪು. *(Can.)* Omlotí; Amrul. *(Beng.).*

P.

454. PANDANUS ODORATISSIMUS, *Linn.*

Kází کا ذ ي; Kadar كدر . *(Arab.)* Kádí کا د ی,
(Pers.) Kévaṛah کیوَرہ——*a variety of,* Kétgi کیتگي *or*
Kédgí کیدگي . *(Hind. and Duk.)* Tázhay-cheḍi தாழைஞ்செடி.
(Tam.) Mogali-cheṭṭu మొగలిచెట్టు; Gájangi గాజంగి;
Gédangi-mogali; గేదంగిమొగలి; Gojjangi గొజ్జంగి; Kétakí
కేతకి. *(Tel.)* Ṭázhá താഴാ; Kaita കൈത. *(Malyal.)* Tále-
márá ತಾಳೆಮರಾ; Kyádage-giḍá ಕ್ಯಾದಗಿಡಾ. *(Can.)* Ketki;
Keyá. *(Beng.)* Kétakí-vrikshaha. *(Sans.)* Kévaḍácha-
jháḍa. *(Mah.)* Kévḍo. *(Guz.)* Veṭṭakayá *or* Veṭṭaka
Ṣataphu; Ṣaṣavá. *(Bur.).*

455. PAPAVER RHŒAS, *Linn. (Red Poppy.)*

Nabátul-ḵhash-ḵhashul-aḥmar نبات الخشخاش الا حمر .
(Arab.) Kókháre-surḵh کو کنار سرخ . *(Pers.)* Lál-póst

لال پوست . *(Hind.)* Lál-*ḳhash-ḳhash*-ká-*jhár* لال خشخش کا جھاڑ . *(Duk.)* *Sh*ivappu-ga*sh*a-ga*sh*á-*ch*eḍi சிவப்புக்கசகசாச்செடி ; *Sh*igappu-póstaká-*ch*eḍi சிகப்புபோஸ்தக்காச்செடி. *(Tam.)* Erra-gasa-gasála-*ch*eṭṭu ఎర్ర గసగసాలచెట్టు ; Erra-pósta-káya-*ch*eṭṭu ఎర్రపోస్తకాయచెట్టు. *(Tel.)* *Cho*-vanna-ka*sh*a-ka*sh*a*ch*-*ch*eṭi ചൊവന്നകശകശച്ചെടി. *(Malyal.)* Kempu-*kh*asa-*kh*asi-giḍá ಕೆಂಪುಖಸಖಸಿಗಿಡ. *(Can.)* Lál-pó*sh*ta ; Lál-pó*sh*tér-gá*ch*h. *(Beng.)* Rakta-póstu-vri*kshaha*. *(Sans.)* Támbaḍa-*kh*asa-*kh*asá-*ch*a-*jh*áḍa. *(Mah.)* Lál-*kh*as-*kh*as-nu-*jh*áḍa. *(Guz.)* *Bh*in-biṇ-amí *or* *Bh-ain*-biṇ-ami *(Bur.)*.

456. PAPAVER SOMNIFERUM, *Roxb.* *(White Poppy.)*

Nabátul-*ḳhash-ḳhásh* نبات الخشخاش . *(Arab.)* Kóknár کوکنار . *(Pers.)* Póst پوست ; *Ḳhash-ḳhásh*-ká-péṛ خشخاش کا پیڑ . *(Hind.)* *Ḳhash-ḳhash*-ká-*jháṛ* خشخش کا جھاڑ . *(Duk.)* Ga*sh*a-ga*sh*á-*ch*eḍi கசகசாச்செடி ; Póstaká-*ch*eḍi போஸ்தக்காச்செடி. *(Tam.)* Gasagasála-*ch*eṭṭu గసగసాలచెట్టు ; Póstakáya-*ch*eṭṭu పోస్తకాయచెట్టు. *(Tel.)* Ka*sh*a-ka*sh*a*ch*-*ch*eṭi കശകശച്ചെടി. *(Malyal.)* *Kh*asa-*kh*asi-giḍá ಖಸಖಸಿಗಿಡ. *(Can.)* Pó*sh*ta ; Pó*sh*tér-gá*ch*h. *(Beng.)* Póstu-vri*kshaha*. *(Sans.)* *Kh*asa-*kh*asá-*ch*a-*jh*áḍa. *(Mah.)* *Kh*as-*kh*as-nu-*jh*áḍa. *(Guz.)* *Bh*in-biṇ *or* *Bh-ain*-biṇ *(Bur.)*.

457. PAPAVER SOMNIFERUM, *Roxb.* *(Seeds of— Poppy Seeds.)*

Bazrul-*ḳhash-ḳhásh* بزر الخشخاش . *(Arab.)* Tu*ḳh*me-kóknár تخم کوکنار ; *Ḳhash-ḳhásh* خشخاش . *(Pers.)* *Ḳhash-ḳhásh* خشخاش . *(Hind.)* *Ḳhash-ḳhash* خشخش .

(Duk.) Gasha-gashá கசகசா. *(Tam.)* Gasa-gasálu గస
గసాలు. *(Tel.)* Kasha-kashak-kuru കശകശക്കുരു. *(Malyal.)*
Khasa-khasi ಖಸಖಸಿ. *(Can.)* Poshtér-bíj ; *Khaskhas.*
(Beng.) Póstu-bíjam. *(Sans.)* *Khasakhasa.* *(Mah.)*
Khaskhas. *(Guz.)* *Bhin-si or Bh-ain-zi.* *(Bur.)*.

458. PAPAVER SOMNIFERUM, *Roxb. Capsules of—Poppy-heads.)*

Qishrul-*khash-khásh* قشرا لخشخا ش . *(Arab.)* Póste-
kóknar پوست كوكنار ; Póste-*khash-khásh* پوست خشخاش .
(Pers.) *Khash-khásh-ké-bóṅḍé* خشخا ش کے بو نڈ ے .
(Hind.) *Khash-khash-ké-bóṅḍé* خشخش کے بو نڈ ے ;
Khash-khash-ká-póst خشخش کا پو ست . *(Duk.)* Gasha-
gashá-tól கசகசாடோல் ; Póstaká-tól போஸ்தகாடோல்.
(Tam.) Gasa-gasála-tólu గసగసాలతోలు ; Póstakáya-tólu
పోస్తకాయతోలు. *(Tel.)* Kasha-kashat-tól കശകശത്തോൽ.
(Malyal.) Khas-khas-nu-póst. *(Guz.)*.

459. PARMELIA PERLATA, *Ach.*

460. PARMELIA PERFORATA, *Ach. Syn.*
LICHEN ROTUNDATUS, *Rott.*

Khirázuṣ-ṣakhar خرا ز الصخر ; Behqul-ḥajar بهقل الحجر .
(Arab.) Gule-sang گل سنگ . *(Pers.)* Patthar-ká-phúl
پتھر کا پھول . *(Hind.)* Phattar-ká-phúl پھتر کا پھول . *(Duk.)*
Kalap-pách-chi கலப்பாச்சி ; Kalap-pú கலப்பு. *(Tam.)*
Ráti-páchi రాతిపాచి ; Ráti-puvvu రాతిపువ్వు. *(Tel.)* Kallu-
huvvu కల్లుహువ్వు. *(Can.)* Sh-ailéyaha. *(Sans.)* Dhonḍécha-
phúla. *(Mah.)* Kiyáv-poéṇ. *(Bur.)*.

With regard to the above Burmese name, see the remarks
under *Gracilaria lichenoides* and *G. confervoides.*

461. PEDALIUM MUREX, *Linn.*

Khasake-kabir خسک کبیر . (*Arab.*) Khasake-kalán خسک کلان . (*Pers.*) Farid-búti فريد بوئي ; Bará-gó*khrú* بڑا کھو کرو . (*Hind.*) Bará-*ghó*krú بڑا کھو کرو ; Hattí-*ghó*krú هتي کھو کرو . (*Duk.*) Peru-neruṇji பெருநெருஞ்சி ; Ánai-neruṇji ஆனைநெருஞ்சி. (*Tam.*) Énuga-palléru-muḷḷu ఏనుగపల్లేరుముళ్ళు ; Pedda-palléru పెద్దపల్లేరు. (*Tel.*) Káṭṭu-neriṇṇil കാട്ടുനെരിഞ്ഞില് ; Ána-neriṇṇil ആനനെരിഞ്ഞില് ; Kákka-muḷḷu കാക്കമുള്ളു. (*Malyal.*) Ánne-galu-giḍá ಅನ್ನೆಗಲುಗಿಡಾ. (*Can.*) Bara-*ghó*kru. (*Beng.*) Hattí-charáṭṭé. (*Mah.*) Moṭṭo-*ghó*kru. (*Guz.*) Ati-neranchi. (*Cing.*) Ṣule-gí. (*Bur.*).

See the remarks under *Cocculus villosus.*

462. PEGANUM HARMALA, *Linn.* (*Seeds of.*)

Ḥurmul حرمل or Ḥarmal حرمل . (*Arab.*) Isband اسبند or Ispand اسپند . (*Pers.*) Isband اسبند . (*Hind. and Duk.*) Ṣhímai-azha-vanai-virai சீமையழவணைவிரை. (*Tam.*) Ṣhíma-góranṭi-vittulu సీమగోరంటివిత్తులు. (*Tel.*) Isband. (*Beng.*).

In some native and other works, *Ispandán* اسپندان is incorrectly used synonymously with the above Arabic, Persian, Hindustani and Dukhni names, but it is the Persian name of *Mustard.*

See the remarks under *Lawsonia alba.*

463. PETROLEUM. (*Rock Oil.*)

Nifṭ نفط ; Qafral-yahúd قفرا ليهود . (*Arab.*) Kafral-yahúd كفرا ليهود . (*Pers.*) Miṭṭí-ká-tél مٹی كاتيل . (*Hind.*) Maṭṭi-ká-tailam مٹی كا تيلم ; Maṭṭi-ká-tél مٹی كاتيل . (*Duk.*) Maṇ-yeṇṇey மண்ணெண்ணெய் ; Maṇ-tayilam மண்தயிலம்.

(Tam.) Manṭi-tayilam మంటతయిలం ; Manṭi-núne మంట నూనె. *(Tel.)* Maṇ-taïlam మంతైలం. *(Malyal.)* Maṇṇu-yaṇṇe మణ్ణయణ్ణె. *(Can.)* Máṭiyá-tail. *(Beng.)* Pruthví-taïlam. *(Sans.)* Maṭṭí-cha-téla. *(Mah.)* Maṭti-nu-tél. *(Guz.)* Yé-ná *or* Yená. *(Bur.)*.

464. PHARBITIS NIL, *Choisy. (Seeds of—Kala-dana.)*

Ḥabbun-níl حب النيل . *(Arab.)* Tuḵhme-níl تخم نيل. *(Pers.)* Kálá-dánah کالا دانه . *(Hind.)* Zirki-ké-bínj ; Káli-zirki-ké-bínj کالی زرکی کے بینج . *(Duk.)* Koḍi-kákkaṭáṇ-virai கொடிகாக்கடாண்விளை ; Jiriki-virai ஜிரிகிவிளை. *(Tam.)* Jiriki-vittulu జిరికివిత్తులు ; Kolli-vittulu కొల్లివిత్తులు. *(Tel.)* Nil-kolomí ; Kálá-dáná. *(Beng.)*.

On account of the word *níl*, which means *Indigo* when used by itself and which is also a part of the name *Nilú-far (Nymphœa)*, entering into the formation of the above Arabic and Persian names *Ḥabbunníl* and *Tuḵhme-níl*, these are occasionally mis-applied to the seeds of *Indigofera tinctoria* and *Nymphœa edulis* or *N. rubra*. See the remarks under *Clitorea ternatea* and *Nigella Indica*; the former with reference to the Dukhni name *Zirkí* and Tamil name *Kúkkaṇáṇ* or *Kúkkaṭáṇ*, and the latter with regard to the Hindustani name *Kálá-dánah.*

465. PHŒNIX DACTYLIFERA, *Linn. (Dried fruits of—Dates.)*

Ḵhurmáe-yábis خرمای یابس . *(Arab.)* Ḵhurmáe-ḵhushk خرمای خشک . *(Pers.)* Khajúr کهجور . *(Hind. and Duk.)* Périch-chaṇkáy பெரிச்சங்காய். *(Tam.)* Karjúru-káya కర్జూరకాయ. *(Tel.)* Ténich-chan-káya തേനിച്ചൻകായ. *(Malyal.)* Kharjúra ಖರ್ಜೂರ. *(Can.)* Khájúr ; Khurmá *(Beng.)* Kharjjúraha. *(Sans)* Kharjúr. *(Mah.)* Khajúr ; Kárék. *(Guz.)* Indi. *(Cing.)* Somblón-zi. *(Bur.)*.

466. PHŒNIX SYLVESTRIS, *Roxb.* *(Wild-date tree.)*

Sandólé-ká-pér سند ولے کا پیڑ . *(Hind.)* Sandólé-ká-jhár سند ولے کا جھاڑ . *(Duk.)* Íshaṇ-cheḍi ஈசஞ்செடி. *(Tam.)* Íta-cheṭṭu ఈతచెట్టు. *(Tel.)* Káṭṭinta കാട്ടിന്ത ; Ínte-cheṭi ഇന്തെന്തചെടി. *(Malyal.)* Janglér-khájúr-gáchh. *(Beng.)* Ṭo-somblóṅ-ẓi. *(Bur.).*

The names of the *vinegar, jaggery, toddy,* and *arrack* of *P. sylvestris* will be found under *Acetum, Saccharum, Toddy,* and *Liquor Spirituous,* respectively.

467. PHYLLANTHUS EMBLICA, *Linn.* Syn. EMBLICA OFFICINALIS, *Gœrtn.* *(Fruits of—Emblic Myrobalans.)*

Amlaj املج . *(Arab.)* Ámelah آمله . *(Pers.)* Áṅvulá آنولا ; Áṅvurah آنور, . *(Hind.)* Áṅvulah آنول . *(Duk.)* Nelli-káy நெல்லிகாய் ; Tóppi தோப்பி. *(Tam.)* Nelli-káya నెల్లకాయ ; Usirike-káya ఉసిరేకాయ ; Ámalakamu అమలకము. *(Tel.)* Ámalakam ആമലകം ; Nelli-káya നെല്ലികായ. *(Malyal.)* Nelli-kăyi ನೆಲ್ಲಿಕಾಯಿ. *(Can.)* Ámlá ; Áṇlá. *(Beng.)* Ámalakam. *(Sans.)* Avaḷá. *(Mah.)* Ámbaḷa. *(Guz.)* Nelli *or* Nellika. *(Cing.)* Zíphiyu-ẓí. *(Bur.).*

The dry fruit of the above plant which is sold in the bazaar, in segments without its nut and seeds, is known under the Arabic and Dukhni names of *Ámelahe-moqash-shar* آمله مقشر and *Áṅval-gaṭṭi* آنول گٹی, respectively.

Nelli is the Tamil word adopted in Telugu, and *Nelli-cheṭṭu* is accordingly applied in the latter language to *P. Emblica* and used synonymously with *Usirika* in Madras and in many other places of Southern India; but it appears from Flora Andhrica that the same name *(Nelli-cheṭṭu)* is given to *Premna esculenta* and *P. latifolia* in some parts of Northern Circars.

Ziphiyu is the Burmese name of *P. Emblica*, but incorrectly applied in Mason's Natural productions of Burmah, to *P. niruri*. *Mi-ziphiyu* is the name of the latter.

468. PHYLLANTHUS MULTIFLORUS, *Willd.*

Kálé-madh-ká-pér كالے مدھ كا پیڑ. *(Hind.)*   Kálé-madh-ká-*jhár* كالے مدھ كا جھاڑ. *(Duk.)*   Karuppu-pilláŋji சருப்புபில்லாஞ்சி; Pilláŋji பில்லாஞ்சி. *(Tam.)*   Nalla-puruguḍu నల్ల పురుగుడు; Puruguḍu పురుగుడు. *(Tel.)*.

Kálí-madh مدھ كالى is the Hindustani and Dukhni name of the fruit of *P. multiflorus*, which means *the black honey*, because the juice of its fruits or the syrup made from them is supposed to be equal to honey. See further remarks about the name under *Fluggea Leucopyrus.*

469. PHYLLANTHUS NIRURI, *Linn.*

Bhuiñ-áñvalah بھوئیں آنولہ. *(Hind.)*   *Bhúiñ-áñvalah* بھوئین آنولہ. *(Duk.)*   Kizhkáy-nelli இழ்காய்நெல்லி; Kizhá-nelli இழாநெல்லி. *(Tam.)*   Néla-usirika నేలవుసిరిక. *(Tel.)*   Kizhá-nelli കീഴാനെല്ലി; Kizhkkáyi-nelli കീഴ്ക്കായിനെല്ലി. *(Malyal.)*   Kiranelli-giḍá ಕಿರನೆಲ್ಲಿಗಿಡಾ. *(Can.)*   Mi-zíphiyu. *(Bur.)*.

See the remarks under *Phyllanthus Emblica* with respect to the Burmese name *Zíphiyu.*

470. PHYLLANTHUS URINARIA, *Linn.*

Lál-*bhuiñ*-áñvalah لال بھوئیں آنولہ. *(Hind.)*   Lál-*bhúiñ*-áñvalah لال بھوئین آنولہ. *(Duk.)*   Shivappu-nelli சிவப்புநெல்லி. *(Tam.)*   Erra-usirika ఎర్రవుసిరిక. *(Tel.)*   *Chiṛu-kizhuká-nelli* ചിറുകീഴുകാനെല്ലി; *Chukanna-kizhá-nelli* ചുകന്നകീഴാനെല്ലി. *(Malyal.)*   Kempu-kiranelli ಕೆಂಪುಕಿರನೆಲ್ಲಿ. *(Can.)*   Mi-ziphiyu-ani. *(Bur.)*.

471. PHYSOSTIGMA VFNENOSUM, *Balfour.* (*Calabar Bean plant.*)

472. PIMPINELLA ANISUM, *Linn.* (*Fruits of— Anise or Ani-seeds.*)

Ráziyánaj رازيانج ; Shamár شمار . (*Arab.*) Ráziyanah والان بزرک ; رازيانه . Bádiyán بادیان ; Váláne-buzarg ; (*Pers.*) Sónf سونف . (*Hind. and Duk.*) Peru\u0146-ṣhíragam பெருஞ்சீரகம்; Ṣhómbu சோம்பு. (*Tam.*) Pedda-jilakara పెద్దజీలకఱ; Sópu సోపు. (*Tel.*) Perin-chírakam പെരിഞ്ചീരകം. (*Malyal.*) Doḍḍa-jírage ದೊಡ್ಡಜೀರಿಗೆ ; Sómpú సొంపె. (*Can.*) Miṭhá-jirá. (*Beng.*) Sómp. (*Mah.*) Mahá-duru ; Déva-duru ; Lokka-duru. (*Cing.*) Samusaba. (*Bur.*).

The native names of these little fruits which are generally known as seeds, are involved in a great confusion in some books. Their correct names are those given in the text, but many of them are often misapplied to several other fruits or seeds, such as the *sweet* and *common Fennel fruits*, *Dill fruits*, and the fruits of *Fœniculum panmorium*, &c. From the great resemblance of the Arabic word *Anísún* انيسون with *Anisum*, *Anise*, or *Aniseed*, they are considered in some books as synonymous. Whether this was the case originally or not, at present, according to all native works, Hakeems and druggists, *Anísún* is not the name of *Aniseed*, but of another fruit or seed which is probably the produce of *Pimpinella (Ptychotis) involucrata*.

Kuppi-cheṭṭu is interpreted *Pimpinella anisum* in Flora Andhrica. It is, however, applied to *Acalypha Indica* in Madras, and considered as synonymous with *Kuppeṇṭa-cheṭṭu*; and in some other places to *Anethum sowa;* but never in any place to *P. anisum*.

The Burmese name in the text, is improperly applied in some books to the fruits or seeds of *Hyoscyamus nigrum* and *Carum ajowan*.

473. PINUS DEODARA, *Roxb.*

Shajratud-dévdár شجرة الديودار ; Ṣanóbarul-hind ; درخت ديودار Darakhte-dévdár (*Arab.*) . صنو برالهند ;

Sanóbare-hindi صنوبرهندي. (*Pers.*)　Kilan-ká-péṛ پیڑ کا کلن; Kilan كلن; Dévdár دیودار. (*Hind.*)　Dévdáru دیودارو. (*Duk.*)　Dévadári-cheḍi செவதாரிசெடி. (*Tam.*)　Dévadári-cheṭṭu దేవదారిచెట్టు.(*Tel.*)　Dévatáramദേവതാരം. (*Malyal.*)　Déva-lári-mará ದೇವದಾರುಮರ. (*Can.*)　Débdáru. (*Beng.*)　Dévadáru-vrikshaha. (*Sans.*)　Dévadárúcha-jháda. (*Mah.*)　Dévdár. (*Guz.*).

Dévdárú is improperly applied to ' *Sethia Indica*' in some Mahratti works.

474.　PINUS DEODARA, *Roxb.* (*Oil of.*)

Kilan-ká-tél کلنکا تیل. (*Hind.*).

475.　PINUS LONGIFOLIA, *Roxb.*

Sanóbarul-hind صنوبرالهند. (*Arab.*)　Sanóbare-hindi صنوبرهندی. (*Pers.*)　Saral-ká-péṛ سرلکاپیڑ; *Chír-ká-péṛ* چیرکاجهاڑ; Saral سرل; (*Hind.*)　Chíṛ-ká-*jháṛ* چیرکاپیڑ. (*Duk.*)　Shuruḷ-dévadári சுருள்தேவதாரி; Shimai-déva-dári சீமைதேவதாரி. (*Tam.*)　Dévadári-cheṭṭu దేవదారిచెట్టు (*Tel.*).

476.　PINUS LONGIFOLIA, (*Resin of.*)

Aalakuṣ-ṣanóbar علک الصنوبر;Ṣamaghuṣ-ṣanóbar صمغ الصنوبر (*Arab.*)　Ṣamaghe-sanóbar صمغ صنوبر. (*Pers.*)　Saral-kí-gónd سرلکیگوند; *Chír-kí-gónd* چیرکیگوند; Ṣanóbar-kí-gónd صنوبرکیگوند; Gandah-barójah گنده بروجه; Gandah-barózah گنده بروزه; Birjí-gónd برجیگوند. (*Hind.*)　Gandah-férózah گندفیروزه. (*Duk.*).

See the remarks under *Olibanum* (*Boswellia thurifera,*) with respect to the word *Gandah-férozah.*

477.　PIPER NIGRUM, *Linn,* (*Berries of—Black Pepper.*)

Filfile-asvad فلفلاسود; Filfile-siyáh فلفلسیاه; Filfile-gird فلفلگرد. (*Pers.*)　Káli-mirch کالیمرچ; Gól-mirch

گل مرچ . *(Hind.)* Káli-mirchi کالي مرچی . *(Duk.)* Miḷagu மிளகு. *(Tam.)* Miriyálu మిరియాలు. *(Tel.)* Kuru-muḷaka കുരുമുളക. *(Malyal.)* Meṇasu ಮೆಣಸು. *(Can.)* Kálá-morich; Gól-morich. *(Beng.)* Maríchi. *(Sans.)* Miré. *(Mah.)* Kálo-mirich; Miri. *(Guz.)* Gam-miris; Kalu-miris. *(Cing.)* Náyukoṇ. *(Bur.)*.

See the remarks under *Embelia ribes.*

478. **PISTACIA KHINJUK,** *Stocks.* ⎱ ⎰ *Galls of.*

479. **PISTACIA CABULICA,** *Stocks.* ⎰

Gule-pistah گل پسته . *(Pers. and Hind.)*.

The Resin of the above plants is named in Arabic and Persian *Kundrún* کند رون or *Kundrúne-talkh* کند رون تلخ which is different from *Kundur* کندر mentioned in Nos. 112 and 113. The meaning of *Gule-pistah* is *flower of Pistacia*, and it is applied to the galls of the above plants from their supposed resemblance to a flower.

480. **PIX LIQUIDA.** *(Tar.)*

Qír قیر . *(Arab.)* Qil قیل . *(Pers.)* Kíl کیل . *(Hind. and Duk.)* Kíl கீல்; Tár தார். *(Tam.)* Kílu కీలు; Táru తారు. *(Tel.)* Kílú ಕೀಲು. *(Can.)* Kíl. *(Cing.)* Tínyuṣi; Kattrá-aṣi. *(Bur.)*.

481. **PLANTAGO ISPAGHULA,** *Roxb. (Seeds of— Spogel Seeds.)*

Bazre-qaṯúná بزر قطونا . *(Arab.)* Isbaghól اسبغول; Isparzah اسپرزه; *Shikam-darídah* شکم دریده . *(Pers.)* Isba-ghól اسبغول . *(Hind.)* Isapghól اسپگهول . *(Duk.)* Iṣhappu-kól-virai ஈசப்புகோல்விதை ; Iskúl-virai இஸ்கோல்விதை. *(Tam.)* Isapagála-vittulu ఇసపగాలవిత్తులు. *(Tel.)* Isabakólu ಇಸಬಕೋಲು. *(Can.)* Eṣhopghól. *(Beng.)* Isabagóla. *(Mah.)* Isapghól. *(Guz.)*.

482. PLUMBAGO CAPENSIS, *Thunb.*

Údah-*chitarmúl* اودہ چترمول ; Údah-*chitarmulam* اودہ چترملم . (*Duk.*) Karuṇ-koḍi-vér கருங்கொடிவேர் ; Karuppu-chittira-múlam கருப்புசித்திரமூலம். (*Tam.*) Nalla-*chitra*-múlam నల్లచిత్రమూలం. (*Tel.*) Karutta-koṭivéli കറുത്തകൊടിവേലി. (*Malyal.*) Nila-*chitramúlá* నీలచిత్రమూలా. (*Can.*) Krishṭṇa-*chitraká*; Nila-*shikha*; Nilágni-*shikha*. (*Sans.*) Údú-*chitra*-múla. (*Mah.*).

483. PLUMBAGO ROSEA, *Linn.*

Shiṭaraje-aḥmar شيطرج احمر . (*Arab.*) *Shítarake*-*surkh* شيترک سرخ . (*Pers.*) Lál-*chitrá* لال چتر ا ; Lál-*chítá* لال چينا ; Lál-*chitarak* لال چيترک . (*Hind.*) Lál-*chitar*-múl لال چترمول ; Lál-*chitar*-mulam لال چترملم . (*Duk.*) *Shivappu*-*chittira*-múlam சிவப்புசித்திரமூலம் ; Koḍimúli கொடிமூலி. (*Tam.*) Erra-*chitra*-múlam ఎర్రచిత్రమూలం. (*Tel.*) Chukanna-koṭuvéli ചുകന്നകൊടുവേലി ; *Chenṭi*-koṭuveli ചെൻടികൊടുവെലി. (*Malyal.*) Kempu-*chitramúlá* ಕೆಂಪುಚಿತ್ರಮೂಲಾ. (*Can.*) Rakto-*chítá*. (*Beng.*) Rakta-*chitraka*; Rakta-*shikha*. (*Sans.*) Támbaḍa-chitramúla. (*Mah.*) Rat-nitúl. (*Cing.*) Kiṇ-*khen*-ni. (*Bur.*).

484. PLUMBAGO ZEYLANICUM, *Linn.*

Shiṭaraj شيطرج . (*Arab.*) *Shitarak* شيترک ; *Shitarah* شينر ہ . (*Pers.*) *Chitrá* چترا ; *Chítá* چينا ; *Chitarak* چيترک . (*Hind.*) *Chitar*-múl چترمول ; *Chitarmul* چترمل . (*Duk.*) Veṇ-*chittira*-múlam வெண்சித்திரமூலம் ; *Chittira*-múlam சித்திரமூலம். (*Tam.*) *Chitra*-múlam చిత్రమూలం ; Agnimáta అగ్నిమాత ; Tella-*chitra*-múlam

తెల్లగచ్చకాయలు. *(Tel.)* Koṭu-véli കൊടുവെലി; Tumpa-koṭu-véli ഇമ്പകൊടുവെലി. *(Malyal.)* Chitra-múlá ಚಿತ್ರಮೂಲ. *(Can.)* Chitá. *(Beng.)* Agni-ṣhikha ; Chitraka-vrikshaha. *(Sans.)* Chitra-múla. *(Mah.)* Sudu-nitul. *(Cing.)* Kiŋ-khen-phiú. *(Bur.).*

485. PLUMBI CARBONAS. *(White Lead.)*

Isfédáj اسفيداج . *(Arab.)* Isfedáb اسفيداب ; Sufédáb اسفيداب . *(Pers.)* Safédah سفيده . *(Hind. and Duk.)* Veḷḷiyya-basvam வெள்ளீயப்பஸ்வம். *(Tam.)* Sisa-bhasmam సీసభస్మం. *(Tel.)* Sísa-bhasma ಸೀಸಭಸ್ಮ. *(Can.)* Sophédá. *(Beng.)* Nága-bhasmá. *(Sans.)* Sísa-bhasma. *(Mah.)* Saphéda. *(Guz.)* Khemá-phiú. *(Bur.).*

Sufédah سفيد is often applied to the *Slaked Lime* in conversation, which is incorrect and should be avoided.

486. PLUMBI OXIDUM. *(Impure Oxide of Lead, or Litharge.)*

Murdá-sanj مرداسنج . *(Arab.)* Murdá-sang مرداسنگ . *(Pers.)* Murdár-sing مردارسنگ . *(Hind. and Duk.)* Mudúrṣhiŋgu முதார்சிங்கு. *(Tam.)* Mudár-sing ముదార్సింగ్. *(Tel.)* Mudár-sinka മുദാർസിങ്ക. *(Malyal.)* Muḍadár-ṣhingi ಮುದದಾರ್ ಶಿಂಗಿ. *(Can.)* Murdár-sing. *(Beng.)* Murdár-sing. *(Guz.).*

487. PLUMBI OXIDUM RUBRUM. *(Red Oxide of Lead, or Red Lead.)*

Isrinj اسرنج ; Usranj اسرنج . *(Arab.)* Sirinj سرنج ; Suranj سرنج . *(Pers.)* Séndúr سيندور . *(Hind. and Duk.)* Chendúram செந்தூரம். *(Tam.)* Chendúramu చెందూరము. *(Tel.)* Chentúram ചെന്തൂരം. *(Malyal.)* Shin-dhúrá ಶಿಂಧೂರಾ ; Chendrá ಚೆಂದ್ರಾ. *(Can.)* Sindúr. *(Beng.)*

Nága-sambhavá ; Sindúraha. *(Sans.)* Sindúr. *(Guz.)* Ṣun.
(Bur.).

488. PLUMBUM. *(Lead.)*

Ánuk آنک . *(Arab.)* Surb سرب . *(Pers.)* Sísá سيسا.
(Hind.) Shísh شيش . *(Duk.)* Íyam ஈயம். *(Tam.)*
Sísamu సీసము. *(Tel.)* Íyam ഈയം. *(Malyal.)* Ṣhísa ಶೀಸ.
(Can.) Sísa. *(Beng.)* Sísakam ; Vangam. *(Sans.)* Sísa.
(Mah.) Kalu-síhu. *(Guz.)* Íyam. *(Cing.)*.

489. POGOSTEMON PATCHOULI, *Pell.* *(Dried Tops of.)*

Pachóli پچولي . *(Hind.)*.

490. POLANISIA (CLEOME) ICOSANDRA, *W. et A. (Seeds of.)*

Jangli-hurhur جنگلي هرهر ; Jangli-hulhul هلهل جنگلي.
(Hind.) Chhórí-ajván چھوري اجوان ; Jangli-hulvul
جنگلي هاول ; Jangli-hulul هلل جنگلي . *(Duk.)* Náy-
vélai நாய்வேளை ; Káttu-kadugu காட்டுகடுகு ; Peru-vélai
பெருவேளை ; Náy-kadugu நாய்கடுகு. *(Tam.)* Kukka-
váminta కుక్క-వామింట ; Kukka-áválu కుక్క-అవాలు ; Néla-
váminta నేలవామింట ; Pedda-váminta పెద్దవామింట. *(Tel.)*
Náyvéla നായ്വേള ; Káttukatuka കാട്ടകടുക ; Náyk-katuka
നായ്കടുക. *(Malyal.)* Hucha-sásavi ಹುಚ್ಚಸಾಸವಿ. *(Can.)*
Ban-hurihuriyá. *(Beng.)* Védamoharyá. *(Mah.)*.

491. POLYNEMUS PLEBEUS. *(Dried Air-bladder of——Isinglass.)*

See the names under *Icthyocolla.* The name of the above
fish in Bengali is *Súl-machh.*

492. POLYPODIUM.

Basfáyij بسفا يج ; Aẓrásul-kalb اضراس الكلب . (*Arab.*)
Khanklí كهنكلى or *Khankáli* كهنكا لى . (*Hind.*) Bisfáyaj
بسفا يج . (*Duk.*).

493. POLYPORUS ANTHELMINTICUS, *Berk.*
(*Bamboo or Worm Mushroom.*)

Va-mo ; *Than-mo.* (*Bur.*).

494. PONGAMIA GLABRA, *Vent.*

Karanj كرنج ; Karan*jh* كرنجھ . (*Hind. and Duk.*)
Puṇgam-maram புங்கமமரம். (*Tam.*) Kánuga-cheṭṭu కానుగ
చెట్టు ; Kaggera కగ్గెర ; Kránuga క్రానుగ. (*Tel.*) Uṇṇa-
maram ഉണ്ണമരം ; Puṇṇam പുന്നം. (*Malyal*) Hónge-
giḍá ಹೊಂಗೆಗಿಡ. (*Can.*) Tamála-vri*ksh*aha. (*Sans.*) Karanja
or Karanj-gá*chh.* (*Beng.*) Karanjícha-*j*háḍa. (*Mah.*)
Karanj-nu-*j*háḍa. (*Guz.*) Magul-karanda. (*Cing.*) Ṣimizu
or Ṭimizu. (*Bur.*).

See the remarks under *Cæsalpinia Bonducella.*

495. POTASSÆ CARBONAS. (*Impure Carbonate of Potash.*)

Jou-khár جوكھار ; Ivak-chhár اوک چھار or *Ouk-
chhár* اوک چھار . (*Hind.*) Jhár-ká-namak جھاڑکا نمک ;
Rák-ká-namak راک کا نمک . (*Duk.*) Maravuppu மரவுப்பு ;
Ṣhámbal-vuppu சாம்பல்வுப்பு. (*Tam.*) Mánu-vuppu మానువు
ప్పు ; Búḍide-vuppu బూడిదెవుప్పు. (*Tel.*) Káram കാരം ;
Pappaṭak-káram പപ്പടക്കാരം; Mara-uppa മരഉപ്പ. (*Malyal.*)
Marada-uppu ಮರದಉಪ್ಪು. (*Can.*) Dáru-lavaṇam. (*Sans.*)
Jháḍicha-miṭha. (*Mah.*).

496. POTASSÆ NITRAS. *(Nitrate of Potash or Saltpetre.)*

Aḳqar ابقر ا. *(Arab.)* Shórah شورد. *(Pers.)* Shóra ا شورا or Shorah شورة. *(Hind. and Duk.)* Poṭluppu பொட்டுப்பு. *(Tam.)* Peṭluppu పెట్లుప్పు; Shúrá-káram శూరకారం. *(Tel.)* Veṭi-uppa വെടിഉപ്പ. *(Malyal.)* Peṭluppu ಪೆಟ್ಲುಪ್ಪ. *(Can.)* Sórá. *(Beng.)* Shóra-míṭha. *(Muh.)* Sóro-khár. *(Guz.)* Poṭ-lunu; Veḍi-lunu. *(Cing.)* Yán-ẓin. *(Bur.)*.

497. POTASSÆ TARTRAS ACIDA. Syn. POTASSÆ BITARTRAS. *(Acid Tartrate of Potash, or Cream of Tartar.)*

Namake-angúr نمك انگور. *(Pers. Hind. and Duk.)* Diráksha-vuppu திராக்ஷவுப்பு. *(Tam.)* Dráksha-vuppu ద్రాక్షవుప్పు. *(Tel.)* Drákshi-uppu ದ್ರಾಕ್ಷಿಉಪ್ಪು. *(Can.)* Dráksha-lavaṇam. *(Sans.)* Drákshi-míṭha. *(Mah.)*.

498. PRUNUM. *(Prunes.)*

Ijás اجاس ا. *(Arab.)* Álú آلو. *(Pers.)* Álú-boḳhárá آلوبخارا. *(Hind. and Duk.)* Álpogáḍá-pazham ஆல் பொகாடாபழம். *(Tam.)* Álpogáḍá-panḍlu ఆల్పొగాడాపండ్లు. *(Tel.)* Álu-bókhárá. *(Beng.)* Álu-bokhára. *(Guz.)* Aálu-paká or Álu-pakárá. *(Bur.)*

499. PSIDIUM PYRIFERUM, *Linn. (Fruit of— White Guava.)*

Amrúde-abyaẓ امرود ابيض ا. *(Arab.)* Amrúde-supéd سفيد سفري آم. *(Pers.)* Sufód-safrí-ám امرود سييد ا. *(Hind.)* Suféd-jám سنيد جام. *(Duk.)* Veḷḷai-goyyá-pazham வெள்ளைகொய்யாபழம். *(Tam.)* Tella-jam-panḍu

తెల్లగోంజు ; Tella-goyyá-pandu తెల్లగొయ్యపండు. *(Tel.)* Veṇ-péra വെൺപെര ; Veṇ-pérakka വെൺപെരക്ക ; Veḷḷa-malák-kappéra വെള്ളമലാക്കപ്പേര. *(Malyal)* Biḷi-shibé-haṇṇu ಬಿಳಿಶಿಬೆಹಣ್ಣು. *(Can.)* *Dhóp-góáchhi-phal* ; *Sádá-piyárá. (Beng.)* Ṣhvéta-amruta-*phalam* ; *Ṣhvéta-bahu-bíja-phalam. (Sans.)* Pán*dh*ara-jámba ; Pán*dh*ara-túp-kél. *(Mah.)* Ujlo-piyára ; Ujlo-péru ; Sap*h*éd-jamrúd. *(Guz.)* Sudu-péra ; Sudu-pera-gaḍi. *(Cing.)* Málaká-*phiú*. *(Bur.)*.

Amrúd امرود is a proper Arabic and Persian name for *Pear*, but in India it is often used for *Guava*.

Véranná is the Malyalim name given to *P. pyriferum* in the Hortus Malabaricus, (Vol. III, Tab. 34,) but it is the name of another plant.

Jám is applied to *Guava* in Dukhni, but in Bengali to the fruit of *Syzigium jambolanum*. The Dukhni name for the latter is *Jámún*.

500. PSIDIUM POMIFERUM, *Linn.* *(Fruit of— Red Guava.)*

Amrúde-aḥmar امرود احمر . *(Arab.)* Amrúde-sur*kh* امرود سرخ . *(Pers.)* Lál-safrí-ám لال سفري آم . *(Hind.)* Lál-jám لال جام . *(Duk.)* Ṣhivappu-goyyáp-pa*zh*am சிவப்பு கொய்யாப்பழம். *(Tam.)* Erra-jám-pandu ఎఱ్ఱజాంపండు ; Erra-goyyá-pandu ఎఱ్ఱగొయ్యపండు. *(Tel.)* *Chem-péra* ചെമ്പെര; *Chem-pérakka* ചെമ്പെരക്ക ; *Chovanna-malák-kappéra* ചൊവന്നമലാക്കപ്പേര. *(Malyal.)* Kempu-*sh*ibé-haṇṇu ಕೆಂಪುಶಿಬೆಹಣ್ಣು. *(Can.)* Lál-góáchhi-phal ; Lál-piyárá. *(Beng.)* Rakta-amruta-*ph*alam ; Rakta-bahu-bíja-*ph*alam. *(Sans.)* Támbaḍa-jámba ; Támbaḍa-túp-kél. *(Mah.)* Lál-piyára ; Lálpéru ; Lál-jamrúd. *(Guz.)* Rat-péra ; Rata-péra-gaḍi. *(Cing.)* Málakí-ní. *(Bur.)*.

See the remarks under the preceding plant.

501. PSORALIA CORYLIFOLIA, *Linn.* *(Seeds of.)*

Búvanchiyán بادو چیان ; Búvchiyán بادنچیان ;
Bávanchi باونجي . *(Hind. and Duk.)* Kárpó-karishi கார்
போகரிஷி ; Kárpuvá-arishi கார்புவாஅரிஷி. *(Tam.)* Bhávanchi-
vittulu భావంచివిత్తులు ; Kálugech-cha-vittulu కాలుగెచ్చవిత్తులు ;
Káru-bógi-vittulu కారుబోగివిత్తులు ; Kála-ginja కాలగింజ. *(Tel.)*
Bávachi ; Hakúch. *(Beng.)* Bávachyá. *(Mah.).*

See the remarks under *Abelmoschus moschatus* with reference
to the name *Mushk-dánah.*

502. PTEROCARPUS MARSUPIUM, *D. C. (Indian Kino tree.)*

Bijésar بجیسر ; Bijésar-ká-per بجیسر کا پیر . *(Hind.)*
Bijesar-ká-*jhár* بجیسر کا جها ڑ . *(Duk.)* Véngai-maram
வேங்கைமரம். *(Tam.)* Végi వేగి ; Végisa వేగిస ; Égisa ఏగిస.
(Tel.) Vénna വെങ്ങ ; Venna-maram വെങ്ങമരം. *(Malyal.)* Pit-shál *or* Pit-sál. *(Beng.)* Gam-málu. *(Cing.).*

In some works on Botany, the above plant is referred to the
Tab. 25, Vol. VI, in the Hortus Malabaricus, but the plant
figured there is neither *P. marsupium,* nor is the Malyalim
name *Karintakarai* 'കരിന്തകരൈ' applicable to it. Although
the leaves in the *Fig.* are *emarginate* and therefore they look
like those of *P. marsupium,* yet the petals are of equal size and
of the same form. Whereas the corolla in the plant under
examination is *papilionaceous.*

503. PTEROCARPUS MARSUPIUM, *D. C. (Gum of—Indian Kino.)*

Dammul-a*kh***vaine-hindi** دم الاخوین هندی . *(Arab.)*
K͟húne-siyávusháne-hindi خون سیاوشان هندي . *(Pers.)*
Hirá-dó*kh***i** هیرا دوکهي ; **Khólar-mandá** کور مندا ا ;
Rang-barat رنگ برت . *(Hind.)* **Nás-ká-dammul-a***kh***vain**
نات کا دم الاخوین . *(Duk.)* **Kándámiruga-mirattam**

காண்டாமிருகநெத்தம். *(Tam.)* Gándámrugam-netturu நாంdாక்ஷுగొనెత்తుడు. *(Tel.)* Véṇṇap-paṣha വെണ്ണപ്പശ. *(Malyal.)*.

See the remarks under *Kino*.

504. PTEROCARPUS SANTALINUS, *Linn.* (*Wood of—Red Sandal-wood.*)

Ṣandale-aḥmar صندل احمر. *(Arab.)* Ṣandale-surkh صندل سرخ. *(Pers.)* Ragat-chandan رگت‌چندن. *(Hind.)* Lál-chandan لال چندن. *(Duk.)* Ṣheṇ-ṣhandanam ஓசெஞ் சந்தனம். *(Tam.)* Erra-gandhapu-chekka ఎఱ్ఱగంధపుచెక్క; Rakta-chandanam ర‌క్తచందనం; Rakta-gandham ర‌క్తగంధం; Kuchandanam కుచందనం. *(Tel.)* Rakta-channanam രക്ത ചന്നനം. *(Malyal.)* Kempu-gandha-chekke ಕೆಂಪುಗಂಧಚೆಕ್ಕೆ. *(Can.)* Rakta-chondon. *(Beng.)* Agaru-gandhakáshṭaha. *(Sans.)* Támbaḍa-chandaṇa; Támbaḍa-gandhácha-chekká. *(Mah.)* Rat-handuṇ. *(Cing.)* Sanḍaku; Naṣa-ni. *(Bur.)*.

In some books, the above Burmese names are improperly applied to *Sandal-wood*.

505. PUNICA GRANATUM, *Linn.*

Shajratur-rummán شجرة الرمان. *(Arab.)* Darakhte-nár درخت نار. *(Pers.)* Anár-ká-pér انار کا پیڑ. *(Hind.)* Anár-ká-jhár انار کا جهاڑ. *(Duk.)* Mádaḷai-ch-chedi மாதளைச்செடி. *(Tam.)* Dánimma-cheṭṭu దానిమ్మచెట్టు; Dáḍima-cheṭṭu దాడిమచెట్టు; Dáḷimba-cheṭṭu దాళింబచెట్టు. *(Tel.)* Mátaḷam-cheṭi മാതളംചെടി. *(Malyal.)* Dáḷimbe-giḍá ದಾಳಿಂಬೆಗಿಡಾ. *(Can.)* Dálim-gáchh. *(Beng.)* Dádima-vrikshaha. *(Sans.)* Dáḷimba-jháḍa. *(Mah.)* Dádam-nu-jháḍa. *(Guz.)* Deluṇ-gahá. *(Cing.)* Ṣale-biṇ or Tali-biṇ. *(Bur.)*.

506. PUNICA GRANATUM *Linn. (Fruit of—Pomegranate.)*

Rummán رمان ; Ráná رانا . (*Arab.*) Anár انار ; Nár نار . (*Pers.*) Anár انار ; Dáram دارّم . (*Hind.*) Anár انار . (*Duk.*) Mádalaip-pazham மாதளம்பழம். (*Tam.*) Dánimma-pandu దానిమ్మపండు ; Dádima-pandu దాడిమపండు ; Dálimba-pandu దాళింబపండు. (*Tel.*) Mátalam-pazham മാതളംപഴം. (*Malyal.*) Dálimbe-káyi ದಾಳಿಂಬೆಕಾಯಿ. (*Can.*) Anár ; Dalim. (*Beng.*) Dádima-phalam. (*Sans.*) Dálimba. (*Mah.*) Dáram ; Dádam. (*Guz.*) Delun *or* Dellun. (*Cing.*) Salé-si *or* Talí-si. (*Bur.*)

The *sweet* and *sour* varieties of *Pomegranate* are distinguished by adding those words to each of the synonymes in the text.

507. PUNICA GRANATUM, *Linn. (Male variety of.)*

Darakhte-gulnár درخت گلنار . (*Pers.*) Gulnár-ká-pér گلنار کا پیر . (*Hind.*) Gulnár-ká-*jhár* گلنار کا جھاڑ ; Gule-anár-ká-*jhár* گل انار کا جھاڑ . (*Duk.*) Pú-madalai பூமாதளை. (*Tam.*) Puvvu-dánimma పువ్వుదానిమ్మ. (*Tel.*) Pú-mádalam പൂമാതളം. (*Malyal.*) Hushi-dálimbe ಹೂಶಿದಾಳಿಂಬೆ. (*Can.*) Mal-delun. (*Cing.*) Gul-anár-nu-*phúl.* (*Guz.*).

508. PYRETHRI RADIX. *(Pellitory of Spain or Pellitory root.)*

Áaqarqarhá عا قرقرحا ; Áudul-qarh عودالقرح ; Áaqar-qarhá عقرقرحا . (*Arab.*) Akalkará اکلکرا . (*Pers.*) Aqal-qara اقلقرا ; Akarkará اکرکرا . (*Hind.*) Aqalqórá اقلقورا . (*Duk.*) Akkirá-káram அக்கிராகாரம். (*Tam.*) Akkára-káram అక్కరకారం ; Ákala-karra ఆకలకర్ర. (*Tel.*) Akki-karuká ആക്കികരുകാ ; Akkilá-káram ആക്കിലാകാരം. (*Malyal.*) Akkalá-karé ಅಕ್ಕಲಕರೆ. (*Can.*) Ákar-kará. (*Beng.*)

Akkal-kará. *(Mah.)* Akar-karo. *(Guz.)* Kúkaij-à or Kúkayà. *(Bur.)*.

509. **PYRUS CYDONIA,** *Linn. Syn.* CYDONIA VULGARIS, *Pers. (Seeds of—Quince seeds).*

Ḥabbus-safarjal حب السفرجل . *(Arab.)* Bihí-dánah تخم آبي ; Beh-dánah به دانه ; Tukhme-ábi بي دانه ; *(Pers.)* Beh-dánah به دانه . *(Hind. and Duk.)* Shimai-mádalai-virai செய்மைமாதளைவிளை. *(Tam.)* Shíma-dálima-vittulu శీమదాడిమవిత్తులు. *(Tel.)* Shíme-dálimba-bíja శీమ దాడింబబీజా. *(Can.)*.

Beh-dánah and *Bé-dánah* being nearly the same in their pronunciation, they are occasionally confounded with each other. The latter is the name of a variety of *Raisins* which are small and seedless, and is often applied to all kinds of *Raisins* without distinction.

510. **PYRRHOSIA HORSFIELDII,** *Blume. (Nut of—Wild-nutmeg).*

Janglí-jáé-phal جنگلی جائ پهل . *(Hind.)* Janglí jáphal جنگلی جا پهل . *(Duk.)* Káṭṭu-jádik-káy காட்டு ஜாதிக்காய். *(Tam.)* Aḍavi-jáji-káya అడవిజాజికాయ. *(Tel.)* Káṭṭu-játik-ká കാട്ടുജാതിക്കാ *(Malyal.)* Ban-jáe-phal. *(Beng.)*.

Q.

511. **QUISQUALIS INDICA,** *Linn, (Rango creeper).*

Rángún-ki-bél رنگون کی بیل . *(Duk.)* Irangún-malli இரங்கூன்மல்லி. *(Tam.)* Rangúnu-malle-cheṭṭu రంగూనుమల్లె చెట్టు. *(Tel.)*.

R.

512. RAIDÆ, *Sp. of.* (*Oil. of—Fish oil.*)

See the names under *Oleum Piscis.*

513. RADIX CHINENSIS, (*China Root*).

Khashabuṣ-ṣiní خشب الصيني ; Aṣluṣ-ṣiní اصل الصيني
(*Arab.*) *Chób-chíní* چوب چيني. (*Pers., Hind., Duk.,
and Beng.*) Chóp-chinni. (*Mah.*) Chób-chinni (*Guz.*).

514. RANDIA DUMETORUM, *Lam.* (*Nut of—Emetic Nut*).

Jouzul-qai جوزالكوثل ; Jouzul-Kouṣal جوزالقي.
(*Arab.*) Mén-phal مين پهل (*Hind.*) Ménḍ-phal مينڈ پهل
Méḍ-phal ميڈ پهل. (*Duk.*) Marukkálaṇ-káy மருக்காளங்
காய். (*Tam.*) Manga-káyalu మంగకాయలు ; Mranga-káyalu
మ్రంగకాయలు ; Mandá-káyalu మండాకాయలు. (*Tel.*) Karaḷik-
káya കരളിക്കായ. (*Malyal.*) Mén-phal. (*Beng.*) ·Kukuru-
mán. (*Cing.*).

One of the above Arabic names, *Jouzulqai* جوزالقي, is
applied to *Strychnos Nux Vomica* in Richardson's Persian and
Arabic Dictionary, Materia Indica, &c., which is a dangerous
error and should be carefully avoided.

515. RAPHANUS SATIVUS, *Linn.* (*Root of—Radish*).

Fujl فجل. (*Arab.*) Turb ترب. (*Pers.*) Múli مولی
(*Hind.*) Mulli ملی. (*Duk.*) Muḷḷáṇgi முள்ளாங்கி. (*Tam.*)
Mullangi మూల్లంగి. (*Tel.*) Mullangi ಮೂಲ್ಲಂಗಿ. (*Can.*) Múlá ;
Múli. (*Beng.*) Móulá or Moulá. (*Bur.*).

516. RHAZYA STRICTA, *Dec.*

Sevar ; Sihar ; Ishvarg: *(Mukráni)*.

517. RHEUM. *(Rhubarb.)*

Rávand راوند . *(Arab.)* **Révand** ريوند . *(Pers.)* **Révand-chíní** ريوندچيني . *(Hind.)* **Révan-chíní** ريوندچيني، . *(Duk.)* **Iréval-chinni** இரேவல்சிண்ணி ; **Manjat-chinak-kizhangu** மஞ்சட்சினக்கிழங்கு. *(Tam.)* **Réval-chinni** రేవల్చిన్ని ; **Pasupu-chína-gadda** పసుపుచీనగడ్డ. *(Tel.)* **Révá-chinnni** రేవాచిన్ని. *(Can.)* **Révan-chini.** *(Beng.)* **Réval-chinní.** *(Mah.)* **Révan-chini.** *(Guz.)*.

518. RHEUM EMODI, *Wall.*

519. RHEUM MOORCROFTIANUM, *Roy.*

520. RHEUM WEBBIANUM, *Roy.*

} *Root of—Indian Rhubarb.*

Rávande-hindí راوند هندي . *(Arab.)* **Révande-hindí** ريوندچيني هندي. *(Pers.)* **Híndí-révand-chíní** ريوندچيني هندي . *(Hind.)* **Nát-kí-révanchíní** نات كي ريوندچيني . *(Duk.)* **Náttu-iréval-chinni** நாட்டு இரேவல்சிண்ணி ; **Náttu-manjat-chínak-kizhangu** நாட்டுமஞ்சட்சினக்கிழங்கு. *(Tam.)* **Náttu-réval-chinni** நாட்டுரேவல்చిన్ని ; **Náttu-pasupu-chína-gadda** నాట్టుపసుపుచీనగడ్డ. *(Tel.)* **Nát-révá-chinni** నాట్రేవాచిన్ని. *(Can.)* **Banglá-révan-chini.** *(Beng.)* **Mulká-cha-révalchinní.** *(Mah.)* **Gámni-révanchini.** *(Guz.)*.

521. RHINACANTHUS COMMUNIS, *Nees.*

Pálak-jóhí پالکجوهي ; **Jóí-páni** جوئيپاني . *(Hind.)* **Kabútar-Ká-jhár** كبوترکاجهاڙ . *(Duk.)* **Nága-malli** நாகமல்லி. *(Tam.)* **Nágamalle** నాగమల్లె. *(Tel.)* **Puzhuk-kolli** പുഴുക്കൊല്ലി ; **Pushpa-kédal** പുഷ്പകെദൽ ; **Nágamallich-chet:**

നാഗമല്ലിച്ചെടി. *(Malyal.)* Nága-mallige ನಾಗಮಲ್ಲಿಗೆ. *(Can.)*
Anitta. *(Cing.)*.

522. RHUS SUCCEDANEA, *Linn. (Galls of.)*

Kákṛásingí كاكڑاسنگي . *(Hind.)* Kákaṛsingí كاكڑسنگي;
or Kákad-singí كاكدسنگي . *(Duk.)* Kákkaṭa-shiṇgi காங்கட
சிங்கி ; Karkáṭaka-shiṇgi கற்காடகஷிங்கி. *(Tam.)* Kákara-
shingi కాకరషింగి. *(Tel.)* Kákaḍa-shingi. *(Mah.)*.

523. RICINUS COMMUNIS, *Linn. (Castor Oil plant.)*

Shajratul-khirvaạ شجرة الخروع . *(Arab.)* Darakhte-
bédanjír درخت بيدانجير . *(Pers.)* Araṇḍká-pér ارنڈ کا پیڑ;
Araṇḍi-ká-pér ارنڈي کا پیڑ . *(Hind.)* Yaraṇḍi-ká-jhár
يرنڈی کا جهار . *(Duk.)* Ámaṇakkam-chcḍi ஆமணக்கம்செடி.
(Tam.) Ámudapu-cheṭṭu ఆముదపుచెట్టు. *(Tel.)* Ávaṇakku
ആവണക്കു. *(Malyal.)* Karaḷa-giḍá ಕರಳಗಿಡ. *(Can.)*
Bhéraṇḍá-gáchh. *(Beng.)* Yeraṇḍa-vrikshaha. *(Sans.)*
Yaraṇḍícha-jháḍa. ¦ *(Mah.)* Yeraṇḍi-nu-jháḍa. *(Guz.)*
Endaru-gahá. *(Cing.)* Keṣú-biṇ. *(Bur.)*.

In Bengali, *Bhéraṇḍá* is the name of *R. communis* and
Eraṇḍa of *Jatropha curcas;* but the latter is the name of the
former plant in Hindustani. This is a source of confusion in
some books, where both names are used synonymously, or confounded with each other.

524. RICINUS COMMUNIS, *Linn. (Seeds of—— Castor Oil Seeds.)*

Khirvaạ خروع ; Bazrul-khirvaạ بزرالخروع . *(Arab.)*
Bédanjír بيدانجير ; Tukhmc bédanjír تخم بيدانجير . *(Pers.)*
Araṇḍ ارنڈ ; Araṇḍi ارنڈی ; Araṇḍ-ké-bínj ارنڈکے بینج;
Araṇḍi-ké-bínj ارنڈي کے بینج . *(Hind.)* Yaraṇḍi يرنڈی;

Yarandi-ké-binj یر نڈ ی کے بیذج .(*Duk.*) Ámauakku-muttu ஆமணக்குமுத்தி ; Ámauakkau-kottai ஆமணக்கண்கொட்டை. (*Tam.*) Ámudapu-vittulu ஆமுடபுவித்துலு. (*Tel.*) Ávauakkin-kuru ആവണക്കിന്‍കുരു. (*Malyal.*) Haralu ಹರಳು. (*Can.*) Bhéraṇḍ or Bhéraṇḍa. (*Beng.*) Yéraṇḍa-bíjam. (*Sans.*) Eraṇḍicha-bíja. (*Mah.*) Yeraṇḍi. (*Guz.*) Endaru or En-daru-aṭṭa. (*Cing.*) Kesu-zi. (*Bur.*).

525. RICINUS COMMUNIS, *Linn.* (*The small-seeded variety of Castor Oil plant*).

Shajratul-khirvaaaus-saghír شجرة الخروع الصغير (*Arab.*) Darakhte-bédanjíre-khurd د رخت بیدانجیر خرد. (*Pers.*) Chhóṭi-araṇḍ-ká-pér چهوتي ابرنڈ کا پیڑ ; *Chhóṭi-araṇḍí-ká-pér* چهوتي ا رنڈ ی کا پیڑ. (*Hind.*) Chiṭlí-yaraṇḍi-ká-*jhár* چهوتي يرنڈي کا جهاڑ ; *Chhóṭi-yaraṇḍi-ká-jhár* چٹلي يرنڈی کا جهاڑ (*Duk.*) Chiṭṭámauakkau-cheḍi சிட்டாமணக்கஞ்செடி. (*Tam.*) Chiṭṭámudapu-cheṭṭu చిట்டமுదపுచెట்டு. (*Tel.*) Cheru-koṭṭá ചെറുകൊട்டാ ; *Chiṭrávauakkam-cheṭi* ചിററാവണക്കംചെടി (*Malyal.*) Chiṭṭa-harala-giḍá ಚಿಟ್ಟಹರಳಗಿಡಾ. (*Can.*) Chhóṭa-Bhéraṇḍá-gáchh. (*Beng.*) Lahana-eraṇḍicha-*jháḍa.* (*Mah.*) Náni-yeraṇḍi-nu-*jháḍa.* (*Guz.*) Punji-endaru-gahá. (*Cing*).

526. RICINUS COMMUNIS, *Linn.* (*Seeds of the Small-seeded variety of Castor Oil plant*).

Khirvaaaus-saghír خروع الصغير ; Bazrul-khirvaaaus-saghír بزر الخروع الصغير ; بید ا نجیر خرد (*Arab.*) Bédanjíre-khurd بید نجیر خرد. (*Pers.*) Tukhme-bédanjíre-khurd تخم بید ا نجیر خرد. (*Pers.*) Chhóṭi-araṇḍ چهوتي ا رنڈ ; *Chhóṭi-araṇḍ-ké-bínj* چهوتي ا رنڈ کے بیذج ; *Chhóṭi-araṇḍi* چهوتي ا رنڈ ی ;

Chhóti-arandi-ké-binj چهوٽي ارنڈى كے بيذج. (*Hind.*)
Chitli-yarandi چٽلي يرنڈ ي ; Chitli - yarandi - ké-binj
چٽلي يرنڈ ي کے بیذج ; Chhóti-yarandí چهو ٽي يرنڈى ;
Chhóti-yarandí-ké-binj چهو ٽي يرنڈ ي کے بیذج. (*Duk.*)
Chittámanakku-muttu சிட்டாமணக்குமுத்த; Chittámanakkan-
kottai சிட்டாமணக்கங்கொடடை. (*Tam.*) Chittámudapu-
vittulu చిట్టామొదపువిత్తులు. (*Tel.*) Chitrávanakkin-kuru ചി
ററാവണക്കിൻകുരു. (*Malyal.*) Chitta-haralu ಚಿಟ್ಟಹರಳು.
(*Can.*) Chhóta-bhérand. (*Beng.*) Lahana-erandicha-bijá.
(*Mah.*) Náni-yerandi. (*Guz.*) Punji-endaru-atta. (*Cing.*).

For the names of *Castor Oil* from the two above varieties of
Ricinus communis, see under *Oleum Ricini*.

527. ROCCELLA FUCIFORMIS, *D. C.*

528. ROCK SALT.

Milhul-hajar ملح ا لحجر ; Milhe-tabarzad ملح طبرز د.
(*Arab.*) Namake-sang نمك سنگ. (*Pers.*) Séndhá-lón
سيند ها لون ; Séndá-lón سيند ا لون ; Séndhá - namak
سيند ا نمك ; Sénda-namak سيند ها نمك. (*Hind.*)
Sóndá-namak سوند ا نمك. (*Duk.*) Induppu இந்துப்பு ;
Indunát-tuppu இந்தநாட்டுப்பு ; Shindu-désha-vuppu சிந்தேச
வுப்பு ; Shóma-nuppu சோமநுப்பு ; Shayindu-lavanam சயி
ந்தலவணம். (*Tam.*) Induppu ఇందుప్పు ; Shayindu-lavanam
సయిందులవణం ; Shindu-désha-vuppu సింధేశవుప్పు ; Chandru-
duppu చంద్రుదుప్పు. (*Tel.*) Intuppa ഇൻടുപ്പ. (*Malyal.*).

529. ROSA CENTIFOLIA, *Linn.* (Hundred-leaved or Cabbage Rose).

Vard ورد ; Varde-ahmar ورد ا حمر ; Vardul-ahmar
ورد الاحمر. (*Arab.*) Gule-surkh گل سرخ ; Gule-guláb گل گلاب.
(*Pers.*) Guláb-ká-phúl گلاب کا پهول ; Guláb-phúl گلاب پهول

(Hind. and Duk.) Irójá-pus*h*pam இரோஜாபுஷ்பம்; Gulúp-pú குலாப்பூ; Irójáp-pú இரோஜாப்பூ. *(Tam.)* Rója-puvvu రోజావువ్వు; Rójá-pus*h*pam రోజావుష్పం; Gulú-puvvu గులావువ్వు. *(Tel.)* Paninir-pus*h*pam പനിനീർപുഷ്പം. *(Malyal.)* Gulábi-huvvu ಗುಲಾಬಿಹುವ್ವು. *(Can.)* Góláp-p*h*úl. *(Beng.)* Gulábácha-p*h*úla. *(Mah.)* Guláb-nu-p*h*úl. *(Guz.)* Rosa-mal. *(Cing.)* Neṣi-poen or Neṇzi-poén. *(Bur.)*.

The names of *Rose-water, Confection* and *Attar* or *Utr* of *Roses*, are as follows:—

Rose Water.

Mául-vard ماءالورد . *(Arab.)* Guláb گلاب ; Aarqe-gule-surk*h* عرق گل سرخ . *(Pers.)* Guláb گلاب . *(Hind. and Duk.)* Panníru பன்னீர். *(Tam.)* Panníru పన్నీరు. *(Tel.)* Pani-nír പനിനീർ. *(Malyal.)* Panníru ಪನ್ನೀರು. *(Can.)* Góláp ; Góláp-páni. *(Beng.)* Guláb ; Pannir. *(Mah.)* Guláb ; Guláb-nu-páṇi. *(Guz.)*.

Confection of Roses.

Julanjabín جلنجبين . *(Arab.)* Gulangabin گلنگبين; Gul-qand گلقند ; Gul-*sh*akar گلشکر . *(Pers.)* Gul-qand گلقند . *(Hind.)* Gulqan گلقن . *(Duk.)* Gul-kandu குல்கந்து ; Rójáp-pú-tittíppu ரோஜாப்புத்திப்பு. *(Tam.)* Gulkandu గుల్కందు. *(Tel.)* Gul-kant ഗുൽകന്ത. *(Malyal.)* Rangu-lámi. *(Cing.)*.

Attar or Utr of Roses.

Aiṭrul-vard عطرالورد ; Aiṭrul-vardul-aḥmar عطرالوردالاحمر. *(Arab.)* Aiṭre-guláb عطرگلاب ; Aiṭre-gule-surk*h* عطرگل سرخ. *(Pers.)* Gulábi-aiṭr گلابی عطر ; Guláb-ká-aiṭr گلاب کا عطر. *(Hind.)* Guláb-ká-aaṭar گلاب کا عطر. *(Duk.)* Guláb-attar

குலாப்அத்தர். *(Tam.)* Gulábi-attaru గులాబీఅత్తరు. *(Tel.)* Panini-rattar പനിനീരത്തൽ. *(Malyal.)* Gulábi-attar గులాబీఅత్తర్. *(Can.)* Guláp-atar. *(Beng.)* Gulábá-cha-atar. *(Mah.)* Guláb-nu-atar. *(Guz.)* Rója-mal-kandum. *(Cing.)*.

530. ROYLEA ELEGANS, *Wall.*

Patkaru. *(Beng.)*.

531. RUBIA CORDIFOLIA, *Linn. (Root of.)*

Fóvvah فو د ; Fóvvahuṣ-ṣabbá-ghin فو ه ا لصبا غين. *(Arab.)* Rúnás رو ناس. *(Pers.)* Majíṭh مجيته ; Manjíṭh منيجنه. *(Hind.)* Manjíṭ منجيت. *(Duk.)* Maṇjiṭṭi மஞ்சிட்டி ; Shevvelli செவ்வெல்லி. *(Tam.)* Maṇjishṭa మంజిష్ట ; Támra-valli తామ్రవల్లి. *(Tel.)* Man-cheṭṭi മഞ്ചട്ടി. *(Malyal.)* Manjushṭá ಮಂಜುಷ್ಠ. *(Can.)* Manjíṭ. *(Beng.)* Kála-méshiká. *(Sans.)* Manjéshṭa. *(Mah.)* Manjiṣṭa ; Velmadata. *(Cing.)*.

  See the remarks under *Oldenlandia umbellata.*

532. RUMEX VESICARIUS, *Linn.*

Ḥummáẓ حما ض or Ḥammáẓ حما ض. *(Arab.)* Turshah ترشه. *(Pers.)* Chúká چوكا. *(Hind.)* Chukkah چكه. *(Duk.)* Shukkáṇ-kirai சுக்காங்கீரை. *(Tam.)* Shukku-kúráku చుక్కుకూరాకు. *(Tel.)* Chukár-sák. *(Beng.)* Kalá-khén-boun. *(Bur.)*.

533. RUTA ANGUSTIFOLIA, *Pers.*

Féjan فيجن. *(Arab.)* Sadáb سداب. *(Pers. and Hind.)* Sadáf سداف. *(Duk.)* Arvadá அர்வடா. *(Tam.)* Sadápa సదాప ; Aruḍu అరుడు. *(Tel.)* Nágadáli-sappu నాగదాళిసప్పు. *(Can.)* Sadápaha. *(Sans.)* Sadáp ; Sitáp. *(Guz.)* Aruda. *(Cing.)*.

S.

534. SACCHARUM OFFICINARUM, *Linn.* *(Sugar-cane.)*

Qaṣabus-sakar قصب السكر ; Qaṣabe-sakar قصب سكر.
(Arab.) Nai-shakar نيشكر. *(Pers.)* Úkh اوكهه ; Gannà گنا.
(Hind.) Gáṇḍá گانڈا. *(Duk.)* Karumbu கரும்பு. *(Tam.)*
Cheruku చెఱుకు ; Árukaṇupula-kranuga అఱకణుపులక్రనుగ ;
Kaṇupula-cheruku కణుపులచెఱుకు. *(Tel.)* Karinpa കരിമ്പ.
(Malyal.) Khabbu ಕಬ್ಬು. *(Can.)* Úk ; Ganna. *(Beng.)*
Ikshuhu. *(Sans '* Úṣ. *(Mah.)* Sérdi ; Naisakar. *(Guz.)*
Úk. *(Cing.)* Kiyán or Kian. *(Bur.)*.

535. SACCHARUM. *(Sugar.)*

Sukkar سكر ; Sakkar سكر. *(Arab.)* Shakar شكر.
(Pers. and Hind.) Shakkar شكر. *(Duk.)* Ṣharukkarai
சருக்கரை. *(Tam.)* Ṣhakkara శక్కర. *(Tel.)* Ṣharkkara
ശക്കര ; Panjasára പഞ്ചസാര. *(Malyal.)* Sakkare ಸಕ್ಕರೆ.
(Can.) Bhúra ; Chiní. *(Beng.)* Ṣharkará ; Panjasáram.
(Sans.) Sákhar. *(Mah.)* Sakkar ; Chíni ; Búra ; Khánd.
(Guz.) Síni ; Sakkere. *(Cing.)* Ṣaghiá or Ṭagiyá. *(Bur.)*.

The following are the names of the varieties of Sugar,
Jaggery, and Sugar-candy, which are commonly met with in the
bazaars of India :—

Sugar.

a. Country Sugar—*Sakkarul-hind* سكر الهند. *(Arab.)*
Shakare-hindí شكر هندي. *(Pers.)* *Lál-shakar* لال شكر. *(Hind.)*
Makhtúmi-shakkar مختومي شكر. *(Duk.)* *Núṣṣu-sharukkarai*
நாட்டுச்சருக்கரை. *(Tam.)* *Núṣṣu-shakkara* నాట్టుశక్కర. *(Tel.)*

Náṭṭu-sharkkara നാട്ടശക്കര ; *Náṭṭu-panjasúra* നാട്ടപഞ്ചസാര.
(Malyal.)   *Náṭ-sakkare* ನಾಟ್ ಸಕ್ಕರೆ. *(Can.)*   *Banglá-chíní.*
(Beng.) *Désha-sharkarú ; Désha-panjasáram. (Sans.) Mulkácha-
súkhar. (Mah.) Gúmni-sakkar ; Gúmni-chíni ; Gúmni-búro ;
Gúmni-khánḍ. (Guz.) Kala-saghiú or Kala-ṭigiyá. (Bur.).*

     b.   **White Sugar**—*Sakkarul-abyaz* سكر الابيض . *(Arab.)*
Shakare-suped سكر سپيد . *(Pers.)*   *Suféd-shakar* سفيد شكر ;
Chíní چيني . *(Hind.)* *Chíní-shakkar* چيني شكر . *(Duk.)* *Chíná-
sharukkarai* சீனாசருக்கரை ; *Vellai-sharukkarai* வெள்ளை சருக்கரை.
(Tam.) *Chíná-shakkara* చీనాషక్కర ; *Tella-shakkara* తెల్లషక్కర.
(Tel.) *Ven-sharkkara* വെൺശക്കര ; *Ven-panjasúra* വെൺ
പഞ്ചസാര. *(Malyal.)* *Biḷi-sakkare* ಬಿಳಿಸಕ್ಕರೆ. *(Can.)*   *Dhúp-
chíní. (Beng.) Shvéta-sharkarú ; Shvéta-panjasáram. (Sans.)
Pándhara-súkhar. (Mah.) Saphéd-sakkar ; Ujlo-chíni ; Ujlo-búro ;
Ujlo-khánḍ. (Guz.) Saghiú-phiú or Ṭagiyá-phiú. (Bur.).*

     c.   **Coarse Sugar**—*Búrá* بورا . *(Hind.)*   *Búrá-shakkar*
بورا شكر . *(Duk.)*   *Búrá-sharukkarai* பூராசருக்கரை. *(Tam.)*
Búrá-shakkara బూరాషక్కర. *(Tel.).*

     d.   **Raw-sugar**—*Ráb-shakkar* راب شكر ;   *Ráb-kí-shakkar*
راب كي شكر . *(Duk.)* *Ráp-sharukkarai* ராப்சருக்கரை. *(Tam.)*
Ráp-shakkara రాప్ షక్కర. *(Tel.).*

     e.   **Loaf-sugar**—*Qand* قند . *(Hind.)*   *Qand-kí-shakkar*
قند كي شكر . *(Duk.)* *Kan-sharukkarai* கன்சருக்கரை. *(Tam.)*
Kan-shakkara కన్షక్కర. *(Tel.).*

<h3 style="text-align:center">Jaggery.</h3>

     a.   **Jaggery** (*of Sugar-cane*)—*Qand* قند . *(Arab.)*   *Kand*
كند *(Pers.)* **Gur** گڑ . *(Hind.)* *Gúṛ* گوڑ . *(Duk.)*   *Vellam*
வெல்லம். *(Tam.)*   *Bellamu* బెల్లము. *(Tel.)*   *Vella* വെല്ല ;
Sharkkara ശക്കര. *(Malyal.)*   *Bella* ಬೆಲ್ಲ. *(Can.)* *Akuru. (Cing.).*

     b.   **Palmyra Jaggery**—*Táṛ-ká-guṛ* تاڑ كا گڑ . *(Hind.)* *Táṛ-
ká-gúṛ* تاڑ كا گوڑ . *(Duk.)* *Panai-vellam* பனைவெல்லம். *(Tam.)*
Táṭi-bellamu తాటిబెల్లము. *(Tel.)* *Pana-vella* പനവെല്ല ; *Pana-
sharkkara* പനശക്കര. *(Malyal.)* *Táḷe-bella* ತಾಳೆಬೆಲ್ಲ. *(Can.)*
Tal-akuru. (Cing.).

c. Cocoanut Jaggery—*Náriyal-ká-gur* ناریل کاگر . *(Hind.)*
Nárél-ká-gúr ناریل کاگوڑ . *(Duk.)* *Tenna-vellam* தென்ன
வெல்லம். *(Tam.)* *Tenkáya-bellamu* ఙొంకాయబెల్లము· *(Tel.)*
Téngá-vella തെങ്ങാവെല്ല ; *Téngá-sharkkara* തെങ്ങാശക്കര. *(Mal-*
yal.) *Kangina-kúyi-bella* ಕಂಗಿನ ಕೂಯಿಬೆಲ್ಲ. *(Can.)* *Púl-akuru.*
(Cing.).

d. Jaggery of Phœnix sylvestris——*Sandólé-ká-gur*
سندولے کاگر . *(Hind.)* *Sandólé-ká-gúr* سندولے کاگوڑ ; *Séndí-*
ká-gúr سیندي کاگوڑ . *(Duk.)* *Ích-cha-vellam* ஈச்சவெல்லம்.
(Tam.) *Íta-bellamu* ఇతబెల్లము. *(Tel.)* *Ínte-vella* ഇന്തെവെല്ല
വെല്ല ; *Ínte-sharkkara* ഇന്തെശക്കര. *(Malyal.)* *Indí-*
akuru. (Cing.).

e. Jaggery of Caryota urens.—*Mari-ká-gur* مازی کاگر .
(Hind.) *Múri-ká-gúr* مازی کاگوڑ . *(Duk.)* *Xúndar-panai-*
vellam கூந்தற்பனை வெல்லம். *(Tam.).*

Sugar-candy.

a. Sugar candy (*of Sugar-cane*)—*Nabút* نبات . *(Arab.)*
Qande-suféd قند سفید ; *Kande-supéd* کند سپید . *(Pers.)* *Misri*
مصري . *(Hind. and Duk.)* *Karkandu* கற்கண்டு. *(Tam.)* *Kala-*
kanda కలకండ. *(Tel.)* *Kalkantu* കല്കണ്ടു. *(Malyal.)* *Kalkanda*
ಕಲ್ಲುಂಡ . *(Can.)* *Misri. (Beng.)* *Súkari. (Cing.).*

b. Palmyra Sugar-candy—*Túr-ki-misri* تاڑكي مصری .
(Hind. and Duk.) *Panai-karkandu* பனைகற்கண்டு. *(Tam.)* *Túti-*
kala-kanda తాటికలకండ. *(Tel.)* *Pana-kalkantu* പനകല്കണ്ടു.
(Malyal.) *Túte-kalkanda* ತಾಟೆಕಲ್ಲುಂಡ . *(Can.)* *Tal-súkari. (Cing.).*

536. SALEP.

Saalab-misri ثعلب مصری ; *Khusyus-saalab* خصي الثعلب ;
Khusyatus-saalab خصية الثعلب . *(Arab.)* *Saalab-misri*
ثعلب مصري . *(Pers., Hind. and Duk.)* *Shálá-mishiri*
சாலாமிஷிரி. *(Tam.)* *Sálá-mnsiri* సాలామిషిరి. *(Tel.)* *Sálá-*
mishri സാലാമിഷ്രി . *(Malyal.)* *Chhálé-michhri. (Beng.)*
Sálama-misri. (Mah.) *Sálammisri. (Guz.)* *Salama-misiri.*
(Cing.) *Sála-misri. (Bur.).*

537. SALICORNIA BRACHIATA, *Roxb.*

Koyalu కోయలు. *(Tel.).*

538 SALICORNIA INDICA, *Willah.*

Umari உமரி. *(Tam.)*   Koyyapippili కొయ్యపిప్పిలి. *(Tel.)*
Jódupalang. *(Beng.).*

539. SALIX CAPREA, *Linn.*

K͟hiláf خلاف . *(Arab.)* Bede-mus͟hk بید مشک.
(Pers.).

540. SALIX CAPREA, *Linn. (Water of.)*

Mául-K͟hiláf ما ا لخلا ف . *(Arab.)* Aarqe-béde-
mus͟hk عرق بید مشک . *(Pers.)* Béde-mus͟hk-ká-aaraq
بید مشک کا عرق . *(Duk.).*

541. SALIX TETRASPERMA, *Roxb.*

Páni-jamá پانی جما . *(Hind.)* Jamti-kí-bél جمتی کی بیل
Jamti-ká pattá جمتی کا پتا . *(Duk.)* Aṭrupálai அற்றுபாலை.
(Tam.) Éṭipála ఏటిపాల. *(Tel.)* Áṭrapála അറ്റാപാല.
(Malyal.) Páni-jomá. *(Beng.).*

542. SALSOLA. (SUAEDA) INDICA.

Ella-kúra ఎల్లకూర. *(Tel.).*

543. SALVADORA WIGHTIANA, *Planch.* · Syn.
S. INDICA, *Wight*; S. PERSICA, *Roxb.*

Arák اراک . *(Arab.)* Darak͟hte-misvák درخت مسواک.
(Pers.) Pílú پیلو . *(Hind.)* Pílú-ká-jhár پیلو کا جهاڑ.
(Duk.) Kalarva களர்வ ; Kárkol-maram கார்கொள்மரம்.
(Tam.) Varagógu వరగోగు. *(Tel.)* Pílú. *(Beng.)* Pílu-
nu-jháḍa. *(Guz.).*

544. SALVADORA INDICA, *Roy.*

Arák اراك . (*Arab.*) Darakhte-misvák درخت مسواك.
(*Pers.*) Bará-pílú برا پيلو . (*Hind.*) Peru-kaḷarvá பெரு
களர்வா ; Kálkoḷ-maram கார்கொள்மரம். (*Tam.*) Pedda-
vara-gógu పెద్దవరగోగు. (*Tel.*) Pílu. (*Beng.*).

545. SALVADORA PERSICA, *Linn.*

Arák ا اراك . (*Arab.*) Darakhte-misvák درخت مسواك.
(*Pers.*) Chhóṭá-pilú چهوٹا پيلو . (*Hind. and Duk.*)
Shiṛu-kaḷarvá சிறுகளர்வா. (*Tam.*) Chinna-varagógu చిన్న
వరగోగు ; Pinna-vara-gógu పిన్నవరగోగు. (*Tel.*) Pílu. (*Beng.*).

546. SANDORICUM INDICUM, *Cav.* (*Wood of.*)

Chandan چندن . (*Duk.*) Shéva-maram சேவமரம்.
(*Tam.*) Chéva-mánu చేవమాను. (*Tel.*) Ṣitto-biṇ *or* Ṭitto-
biṇ. (*Bur.*).

In Hindustani *Chandan* is one of the designations of *Sandal-
wood*, but in Dukhni it is applied to the inner wood of any
plant, which is red or reddish black; particularly to that of
the above tree.

**547. SANTALUM ALBUM, *Linn. Syn.* SIRIUM
MYRTIFOLIUM, *Linn.* (*Wood of—Sandal-wood.*)**

Ṣandale-abyaẓ صندل ابيض . (*Arab.*) Ṣandale-supéd
صندل سپيد . (*Pers.*) Chandan چندن ; Suféd-chandan
سفيد چندن . (*Hind.*) Ṣandal صندل . (*Duk.*) Shandanak-
kaṭṭai சந்தனக்கட்டை. (*Tam.*) Gandhapú-chekka గంధపు
చెక్క. (*Tel.*) Chandana-muṭṭi ചന്ദനമുട്ടി. (*Malyal.*)
Gandhadá-chekke ಗಂಧದ ಚೆಕ್ಕೆ. (*Can.*) Chondon ; Sádá-
chondon ; Sandal. (*Beng.*) Shri-gandha-káshṭaha. (*Sans.*)
Gandhácha-kóḍa. (*Mah.*) Súkéṭ. (*Guz.*) Sudu-handuṇ ;
Handuṇ. (*Cing.*) Naṣaphiyu ; Sandakú. (*Bur.*).

The following are the names of the essential Oil of Sandal-wood.

Aitre-ṣandal سندل صطر. (Pers.) Sandal-ká-ṣitr سندال كاعطر. (Hind.) Sandal-ká-ṣaṭar صندل كا عطر. (Duk.).

548. SAPINDUS EMARGINATUS, Vahl. (Nut of—Soap-nut.)

Findaqe-hindí فندق هندي or Fandaqe-hindí فندق هندي; Bandaqe-hindí بند ق هندي. (Arqb.) Ratah ر ته. (Pers.) Riṭhá ریتها or Riṭhah ریتهه. (Hind. and Duk.) Ponnán-koṭṭai பொன்னுங்கொட்டை. (Tam.) Kunkuḍu-káyalu కుంకుడు కాయలు; Kúkuḍu-káyalu కూకుడు కాయలు. (Tel.) Ur-vanjik-káya ഉർവഞ്ഞിക്കായ; Punnan-koṭṭa പുന്നങ്കൊട്ട. (Malyal.) Knkaṭe-káyi ಕಂಕಟೆಕಾಯಿ. (Can.) Riṭhá. (Beng.) Arishṭa-phalam. (Sans.) Riṭhá. (Mah.) Arítha (Guz.) Miávmeṇ-sue-khé-ṣí or Me-áv-me-sue-kha-ti. (Bur.).

The meaning of the above Burmese name is *the fruit of Monkey's blood*, and it is applied to *Soap-nut* from its supposed resemblance to the blood of a Monkey. See the remarks under *Acacia concinna*.

549. SAPO. (Soap.)

Ṣábún صابون. (Arab. Pers. and Hind.) Ṣhabbu சபு. (Tam.) Sabbu సబ్బు. (Tel.) Sábún. (Beng.) Sábún. (Guz.) Ṣuppiya. (Bur.).

550. SARSÆ RADIX. (Sarsaparilla or Jamaica Sarsaparilla.)

Aushbah عشبه; Aushbahe-maghrabí عشبه مغربي. (Arab. and Pers.) Aushbah عشبه; Sálsá سالسا. (Hind.) Aushbah عشبه. (Duk.) Shimai-nannári சீமைநன்னாரி; Ṣharaṣha-vér சாரசவேர். (Tam.) Sína-sugandhi-pála ಸೀಮ

కుంరం; Sárasa-véru సారసవేరు *(Tel.)* Narutinti നറ
ുതിന്തി. *(Malyal.)* Chhálchhá or Sálsá. *(Beng.)* Ushbo;
Ushbo-magrabi. *(Guz.)* Raṭa-irimusu. *(Cing.)*.

The *Country* and *Jamaica Sarsaparilla* are generally found
in books under the same designations, but they have distinct
names, which will be found in this Catalogue under their respective heads.

See the remarks under *Solanum rubrum* and *Hemidesmus
Indicus*, with respect to the Hindustani name *Makó* مکو or *Makóí*
مکوی.

551. SCAMMONIUM. *(Scammony.)*

Saqmúniya سقمونیا; Maḥmúdah محمود د. *(Arab.
Pers. and Hind.)* Shakamúniyá சகமுனியா; Mámúdá
மாமூதா. *(Tam.)* Shakumuniyá శకుమునియా; Mámúdá
మామూదా. *(Tel.)*.

552. SCILLA. *(Squill.)*

Isqil اسقیل; Ạanṣal عنصل: Baṣlul-fár بصل الفار;
Baṣlul-bar بصل البر. *(Arab.)* Piyáze-dashti پیاز دشتی;
Piyáze-mósh پیاز موش. *(Pers.)* Viláyatí-kándá ولایتی کاندا;
Viláyatí-jánglí-piyáz ولایتی جنگلی پیاز. *(Hind.)* Vilá-
yatí-janglí-piyáz ولایتی جنگلی پیاز; Viláyatí-kandrá
ولایتی کندرا. *(Duk.)* Shímai-nari-veṇgáyam சீமைநரி
வெங்காயம். *(Tam.)* Shíma-nakka-vulligaḍḍa సీమనక్క-వుల్లి
గడ్డ. *(Tel.)* Shíma-káṭṭuḷḷu ശീമകാട്ടുള്ളി. *(Malyal.)*
Síme-aḍavi-iruḷḷi ಸೀಮೆಅಡವಿಇರುಳ್ಳಿ. *(Can.)* Biláti-janglí-
piáj. *(Beng.)* Raṭa-val-lúnu. *(Cing.)* Ṣimbo-to-keṣúń.
(Bur.).

See the remarks under *Urginea Indica*.

553. SCINDAPSUS (POTHOS) OFFICINALIS, Schott. (Berries of.)

Gaj-piplí گج پیپلي ; Baṛi-piplí بڑی پیپلی . (Hind.) Hatti-piplí ھتی پیپلي . (Duk.) Atti-tippili அத்திதிப்பிலி ; Ánait-tippili ஆனைத்திப்பிலி. (Tam.) Énuga-pippaḷḷu ఎనుగ పిప్పళ్ళు; Gaja-pippaḷḷu గజపిప్పళ్ళు. (Tel.) Atti-tippili അത്തിതിപ്പിലി. (Malyal.) Doḍḍa-hipalli ದೊಡ್ಡಹಿಪಲ್ಲಿ. (Can.) Goj-piplí. (Beng.) Gaja-pippali. (Sans.) Thóra-pimpli. (Mah.) Motto-pipér. (Guz.)

554. SECAMONE EMETICA, R. Br.

555. SEMECARPUS ANACARDIUM, Linn. (Nut of—Marking nut.)

Ḥabbul-faḥm حب ا لفهم ; Ḥabbul-qalb حب القلب ; Inqardīyá انقرد یا . (Arab.) Biládur بلادر . (Pers.) Bhélá بهیلا ; Bhiláván بهیلاوان . (Hind.) Bhiláván بهلوان . (Duk.) Shén-kottai சேம்கொட்டை ; Shérán-kottai சேரான்கொட்டை. (Tam.) Jiḍi-vittulu జిడివిత్తులు; Tummeda-mámidi తుమ్మెదమామిడి; Bhallátamu భల్లాతము ; Bhallátakí భల్లాతకీ. (Tel.) Chérunkuru ചെരുങ്കുരു; Ténprákka തെന്പ്രാക്ക. (Malyal.) Cérú ಗೇರು. (Can.) Bhélá; Bhélvá. (Beng.) Bhallátakí-bíjam. (Sans.) Bibá. (Mah.) Bhilámu (Guz.) Shén-kotte. (Cing.) Khi-si. (Bur.).

See the remarks under Anacardium occidentale.

556. SENNA. (Alexandrian Senna.)

Saná سنا ; Saná-makkí سنا مکي . (Arab. Pers. and Hind.) Sunná-makki سنا مکي . (Duk.) Shúrattu-nilá-tatai சூரத்துநிலாவரை ; Shimai-nilávarai சிமைநிலாவரை.

(Tam.) Shúrattu-tangédu རུང་ཚོགས; Shína-tangédu ᱩᱵᱟᱴᱜᱩ. *(Tel.)* Néla-ávarke-gidá ᱱᱮᱞᱟᱣᱟᱨᱠᱮᱜᱤᱫ. *(Can.)* Súná-makkí *or* Shúná-mu-khí. *(Beng.)* Súná-mukhi. *(Mah.)* Súua-mukhi. *(Guz.)* Raṭa-sana-kola. *(Cing.).*

557. **SESAMUM INDICUM,** *Linn. (Jinjili Oil plant—Seeds of.)*

Simsim سمسم. *(Arab.)* Kunjad كنجد. *(Pers.)* Til تل. *(Hind. and Duk.)* Elḷu எள்ளு. *(Tam.)* Nuvvulu నువ్వులు. *(Tel.)* Elḷu എള്ള് ; Kárelḷu കാരെള്ള് ; Chiṭralḷu ചിത്രെള്ള്. *(Malyal.)* Yaḷḷu ಯಳ್ಳು. *(Can.)* Til; Ghoṣhya-á. *(Beng.)* Tilaha. *(Sans.)* Tiḷa. *(Mah.)* Til (*Guz.*) Talla or Talla-aṭṭa. *(Cing.)*

558. **SESAMUM INDICUM,** *Linn. (Oil of—Jinjili-Oil.)*

Shíraj شيرج ; Dhónul-ḥal د هن ا لحل ; Dhónus-sim-sim د هن ا لسمسم. *(Arab.)* Róghane-kunjad رو غن كنجد ; Róghane-shírin رو غن شيرين. *(Pers.)* Til-ká-tél تل كا تيل ; Bárik-tél بارِيك تيل. *(Hind.)* Miṭhá-tél ميٹها تيل ; Miṭṭhá-tél مٹها تيل. *(Duk.)* Nal-leṇṇey நல்லெண்ணெய். *(Tam.)* Manchi-núne మంచినూనె. *(Tel.)* Nalleṇṇá നല്ലെണ്ണ. *(Malyal.)* Vaḷḷe-yaṇṇe ಎಳ್ಳೆಣ್ಣೆ. *(Can.)* Tila-tailam. *(Sans.)* Chokhóṭa-téla. *(Mah.)* Míṭho-tél ; Míṭhu-tél. *(Guz.)* Talla-tel. *(Cing.)* Nahu-si. *(Bur.).*

559. **SESBANIA ÆGYPTICA,** *Pers.*

Jét جيت ; Rásin راسن. *(Hind.)* Ravásing رواسنگ ; Ravá-sin رواسن. *(Duk.)* Chempai செம்பை. *(Tam.)* Sómanti సోమంతి. *(Tel.)* Chempa ചെമ്പ. *(Malyal.)* Jét. *(Beng.)* Rájam. *(Sans.).*

560. SEVUM. *(Suet.)*

Samín سمين ; Shaḥm شحم . *(Arab.)* Paiyah پیه .
(Pers.) Charbi چربي . *(Hind. and Duk.)* Kozhuppu
கொழுப்பு. *(Tam.)* Kovvu కొవ్వు. *(Tel.)* Kobbu ಕೊಬ್ಬು.
(Can.) Chorbhi ; Chikná. *(Beng.).*

561. SHOREA ROBUSTA, *Roxb.* *(Resin of.)*

Qanqahar قنقهر ; Qíqahar تيقهر . *(Arab.)* Laạle-moạab-
bari لعل معبرى . *(Pers.)* Rál رال ; Dhúná دهونا ;
Dhonah دهونه ; Ḍámar دٙامر . *(Hind.)* Rál رال . *(Duk.)*
Kuṇgiliyam குங்கிலியம். *(Tam.)* Guggilamu గుగ్గిలము. *(Tel.)*
Kungiliyam കുങ്കിലിയം. *(Malyal.)* Guggaḷá ಗುಗ್ಗುಳ. *(Can.)*
Dhuná ; Rál. *(Beng.)* Guggilam ; Koushi-kaha. *(Sans.)*
Rája ; Guggiḷu. *(Mah.)* Dummala. *(Cing.).*

In Shakespears' and other Hindustani Dictionaries, &c., *Súl*
سال is applied to *Shorea robusta*, probably from the latter being
called *Saul-tree* in English in some books. *Súl,* however, is a
correct Persian name of *Tectona grandis (Teak-tree).* *Rál* رال
is the name of the *Resin* of *S. robusta.*

562. SIDA ACUTA, *Burm.*

Malai-táṇgi மலைத்தாங்கி; Pon-muṣhaṭṭai பொன்முசட்டை;
Vaṭṭa-tirippi வட்டதிரிப்பி. *(Tam.)* Chiṭimuṭi చిటిముటి;
Muttavapulagam ముత్తవపులగం. *(Tel.)* Malatáṇṇi മലതാണ്ണി;
Cheṛuparuva ചെറുപരുവ. *(Malyal.)* Korétá. *(Beng.)*
Sirivadi-babila. *(Cing.).*

563. SIDA RETUSA, *Linn.*

Ḥulbahe-barrí حلبه برى . *(Arab.)* Shanblide-barrí
شنبليدبري ; Shamlite-dashtí شمليت دشتي . *(Pers.)*
Jangli-méthi جنگلي ميتهي . *(Hind. and Duk.)* Mayir-

mánikkam மயிர்மாணிக்கம். (*Tam.*).Mayilu-mánikyam మయిలు
మాణిక్యం. (*Tel.*) Mayir-mánikkam മയിര്‍മാണിക്കം ; Karun-
toṭṭi കറുന്തൊട്ടി. (*Malyal.*) Bon-méthí. (*Beng.*) Koṭi-
káṇ-babila ; Maïr-mánikam. (*Cing.*).

A few years ago, Dr. Bidie had an occasion to examine a
small plant sent to him under the Tamil name *Mayir-mánikkam,*
and it proved to be *S. retusa.* The same name is adopted, with
a slight alteration in several languages, viz., Telugu, Malyalim,
Cingalese, &c., and the plant is more readily recognised by that
name than any other.

The *Fig.* in the Hortus Malabaricus (Vol. x, Tab. 18),
corresponds exactly with *S. retusa,* but the Malyalim name
assigned to it in that work, ' *Karun-toṭṭi,* is very doubtful one.
So is also the case with the Cingalese name, *Koṭi-káṇ-babila.*

564. **SINAPIS JUNCEA,** *Linn.* ⎫   *Seeds of—*
                                           ⎬   *Indian*
565. **SINAPIS RAMOSA,** *Roxb.* ⎭   *Mustard.*

Ḳhardal خردل . (*Arab.*) Sipandán سپندان or Ispandán
اسپندان . (*Pers.*) Rái رائي or Ráyán رايان . (*Hind.*
and Duk.) Kaḍugu கடுகு. (*Tam.*) Áválu ఆవాలు. (*Tel.*)
Kaṭuka കടുക. (*Malyal.*) Sásave ಸಾಸವೆ. (*Can.*) Rái. (*Beng.*)
Sarshaphaha. (*Sans.*) Moharé. (*Mah.*) Ráyi. (*Guz.*)
Abbé. (*Cing.*) Muṇṇiyén-zi. (*Bur.*).

See the remarks under *Peganum Harmala.*

566. **SINAPIS DICHOTOMA,** *Roxb.* ⎫
                                             ⎬ *Oil of.*
567. **SINAPIS GLAUCA,** *Roxb.* ⎭

Sarsón-ká-tél سرسون كا تيل . (*Hind.*) Ráyán-ká-tél
رايان كا تيل . (*Duk.*) Sarsho-teḷ. (*Beng.*).

568. **SMILAX GLABRA,** *Roxb.*

Baṛi-chób-chíní بڑى چوب چينى . (*Hind.*) ' Húrina-
*sh*úk-china.' (*Beng.*).

569.   SMILAX LANCEÆFOLIA, *Roxb.*

Hindi-chób-chiní هندي چوب چيني . *(Hind.)* 'Gutca-shúk-china.' *(Beng.)*.

570.   SMILAX OVALIFOLIA, *Roxb*

Jangli-aushbah جندی عشبه . *(Hind.)* Malait-támarai மலைத்தாமரை. *(Tam.)* Konda-támara ; Kistapa-támara ; Konda-guruva-tige ; Si-tapa-chettu ; Konda-dantena ; Kummara-baddu . *(Tel.)* Kal-támara ; Kari-vilánti . *(Malyal.)* Kúku. *(Bur.)*.

Komárika or ' Koomarika' and Kumárí are Cingalese and Bengali synonymes of a species of *Aloe* (*A. Indica*), but the former is found applied to *S. ovalifolia* in the Hortus Suburbanus Calcuttensis and other works, which is not correct

571.   SMILAX. *Sp. of.*
' Tsein-apho.' *(Bur.)*.

572.   SODÆ BIBORAS. *(Biborate of Soda or Borax.*

Bóraq بورق ; Milhus-sághah ملح الصاغه . *(Arab.)* Tinkár تنكار or Tankár تنكار . *(Pers)* Soháge سهاگا ; Tinkál تنكال . *(Hind)* Sohágah سهاگه . *(Duk.)* Veṇ-káram வெண்காரம். *(Tam.)* Elegáram . *(Tel.)* Ponkáram ; Veḷḷa-káram . *(Mal-yal.)* Biligára . *(Can.)* Sohágá. *(Beng.)* Vengá-ram ; Puskara. *(Cing.)* Lakhiya or Let-khya. *(Bur.)*.

573.   SODÆ CARBONAS. *(Impure Carbonate of Soda.)*

Qili قلي ; Milhul-qili ملح القلي *(Arab.)* Shikhár شخار ; Tine-gáqur طلين كاذر . *(Pers.)* Sajjí سجي ; Sajji-

mitti منّی ; Sajji-khár سجی کهار . (Hind.) Chour-
ki-matti چوڑ کا منّی ; Chour-ká-namak چوڑ کي منّی .
(Duk.) Shach-chi-káram சக்கிகாரம். (Tam.) Lota-
sach-chi లోటసచ్చి. (Tel.) Chhobji-máti. (Beng.) Sarjiká-
kshará. (Sans.) Sajjekhára. (Mah.).

574. SODÆ SULPHAS. (Crude Sulphate of Soda.

Khárá-lón. (Hind.) Khári-nún. (Beng.).

575. SODII CHLORIDUM. (Chloride of Sodium or Common Salt.)

Milh ملح ; Milhul-aajin ملح العجين . (Arab.) Namak
نمک ; Namakekhurdaní نمک خوردني ; Namake-taaám
نمک طعام . (Pers.) Lón لون ; Namak نمک . (Hind.)
Namak نمک ; Nimak نمک or Nammak نمک . (Duk.)
Uppu உப்பு. (Tam.) Lavaṇam లవణం ; Uppu ఉప్పు. (Tel.)
Uppa ಉಪ್ಪ ; Livaṇim ലവണം. (Malyal.) Uppu ಉಪ್ಪು.
(Can) Nún ; Nimok. (Beng.) Lavaṇam. (Sans.) Miṭha.
(Mah.) Miṭhú. (Guz.) Lunu. (Cing.) Ṣa. (Bur.).

576. SOLANUM INDICUM, Linn. (Fruit or Berry of.)

Muḷḷi முள்ளி ; Pappara-muḷḷi பப்பரமுள்ளி. (Tam.)
Káka-máchi కాకమాచి ; Tella-mulaka తెల్లములక. (Tel.) Cheru-
chunta ചെറുചുണ്ട. (Malyal.) Bayá-kúr. (Beng.) Tibbatu.
(Cing.).

The Dukhni and Mahratti names Kólsá-ká-jhár and 'Kólusi-ryácha-phala' are erroneously applied to this plant in some works.

577. SOLANUM JACQUINI, Willd. (Fruit or Berry of.)

Hadaqe-barrí حدق بری . (Arab.) Bádanjáne-barrí
بادنگان بری ; Bádangáne-barrí بادنجان بری . (Pers.)

Bhatkatyá بهتكتيا ; Bhatkatái بهت كتا ني ; Katái كتا ني ;
Réngni رينگني ; Janglí-baigan جنگلي بيگن . (Hind.)
Ḍórlá دّور لا . (Duk.) Kaṇḍaṇ-kattiri கண்டங்கத்திரி. (Tam.)
Vákuḍu వాకుడు ; Nela-mulaka నెలముల. (Tel.) Kaṇṭam-
kattiri കണ്ടംകത്തിരി. (Malyal.) Nelagullá నెలగుళ్ళ.
(Can.) Jongli-baigon ; Káṅṭá-karí. (Beng.) Kaṇṭakáriká.
(Sans.) Dórali. (Mah.) Ringni ; Vaingni. (Guz.) Kaṭu-
valbaṭu. (Cing.) Khayán-kazo. (Bur.).

Khayan is the Burmese name for S. melongena, but it is
given in some books to S. jacquinii. To render it applicable
to the latter, Kazo should be added to it.

578. SORGHUM VULGARE, Pers. (Grains or Seeds of.)

Ẓurrat ذرت . (Arab.) Jávrase-hindí جاورس هندي
(Pers.) Javár جوار . (Hind.) Javári جواری ; Jári
جاری . (Duk.) Chólam சோளம். (Tam.) Zonnalu
జొన్నలు. (Tel.).

579. SOYMIDA FEBRIFUGA, Juss. (Rohun Tree.)

Róhan روهن ; Róḥán روحان . (Hind.) Shém-
maram சேம்மரம். (Tam.) Chéva-mánu చేవమాను ; Sómida-
mánu సోమిదమాను ; Súmi సూమి. (Tel.) Róhan. (Beng.)
Patránga. (Sans.).

580. SPHÆRANTHUS HIRTUS, Willd.

Kamázariyús كمازريوس or Kamázariyús كما د ريوس .
(Arab.) Kamádariyús كماد ريوس . (Pers.) Muṇḍi
منڈي . (Hind.) Múndí موندّي . (Duk.) Kóṭṭak-karaṇḍai
கோட்டக்கரந்தை. (Tam.) Bóḍa-tarapu బోడతరపు. (Tel.)
Minángaṇṇi മിനാങ്ങണ്ണി ; Aṭakká-maṇi അടക്കാമണി.
(Malyal.) Muṇḍi. (Beng.).

581. SPONDIAS MANGIFERA, *Pers.*

Darakhte-maryam درخت مريم . (*Pers.*) Ámré-ká-pér ; آمريكا پير . (*Hind.*) Maryam-ká-*jhár* مريم كا جهاز . (*Duk.*) Mari-máy-chedi மரிமாஞ்செடி. (*Tam.*) Ivura-mámidi ఇవురమామిడి ; Ambála-chettu అంబాలచెట్టు ; Sítavrukshamu శీతవృక్షము ; Pita-vrukshamu పీతవృక్షము. (*Tel.*) Anpázham ആമ്പഴം. (*Mal-yal.*) Amatemará ಅಮಟೆಮರಾ. (*Can.*) Ámrá-gáchh. (*Beng.*) Ambácha-*j*káda. (*Mah.*) Gue-bin. (*Bur.*).

582. SQUALUS CARCHARIAS, *Linn.* (*White Shark.*)

Suféd-shórah-mach-chhi سفيد شور ۵ مچهی . (*Duk.*) Pál-shorá-mín பாச்சொருமீன். (*Tam.*) Tella-sorá-chepa తెల్లసొరాచేప. (*Tel.*).

583. SQUALUS CARCHARIAS, *Linn.* (*White Shark—Oil of.*)

See the names under *Oleum Piscis.*

584. STANNUM. (*Tin.*)

Qalaí قلعي ; Rasás رصاص . (*Arab.*) Arziz ارزيز ; Arzír ارزير . (*Pers.*) Rángá رانگا . (*Hind.*) Katthil كتهيل . (*Duk.*) Velliyam வெள்ளியம். (*Tam.*) Vendi-sísam వెండిసీసం. (*Tel.*) Velliyam വെള്ളിയം. (*Malyal.*) Ráng or Rángá. (*Beng.*) Rángá. (*Sans.*) Síhu. (*Guz.*) Sudu-íyam. (*Cing.*).

On account of the English word *tin* being commonly in use for the thin plates of *Iron* covered with *Tin*, the vernacular names of the former (plates) are generally misapplied to the latter (*Tin*). The names I have inserted above in the text are the correct names of the metal *Tin* or *Stannum.*

585. STRYCHNOS COLUBRINA, *Linn.*

Nàgamusaḍi నాగముసడి. (*Tel.*) Módira-káṇṇiram മോദിരകാഞ്ഞിരം. (*Malyal.*).

586. STRYCHNOS NUX VOMICA, *Linn.* (*Seeds of—Nux Vomica.*)

Iɡáráqí ' اذاراقي ; Ḵhánequl-kalb خانق الكلب (*Arab.*) Fulúse-máhi فلو س ما هي ; Qátilul-kalb قا تل الكلب ; Kochólah كچولہ . (*Pers.*) Kuchlá كچلا . (*Hind.*) Kuchlah كچلہ ; Kuchlé-ké-binj كچلى كے بينج . (*Duk.*) Eṭṭik-koṭṭai எட்டிக்கொட்டை. (*Tam.*) Mushṭi-vittulu ముష్టివిత్తులు ; Muṣhiḍi ముషిడి. (*Tel.*) Káṇṇi-rak-kuru കാഞ്ഞിരക്കുരു. (*Malyal.*) Mushṭi-bíjá ముష్టిబీజా. (*Can.*) Kuchlá. (*Beng.*) Mushṭi-bijam ; Vishamushṭi-bijam. (*Sans.*) Kuchla. (*Mah.*) Kuchlá. (*Guz.*) Goḍa-kaduru-aṭṭa *or* Koda-kaduru-aṭṭa. (*Cing.*) Khabóṅ. (*Bur.*).

From the similarity of the Burmese words Khabóṅ and Khamóṅ, they are confounded with each other in some books, and used synonymously in some others (Mason's Natural Productions of Burmah, &c.) It is a serious confusion, because the latter is the name of *S. potatorum*, the seeds of which are used in large doses as an emetic, &c. ; while the former is the name of *S. Nux vomica*, the nut of which, though a medicine in very minute doses, is highly poisonous in larger quantities.

An error very like the above is also found in the Materia Indica and Richardson's Dictionary, viz., the Arabic name of the nut of *Randia dumetorum* (*Jouzal-qai* جوز القي), which means *Emetic Nut*, is applied to *S. Nux vomica*.

Besides the above, the Telugu, Sanscrit and Tamil names *Katakamu, Kataka* and *Kadilikam*, &c., are used in some works for the nut of *S. N. vomica*, and in a few others for that of *S. potatorum*. This is a source of dangerous confusion, and I have therefore omitted the names from the text under both plants.

587. STRYCHNOS POTATORUM, *Linn. (Seeds of—Clearing-nut.)*

Nirmalí نرملي . (*Hind.*) Chil-binj چل بینج . (*Duk.*) Tétrán-koṭṭai தெற்றங்கொட்டை. (*Tam.*) Chilla-ginjalu చిల్లగింజలు. (*Tel.*) Tétrán-parala തെറ്റാമ്പരല ; Tétrán-koṭṭa തെറ്റാന്‍കൊട്ട. (*Malyal.*) Chilli-bijá ಚಿಲ್ಲಿಬೀಜ. (*Can.*) Nirmalí. (*Beng.*) Nirmali. (*Mah.*) Nir-maḷi. (*Guz.*) Ingini-aṭṭa. (*Cing.*) Khamón ; Kamou-yeki. (*Bur.*).

See the remarks under *S. Nux vomica.*

588. STYRAX. (*Solid Storax.*)

Iṣṭarak اصطرک ; Méaahe-yábisah ميعة يابسه . (*Arab.*).

589. SUCCINUM. (*Amber*).

Qarnul-baḥar قرن البحر ; Miṣbáḥurrúm مصباح الروم ; Inqiṭriyún انقطريون . (*Arab.*) Kahruba كهربا . (*Pers. and Hind.*) Kapúr كپور . (*Duk.*) Karpúra-maṇi கர்ப்பூரமணி. (*Tam.*) Karpúra-púsa కర్పూరపూస. (*Tel.*) Páyiṅ or Payeṅ. (*Bur.*).

The above Dukhni name *Kapúr* كپور is often confounded with *Kápúr* كاپور, which is the name of *Camphor* in the same language. See the remarks under *Camphor.*

590. SULPHUR.

Kibrít كبريت . (*Arab.*) Gógird گوگرد (*Pers.*) Gandhak گندهک . (*Hind.*) Gandak گندک . (*Duk.*) Gandakam கந்தகம். (*Tam.*) Gandhakam గంధకం. (*Tel.*) Gantakam ഗന്തകം. (*Malyal.*) Gandhaká ಗಂಧಕ. (*Can.*) Gandrok. (*Beng.*) Gandhakáha. (*Sans.*) Gandhak (*Mah.*) Gandhak. (*Guz.*) Gandakam. (*Cing.*) Kán. (*Bur.*).

There are several varieties of *Sulphur* sold in the bazaars of Southern India. With the exception of two, they are not, as far as I am aware of, known by any particular English name. Their native names are as follows :—

    a.   Stick or Roll Sulphur—*Bárút-ki-gandak* باروت کی گندک. (Duk.) *Bána-gandakam* பாணகந்தகம்; *Kuḷá-gandakam* குளா கந்தகம். (Tam.) *Bána-gandhakamu* బాణగంధకము; *Kuḷá-gandha-kamu* కుళాగంధకము. (Tel.).

    b.——*Amilahsár-gandhak* آمله سار گند هک. (Hind.) *Ánvlahsár-gandak* آ نوله سار گندک. (Duk.) *Nellik-káy-ganda-kam* நெல்லிக்காய்கந்தகம். (Tam.) *Nellikáya-gandhakam* నెల్లికాయగంధకం. (Tel.) *Ámalaka-gantakam* ആമലകഗന്തകം. (Malyal.) *Nelli-gandhakú* ನೆಲ್ಲಿಗಂಧಕ. (Can.) *Amlasa-gandrok.* (Beng.) *Ámalaka-gandhakaha.* (Sans.) *Araḷá-gandhak.* (Mah.) *Ámbaḷa-gandhak.* (Guz.) *Nelli-gandakam.* (Cing.).

    c.   Native Sulphur—*Kach-chí-gandak* کچّی گندک. (Duk.) *Pach-ch-ai-gandakam* பச்சைகந்தகம். (Tam.) *Pach-chi-gandha-kam* పచ్చిగంధకం. (Tel.) *Pach-cha-gantakam* പച്ചഗന്തകം. (Malyal.)

    d.——*Dál-gandak* دال گندک. (Duk.) *Paruppu-gandakam* பருப்புகந்தகம். (Tam.) *Pappu-gandhakamu* పప్పుగంధకము. (Tel.) *Paruppu-gantakam* പരുപഗന്തകം. (Malyal.)

The Stick or Roll Sulphur is the same what is described in some books under that name.

The second variety (*b*) occurs in crystalline pieces like those of Alum. It is of bright yellow color with a shade of green. It is the purest of all the varieties of Sulphur met with in the Indian bazaars, and the one generally used in medicine. Its color is some what like that of the ripe fruit of *Phyllanthus Emblica* (*Emblic Myrobalans*), hence the meaning of all its names.

The third (*c*) is the worst kind of Sulphur in the bazaar. It is very impure, hard, and generally whitish yellow in color. It corresponds with the 'Native Sulphur' mentioned in some books.

The fourth variety (*d*) is of the brightest yellow color. It is found in small pieces, some of which are thin and concave, some flat and irregular, and some round like a shot, &c. This Sulphur is named as *Dál-gandak*, &c., in allusion to the resemblance it bears in form and color to the half seeds (without husk) of *Cajanus Indicus,* sold in the bazaar under the name of *Dál* لال, &c.

In addition to the above, there is another substance called *Red Sulphur* in native languages, as follows :—

Kibrite-aḥmar كبريت ا حمر .. *(Arab.)* Gógirde-surkh گوگرد سرخ . *(Pers.)* *Lál-gandhak* لال گندھک . *(Hind.)* *Lál-gandak* لال گندک . *(Duk.)* Kózhit-talai-gandakam கோழித்தலைகந்தகம். *(Tam.)* Erra-gandhakamu ఎఱ్ఱగంధకము. *(Tel.)* Choranna-gantakam പൊവന്നഗന്തകം. *(Malyal.)* Kempu-gandhakú ಕೆಂಪುಗಂಧಕ- *(Can.)* Lál-gandrok *(Beng.)* Rqkta-gandhakaha. *(Sans.)* Támbaḍa-gandhak. *(Mah.)* Lál-gandhak. *(Guz.).*

This substance is found in small and highly crystalline, flat or irregular pieces, of purple or brick-dust color. I think it is a sulphuret of some metal, but what the latter is have not yet found out. This Sulphur or Sulphuret burns with a faint blue flame, and emits a slight smell of Sulphur*.

591. SYZIGIUM JAMBOLAUM, *D. C. (Fruit of.)*

Jámun حامن *(Hind.)* **Jámún** جامون . *(Duk.)* **Nágap-pazham** நாகப்பழம். *(Tam.)* **Nérédu-pandu** నేరేడు పండు. *(Tel.)* **Ṇa-valin-pazham** ഞാവളിൻപഴം ; **Návaḷ-pazham** ഞാവൽപഴം. *(Malyal.)* **Nerale-haṇṇu.** ನೇರಳೆ ಹಣ್ಣು. *(Can)* **Jám** ; **Jám-gúlá** ; **Kálá-jám.** *(Beng.)* **Jambú-phalam.** *(Sans.)* **Jámbaḷáphal.** *(Mah.)* **Jáanbu.** *(Guz.)* **Navva-geḍi.** *(Cing.)* **Ṣabi-e-si** *or* **Sabyezi.** *(Bur.).*

See the remarks under *Psidium pyriferum.*

---

* It is very frequently resorted to by native Alchymists, and is said to be the chief ingredient used by them in preparing the artificial gold and silver ?

T.

592. TACCA PINNATIFIDA, *Forsk.*

Bará-kandá بڑا كند ا . *(Duk.)*   Periya-karuṇaik-
kizhaṇgu பெரியக் கருணைக் கிழங்கு. *(Tam.)* Pedda-kanda-gaḍḍa
పెద్దకందగడ్డ. *(Tel.)* Ćhane-kizhaṇṇa ചനെകിഴങ്ങ . *(Malyal.)* Pánkhadé ; Touta. *(Bur.)*.

593. TAMARINDUS INDICA, *Linn.* *(Pod or Fruit of—Tamarind.)*

Tamare-hindi تمر هندي ; Ḥumar حمر ; Ḥúmar حومر ;
Ṣabárá صبا را . *(Arab.)* Anbalah انبله ا. *(Pers.)* Anbli
انبلي ا . *(Hind.)* Amli ا ملي ; Amlí-ká-bóṭ بوٹ كا ملي ;
Ambli امبلي . *(Duk.)*   Puḷiyam-pazham புளியம்பழம்.
(Tam.) Chinta-paṇḍu చింతపండు. *(Tel.)* Puḷiyam-pazham
പുളിയമ്പഴം. *(Malyal.)*   Huṇaṣhé-haṇṇu ಹುಣಸೆಹಣ್ಣು.
(Can.) Téñtúl ; Tintúri ; Ámli ; Tétai. *(Beng.)* Téntrání-
phalam. *(Sans.)* Chinch. *(Mah.)* Ámbli. *(Guz.)* Siyam-
bula. *(Cing.)* Magi. *(Bur.)*.

Chinchá جنجا is the Dukhni name of *Tamarind-stone* which
is also used in medicine by natives.

The red variety of Tamarind which is occasionally met with
in Southern India, is recognised by the addition of the word
red to its ordinary names.

594. TAMARIX GALLICA, *Linn.*

Aṣl اثل ; Ṭarfá طرفا . *(Arab.)* Gaz گز ; Daraķhte-
gaz درحت گز ; Shór-gaz شور گز . *(Pers.)* Jháv جهاو ·
(Hind. and Duk.) Áṭru-shavukku-maram அத்துசவுக்கு

மரம்; Kóṭa-ṣhavukku-maram கோடசவுக்குமரம்; Shiṛu-ṣhavukku-maram சிறுசவுக்குமரம். *(Tam.)* Éru-saru-mánu ఏరుసరుమాను; Shiri-saru-mánu శిరిసరుమాను. *(Tel.)* Jháv. *(Beng.)* Jháv-nu-jháḍa. *(Guz.).*

Át-alari is the Tamil name commonly in use in Southern India for *T. Gallica* or *T. Orientalis*, but the meaning of it is *the river Aḷari* or *Nerium odorum.* As the name is apt to be confounded with some variety of the latter very poisonous plant, I have omitted it from the text.

595. TAMARIX GALLICA, *Linn. (Galls of——Tamarix Galls.)*

Ṣamaratul-aṣl ثمرة الاثل; Ṣamaratuṭ-ṭarfá ثمرة الطرفا; Habbul-aṣl حب الاثل; Aaẓbah عذبه; Jazmázaj جزمازج *(Arab.)* Gazmázaj گزمازج; Gazmázak گزمازک; *(Hind.)* Gazmájú گزماز. *(Pers.)* Baṛi-máiṅ بڑيمائين . *(Hind.)* Baṛi-máí بڑيمانی . *(Duk.).*

There is a common notion in the bazaars of Madras, that the galls known under the above vernacular names are the produce of *Prosopis spicigera*, and not of any species of *Tamarix*, hence their Tamil and Telugu synonymes *Vannik-káy* வன்னிக்காய் and *Jimmi-káya* జిమ్మికాయ. I have examined the plant *(P. Spicigera)* in all seasons during the last 2 years, and found it to produce no galls whatever.

596. TAMARIX GALLICA, *Linn. (Manna of.)*

Gaz-anjabíṅ گز انجبين . *(Arab.)* Gaz-angabíṅ گز انگبين . *(Pers.).*

597. TAMARIX ORIENTALIS, *Vahl. Syn.* T. FURAS, *Ham.*

Aṣlul-aḥmar اثل الاحمر; Ṭarfáe-aḥmar طرفا احمر . *(Arab.)* Gaze-surkh گزسرخ . *(Pers.)* Lál-jháv لال جهاو . *(Hind. and Duk.)* Shivappu-áṭru-ṣhavukku-maram சிவப்

புஒற்றுசவுக்குமரம் ; Shivappu-kóṭa-ṣhavukku-maram இவப்
புடொாடசவுக்குமரம் ; Shivappu-ṣhiṛu-ṣhavukku-maram இவப்
புஇறுசவுக்குமரம். (*Tam.*) Erra-érusaru-mánu அஇயிகூஷௌ
கானு ; Erra-ṣhiri-saru-mánu அஇஷௌஷௌகானு. (*Tel.*) Rakta-
jháv. (*Beng.*) Lál-jháv-nu-jháḍa. (*Guz.*).

See the remarks in No. 594.

598. TAMARIX ORIENTALIS, *Vahl.* (*Galls of— Tamarix Galls.*)

Ṣamaratul-aṣal نَمرة الاثل ; Ḥabbul-aṣal حب الاثل
(*Arab.*) Gazmázak گزمازک ; Gazmázú گزمازو. (*Pers.*)
Chhóṭi-máiṅ جهوٹی مائین. (*Hind.*) Chhóṭi-máḷ
(*Duk.*).

See the remarks in No. 595.

599. TECTONA GRANDIS, *Linn.* (*Teak-tree.*)

Sáj ساج. (*Arab*) Sál سال. (*Pers.*) Sákhú ساکهو ;
Ságún ساگون. (*Hind.*) Sagván ساگوان. (*Duk.*) Tékku-
maram தேக்குமரம். (*Tam.*) Tóku-mánu தேகுமானு. (*Tel.*)
Tékka-maram തേക്കമരം. (*Malyal.*) Ságách. (*Guz.*).

See the remarks under *Shorea robusta.*

600. THEA. (*Tea.*)

Ṣáé صاى or Ṣáe صاء. (*Arab.*) Cháye چاے
(*Pers. and Hind.*) Chá چا. (*Duk.*) Té-ilai தேஇலை.
(*Tam.*) Téyáku தேயாகு. (*Tel.*) Chápátá ; Chánhá-
pátá. (*Beng.*) Chá. (*Guz.*) Té-kola. (*Cing.*) Laphe-
kháv. (*Bur.*).

601. TEPHROSIA PURPUREA, *Pers.*

Sarphóṅká سر پهونکا. (*Hind.*) Hunnáli هنالي ;
Janglí-kulthí جنگلي کلتهي. (*Duk.*) Koḷḷuk-káy-véḷai கொ

ஞ்கிகாட்டேலை. (*Tam.*) Vempali ౙంపరి. (*Tel.*) Ko-
zhiṇṇila കൊഴിഞ്ഞില. (*Malyal.*) Bon-nil-gáchh. (*Beng.*).

602. TEREBINTHINÆ OLEUM, (*Turpentine Oil*).

Dhónur-rátinaj دهن الراتينج ; *Dhónur-rátíyánáj*
روغن راتيانه . (*Arab.*) Róghane-rátíyánah دهن الراتيانج
(*Pers.*) Gandhá-barójé-ká-tél كندها بروجي كا تيل . (*Hind.*)
Gandah-féró́zé-ká-tél كند، فيروزے كا تيل ; Káfár-ká-
tailam كافور كا تيل . (*Duk.*) Káfúr-ká-tél كا فوركا ثيلم ;
Karppúrat-tailam கர்ப்பூரதைலம். (*Tam.*) Kar-púra-
tailam కర్పూరతైలం. (*Tel.*) Karppúra-tailam കർപ്പൂര
തൈലം. (*Malyal.*) Karapúradɔ-tailɔ̀ ಕರ್ಪೂರದ ತೈಲ.
(*Can.*) Kapúrér-tail. (*Beng.*) Karpúra-tailam. (*Sans.*)
Kápúrácha-tela. (*Mah.*) Kapúrnu-tél ; Tarpintan. (*Guz.*)
Kapuru-tel. (*Cing.*). Piyo-ṣí. (*Bur.*).

Except the Arabic and Persian, the meaning of all other
above names is *the oil of Camphor*, and they are applied to the
oil of *Turpentine* merely on account of the resemblance of its
smell to that of *Camphor*.

603. TERMINALIA BELLERICA, Roxb. (*Fruit of—Belleric Myrobalans*).

Balílaj بليلج (*Arab.*) Balílah بليله . (*Pers.*) *Bharlá* بهرلا ;
Bh-airá بهيرا ; *Bh-airah* بهيره . (*Hind.*) Balṛá بلڑا
Balḍá بلڈا . (*Duk.*) Tánṛik-káy தான்றிக்காய். (*Tam.*)
Tándra-káya తాండ్రకాయ. (*Tel.*) Táṇi താണി. (*Malyal.*)
Tári-káyi ತಾರಿಕಾಯಿ. (*Can.*) Bohorá. (*Beng.*) Béhadá.
(*Mah.*) Bulu. (*Cing.*) Phánkhá-si or Phángá-si. (*Bur.*).

604. TERMINALIA CATAPPA, Linn. (*Nut of—Indian Almond*).

Bádáme-hindí بادام هندى . (*Pers.*) Hindi-bádám
هندى بادام ; Janglí-bádám جنگلي بادام . (*Hind. and*

.(*Duk.*) Náttu-vádam-koṭṭai நாட்டுவாதம்கொட்டை. (*Tam.*)
Náttu-bádam-vittulu నాట్టుబాదంవిత్తులు. (*Tel.*) Náttu-bádam
നാട്ടുബാദം ; Koṭṭa-kuru കൊട്ടക്കുരു. (*Malyal.*) Nát-
bádámi ನಾಟ್ ಬಾದಾಮಿ. (*Can.*) Banglá-badám. (*Beng.*)
Inguḍi-*ph*alam ; Deṣha-bádámitte. (*Sans.*) Náṭ-bádám.
(*Mah.*) Náṭ-ni-badám. (*Guz.*) Koṭamba (*Cing.*).

The Malyalim names found in the Hortus Malabaricus
(Vol. IV., Tab. 3 and 4) are not generally recognisable. See
the remarks under *Amygdala* in page 46.

605. **TERMINALIA CHEBULA,** *Retz.* (*Fruit of—*
Chebulic myrobalans).

Halílaj هليلج ; Halílaje-aṣfar هليلج اصفر . (*Arab.*)
Halilah هليله ; Halílahe-zard هليلة زرد . (*Pers.*) Haṛ هڙ ;
Pílé-haṛ پيلى هڙ ; Haṛ-pílé هڙپيلى ; Harrá هڙڙا . *Hind.*)
Halṛá هلڙا ; Haṛlá هڙلا ; Pílá-halṛá پيلا هلڙا ; Halḍá هلڏا.
(*Duk.*) Kaḍuk-káy கடுக்காய் (*Tam.*) Karakkáya కరక్కాయ
లు. (*Tel.*) Kaṭukká కటుక్కా. (*Malyal.*) Aḷalc-káyi അള
ലെക്കായ. (*Can.*) Háritakí ; Hórá. (*Beng.*) Haritaki-
*ph*alam. (*Sans.*) Hiraḍá. (*Mah.*) Haṛle ; Pílo-haṛle.
(*Guz.*) Aralu. (*Cing.*).

When the young fruits of *T. chebula* are dried, they become
black or brown in colour, and the names applied to them are
different from those in use for the ripe fruits of the same plant.
They are—

Halílaje-asvad هليلة اسود . (*Arab.*) *Halilahe-siyáh* هليلة سياه
(*Pers.*) *Bál-haṛ* بال هڙ ; *Zangí-haṛ* زنگى هڙ ; *Kále-haṛ* كالى هڙ .
(*Hind.*) *Bál-halṛé* بال هلڙے ; *Zangí-halṛé* زنگي هلڙے ; *Kálé-halṛé*
كالى هلڙے . (*Duk.*) *Kaḍuk-káy pinji* கடுக்காய்பிஞ்சி. (*Tam.*)
Pinda-karak-káya పిండకరక్కాయ (*Tel.*) *Kaṭukká-pinji* కటుక్కా
పింజి. (*Malyal.*) *Aḷalc- pinda* അളെപിണ്ട. (*Can.*).

The following are the names of the gall-like excrescences found on the leaves and young branches of *T. chebula.*

Halṛé-ké-phúl هلرے کی پهول. *(Duk.) Kaduk-káy-pú* கடுக்காய்ப்பூ. *(Tam.) Karak-káya-puvvalu* கரக్కాయపువ్వలు. *(Tel.) Kaṭukká-pú* കടുക്കാപൂ. *(Malyal.) Aḷale-huvvu* ಅಳಲೆಹುವ್ವು. *(Can.) Haritaki-phúl* *(Beng.) Haritaki-pushpam. (Sans.) Hiraḍa-phúla.* *(Mah.) Harle-phúl; Pilv-harle-phúl. (Guz.) Aralu-mal (Cing.).*

These excrescenses are incorrectly considered as flowers of the plant; hence the meaning of the above names.

606. TERMINALIA GLABRA, *W. et A.*

Arjan ارجن ۱; Arjan-ká-péṛ ارجن کا پیڑ. *(Hind.)* Veḷḷai-maruda-maram வெள்ளைமருதமரம். *(Tam.)* Tella-maddi-cheṭṭu తెల్లమద్దిచెట్టు; Maddi-cheṭṭu మద్దిచెట్టు. *(Tel.)* Veḷḷa-maruta വെള്ളമരുത; Pulla-maruta പുള്ളമരുത. *(Malyal.).*

607. TERMINALIA TOMENTOSA, *W. et A.*

Ásan آسن. *(Hind.)* Janglí-karanj جنگلی کرنج. *(Duk.)* Karuppu-maruta-maram கருப்புமருதமரம். *(Tam.)* Nalla-maddi-cheṭṭu నల్లమద్దిచెట్టు. *(Tel.)* Karu-maruta കരുമരുത. *(Malyal.)* Áṣhán; Piyá-ṣhál. *(Beng.).*

608. TETRANTHRA ROXBURGHII, *Nees.* (Wood of.)

Magháṣe-hindí مغاث هندی. *(Arab.)* Kilz كلز. *(Pers.)* Maidá-lakṛi میدا لکڑی. *(Hind. and Duk.)* Muṣhaippé-yeṭṭi முஷைப்பேயெட்டி; Maidá-lakṭi மைதாலக்டி; Piṣhin-paṭṭai பிஷின்பட்டை. *(Tam.)* Naramámidi నరమామిడి; Meda మెడ *(Tel.)* Kukur-chitá. *(Beng.)* Maidá-lakaḍi. *(Mah.).*

609. THALICTRUM FOLIOLOSUM, *D. C.* *(Root of.)*

Pílí-jaṛí پیلي جڑي . *(Hind.)*.

610. THESPESIA POPULNEA, *Corr.*

Páras-pípal پارس پیپل . *(Hind.)* Páras-pippal پارس پپل . (*Duk.*) Púraṣha-maram புரசமரம். (*Tam.*) Gangarénu-cheṭṭu గంగరేను చెట్టు. *(Tel.)* Púvvaraṣha പൂവ്വരശ. *(Mal-yal.)* Pórash. *(Beng.)* Pársácha-jháḍa. *(Mah.)* Párasa-píplo. *(Guz.)* Gansurí-gahá. *(Cing.)*.

611. THEVETIA NERIIFOLIA, *Juss.* *(The Exile or yellow Oleander.)*

Pílá-kanér پیلی پہول کاکنیر ; Píle-*phúl*-ká-kanér پیلا کنیر . (*Duk.*) Pach-ch-ai-alari பச்சைஅலரி ; Tiruvách-chip-pú திருவாச்சிப்பு. *(Tam.)* Paçh-çha-gannéru పచ్చగన్నేరు. *(Tel.)* Pach-cha-arali പച്ചഅരലി. *(Malyal.)* Molamiyái-pán. *(Bur.)*.

612. TIARIDIUM INDICUM, *Lehm.*

Háthí-shúrá ہاتھي شورا . *(Hind.)* Bich-chhú-ké-dánk-ká-pattá بچھو کی ڈانک کا پتا . *(Duk.)* Tét-koḍukki தேட்கொடுக்கி. *(Tam.)* Télumaṇi-cheṭṭu తేలుమణిచెట్టు ; Nága-danti నాగదంతి. *(Tel.)* Tél-koṭukka തെൽകൊടുക്ക ; Teḷiyaṇṇi തെളിയണ്ണി. *(Malyal.)* Háti-shurá. *(Beng.)* Nágadanti. *(Sans.)*.

613. TINOSPORA CORDIFOLIA, *Miers.* **Syn. Cocculus cordifolius,** *D. C.* *(Gulancha.)*

Giló گلو . *(Arab.)* Gul-bél گل بیل . *(Pers.)* Gulanchá Gul-bél گل بیل . *(Hind.)* Gul-bél گل بیل . (*Duk.*) گلنچا ; Shindil-koḍi சிந்தில்கொடி. *(Tam.)* Tippa-tíge తిప్పతీగ ;

Gaḍúchi గడూచి. *(Tel.)*   Amruta അമൃത ; *Chiṭrámruta* ചിറാമൃത. *(Malyal.)* Amruta-baḷḷi അമൃతബള్ళి. *(Can.)* Gulanchá. *(Beng.)* Sómavalli ; Gaḍúchi. *(Sans.)* Gulavélí. *(Mah.)* Gulvél. *(Guz)* Rasakinda *(Cing.)* Ṣinza-manne or Singo-moné. *(Bur.)*.

An Extract of this plant, which is in common use of the Hakeems, is known by the following names : —

Satte-giló ست گلو . *(Pers. and Hind.)*   *Gul-bél-ká-sat* گل بیل کا ست : *(Duk.)* Shíndal-sharukkarai சிந்தல் சருக்கரை. *(Tam.)* Tippa-sattu తిప్పసత్తు. *(Tel.)* Palo. *(Beng.)*.

It looks like a flour and tastes bitter. It chiefly consists of an amylaceous substance with a bitter principle.

614. TODDALIA ACULEATA, *Pers. (Berries of.)*

Janglí-kálí-mirch جنگلي كا لي مرچ . *(Hind.)* Janglí-kálí-mirchí جنگلي كا لي مرچي . *(Duk.)* Miḷakaṛanai மிளகரணை. *(Tam.)* Mirapa-kándra మిరపకాండ్ర ; Konda-kasinda-cheṭṭu కొండకసిందచెట్టు. *(Tel.)* Toṭali തൊടലി ; Muḷaka-táṇi ഉളകതാണി ; Kákka-toṭali കാക്കതൊടലി. *(Malyal.)* Kudu-miriṣh. *(Cing.)*.

See the remarks under *Zizyphus jujuba.*

615. TODDY.

Tárí تا ري . *(Pers,)* Séndi سيندي ; Tárí تا ري . *(Hind. and Duk.)* Kaḷḷu கள்ளு. *(Tam.)* Kallu కల్లు. *(Tel.)* Henḍa ಹೆಂಡ *(Can.)* Rá. *(Cing.)*.

Toddy was originally derived from the Hindustani word *Tárí* تا ري, which is the name of the intoxicating juice obtained from *Palmyra Tree (Borassus flabelliformis)*; but according to the present usage, it is applied in English to every juice drawn from a plant and used as a drink.

There are many kinds of *Toddy* in India, and they are named according to the plants from which they are produced. The following are the names of some of the varieties of *Toddy* in Southern India :—

  a. Toddy of Borassus flabelliformis or Palmyra Toddy.— *Tári* تاري *(Pers.)* *Tári* تاڑی *(Hind. and Duk.)* *Panan-kallu* பனங்கள்ளு. *(Tam.)* *Táṭi-kallu* తాటికళ్లు. *(Tel.)* *Tat-rá.* *(Cing.).*

  b. Toddy of Phœnix Sylvestris.— *Séndhí* سیندهی. *(Hind.)* *Séndí* سیند ي. *(Duk.)* *Ích-chan-kallu* ஈச்சங்கள்ளு. *(Tam.)* *Íta-kallu* ఈతకళ్లు. *(Tel.)* *Indí-rá.* *(Cing.).*

  c. Toddy of Cocos nucifera or Cocoanut Toddy— *Tárye-nárgil* تاري ناريگیل. *(Pers.)* *Náréli* ناریلی. *(Hind.)* *Nárél-ki-tá i* ناریل کی تاڑی ; *Nárél-ki-séndi* ناریل کی سیندي. *(Duk.)* *Téngú-kallu* தெங்காகள்ளு ; *Tennan-kallu* தென்னங்கள்ளு. *(Tam.)* *Ṭenkáya-kallu* టెంకాయకళ్లు. *(Tel.)* *Pál-rá.* *(Cing.).*

  d. Toddy of Caryota Urens— *Múri-ki-séndí* ماڑی کی سیندي ; *Múri-ki-tári* ماڑی کی تاڑي. *(Duk.)* *Kúndar-panan-kallu* கூந்தற்பனங்கள்ளு. *(Tam.).*

  e. Toddy of Azadirachta Indica or Morgosa Toddy— *Nimb-ká-nírá* نیم کانیرا ; *Nim-ká-nírá* نیمب کا نیرا. *(Hind.)* *(Duk.)* *Véppan-kallu* வேப்பங்கள்ளு. *(Tam.)* *Vépa-kallu* వేపకళ్లు. *(Tel.)* *Nimba-rá.* *(Cing.).*

  f. Toddy of Ficus glomerata— *Gullér-ká-nírá* گلیر کا نیرا. *(Hind.)* *Gullar-ká-nírá* گلر کانیر ا. *(Duk.)* *Attik kallu* அத்திக்கள்ளு. *(Tam.)* *Atti-kallu* అత్తికళ్లు. *(Tel.)* *Atti-rá.* *(Cing.).*

The Hindustani and Dukhni name *Nírá* نیرا is applied to those *Toddies* which do not possess intoxication, and also to all *Toddies* when they are fresh and not yet began to ferment. For example, *Tari-ká-nírá* تاڑي کا نیرا is the *Palmyra Toddy* before it begins to ferment, in which condition it is found early in the morning before the sun-rise.

616. TRAPA BISPINOSA, *Roxb. (Fruit of.)*

Singárá سنگاڑا ; Singhárah سنگھاڑہ ; Páni-*phal* یانی پھل . *(Hind. and Duk.)* Panri-mottai பன்றிமொட்டை ; Panni-móndán-kizhangu பண்ணிமோந்தான்கிழங்கு. *(Tam.)* Pandi-gadda పంది గడ్డ ; Parike-gadda పరికెగడ్డ. *(Tel.)* Páni-*phal. (Beng.).*

617. TRAGACANTHA. *(Tragacanth or Gum Tragacanth.)*

Kaşérá كثيرا ; Şamaghul-qaşşád صمغ القتاد or Samaghul-qattád صمغ القتاد . *(Arab.)* Katérá كتيرا ; Zól zadah زول زدہ . *(Pers.)* Katérá كتيرا ; Katérá-gónd كتيراگوند . *(Hind. and Duk.)*

In the bazaars of S. India, *Tragacanth* is generally and incorrectly known as the *gum of Almond;* whence its Tamil and Telugu synonymes, *Búdam-pişhin* பாதம்பிசின் and *Búdam-banka* బాదంబంక.

618. TREAK FAROOK.

Tiryáqul-fárúq تریاق الفاروق or Tiryáqe-fárúq . *(Arab.)* Tiryáke-fárúq تریاق فاروق ; Tiryáqe-akber تریاق اکبر . *(Pers.)* Tiryáqe-fárúq تریاک فاروق . *(Hind.)* Tiryá-fárúq تریا فاروق . *(Duk.).*

619. TRIBULUS LANUGINOSUS, *Linn.*

Bastítáj بستیتاج ; Khasak خسک . *(Arab.)* Kháre-khasak خار خسک . *(Pers.)* Gókhrú گوکھرو . *(Hind.)* Ghókrú گھوکرو . *(Duk.)* Nerunji நெருஞ்சி. *(Tam.)* Palléru-mullu పళ్ళేరుముళ్ళు ; *Chiru-palléru* చిరుపళ్ళేరు. *(Tel.)* Nerinjil നെരിഞ്ഞില്‍. *(Malyal.)* Negalu-gidi ನೆಗಲುಗಿಡಿ. *(Can.)* Vanasrangátá ; Gokhurhú ; Trikantaka-vallí. *(Sans.)* Ghókarú ; Charátté. *(Mah.)* Gókhru. *(Guz.)* Neranchi or Neranji. *(Cing.)* Sule-anén. *(Bur.).*

620. TRICHOSANTHES CORDATA, *Roxb.*

621. TRICHOSANTHES CUCUMERINA, *Linn.*

Jangli-chi-chóndá جنگلي چچوند ا . *(Hind.)* Káttup-pépuḍal காட்டுப்பெய்புடல்; Péy-puḍal பேய்புடல். *(Tam.)* Aḍavi-poṭla అడవిపొట్ల; Chédu-poṭla చేదుపొట్ల; Paṭólamu పటోలము. *(Tel.)* Kaippam-paṭólam കൈപ്പംപടോലം; Paṭavaḷam പടവളം; Pépaṭolam പെപടോലം. *(Malyal.)* Beṭṭada-paḍavalá ಬೆಟ್ಟದ ಪಡವಲ. *(Can.)* Ban-chi-changá. *(Beng.)* Ráṇácha-paḍavaḷi. *(Mah.)* Tó-pelen-moye. *(Bur.)*.

622. TRICHOSANTHES NERVIFOLIA, *Linn.*

Syn. T. DIOICA, *Roxb.*

Parvar پرور; Palval پاول . *(Hind.)* Kombu-puḍalai கொம்புபுடலை. *(Tam.)* Kommu-poṭla కొమ్ముపొట్ల. *(Tel.)* Paṭólam പടോലം. *(Malyal)* Potól. *(Beng.)*.

623. TRICHOSANTHES PALMATA, *Roxb.*

Anbaghól نبغو ل ا; Ḥanẓale-aḥmar حنظل احمر . *(Arab.)* Ḥanẓale-surkh حنظل سرخ . *(Pers.)* Lál-indráyan لال اندراون ; لال اندراين . *(Hind.)* Lál-indrávan Gúdá-pandú گودا پندرو . *(Duk.)* Koraṭṭai கொரட்டை; Shavari-pazham சவரிபழம். *(Tam.)* Avvagúda-pandu అవ్వగూడపండు; Ábuvva అబువ్వ. *(Tel.)* Avagude-haṇṇu ಅವಗುಡೆಹಣ್ಣು. *(Can)* Kavanḍala. *(Mah.)* Titta-hoṅdala. *(Cing.)*.

624. TRIGONELLA FŒNUM-GRÆCUM, *Roxb.* (Seeds of.)

Ḥulbah حلبه . *(Arab.)* Shanbalíd شنبليد; Shamlít شمليت; Shamlíz شمليز . *(Pers.)* Méthí ميتهي . *(Hind. and Duk.)* Vendáyam வெந்தயம். *(Tam.)* Mentulu మెం

கூல. *(Tel.)* Uluva உளுவ ; Ventayam വെന്തയം. *(Malyal.)* Ménthyá ಮೆಂಥ್ಯ. *(Can.)* Méthi. *(Beng.)* Méthí. *(Sans.)* Méthí. *(Mah.)* Méthí. *(Guz)* Uluva. *(Cing.)* Pe-nán-ṭa-zi. *(Bur.)*.

625. TRITICUM VULGARE. *Vill. (Seeds or Grains of—Wheat.)*

Ḥinṭah حنطه . *(Arab.)* Gandum گندم . *(Pers)* Géhún گیهوں . *(Hind.)* Gehún گېهوں . *(Duk.)* Gódumai கோதுமை. *(Tam.)* Gódumulu గోధుమలు. *(Tel.)* Kótanpam കോതമ്പം. *(Malyal.)* Gódhi ಗೋಧಿ. *(Can.)* Giún. *(Beng.)* Yavá. *(Sans.)* Gahung. *(Mah.)* Ghavum. *(Guz.)* Tiringu. *(Cing.)* Giyonsabú. *(Bur.)*.

626. TYLOPHORA ASTHMATICA, *W. et A.* *(Country Ipecacuanha plant.)*

Janglí-pikván جنگلي پكوان ; Antamúl انتمول . *(Hind.)* Pit-káṛi پت کاڑي . *(Duk.)* Nach-churuppán நச்சுருப் பான் ; Naṇja-murich-chán நஞ்சமுரிச்சான் ; Náy-pálai நாய் பாலை ; Péyp-pálai பேய்ப்பாலை. *(Tam.)* Verri-pála వెఱ్ఱిపాల ; Kukka-pála కుక్కపాల. *(Tel.)* Valli-pála വള്ളിപ്പാല. *(Malyal.)* Anto-mul. *(Beng.)* Bin-nuga. *(Cing.)*.

See the remarks under *Hemidesmus Indicus.*

627. TYPHONIUM ORIXENSE, *Schott.*

Karuṇaik-kizhaṇgu கருணைக்கிழங்கு ; Kár-karuṇaik-kizhaṇgu கார்கருணைக்கிழங்கு. *(Tam.)* Kanda-gadda కంద గడ్డ ; Durada-kanda-gadda దురదకందగడ్డ. *(Tel.)* Chéna ചേന. *(Malyal.)* Ghéṭ-kochu. *(Beng.)*.

U

628. UNCARIA GAMBIR, *Roxb.* (*Wood of*)

Ankuḍu-karra అంకుడుకఱ్ఱ. (*Tel.*)   Gambir. (*Malay.*)

629. URGINEA INDICA, *Kunth.* Syn. Scilla indica, *Roxb.* (*Bulb of—Indian Squill.*)

Isqíle-hindí سقيل هندي ا ; Aanṣale-hindí عنصل هندي ; Baṣlul-fáre-hindí بصل الفار هندي ; Baṣlul-barre-hindí بصل البر هندي . (*Arab.*)   Piyáze-dashtié-hindí پياز دشتئ هندى ; Piyáze-móshe-hindí پياز موش هندى . (*Pers.*)   Kándá كاندا ; Jangli-piyáz جنگلي پياز . (*Hind.*)   Jangli-piyáz جنگلي پياز ; Kandrá كندرا . (*Duk.*)   Nari-veṇgáyam நரிவெங்காயம். (*Tam.*)   Nakka-vulli-gaḍḍa నక్కఉల్లిగడ్డ. (*Tel.*)   Káṭṭulli കാട്ടുള്ളി. (*Malyal.*)   Aḍavi-irulli ಅಡವಿಇರುಳ್ಳಿ. (*Can.*)   Jongli-piaáj ; Ban-piaáj. (*Beng.*)   Vana-palándam. (*Sans.*)   Ráṇácha-kándé. (*Mah.*)   Jangli-kánda. (*Guz.*)   Val-lúnú. (*Cing.*)   To-keṣúṅ ; Tankaet-tva. (*Bur.*).

The Arabic and Persian names applied in books to the bulb of both *U. Indica* (*Indian Squill*) and *U. Scilla* (*Squill*) are generally the same; but to render them correctly applicable to the former the affix *Country* or *Indian* should be added to each of them.

Kándá is correctly the Hindustani name of *Indian Squill,* but is found applied in several books to *Onion.*

In some works (Materia Indica, &c.,) *Ledebouria hyacinth-oides* is confounded, under the name of *Erythronium Indicum* (*Rott.*), with *Scilla* (*Urginea) Indica,* and the vernacular names of the latter are applied to the former. These names, however, will not be properly applicable to *L. hyacinthoides* unless the prefix *small* or *lesser* is added to them, as is the case with the names under that plant in this Catalogue.

There is the same confusion about these drugs in the bazaar, where they are generally sold under the same names. But there is enough of difference between them to distinguish them, as follows:—

<table>
<tr><td>

Bulb of U. Indica.

1. It is a *tunicated* bulb, consisting of fleshy coats, which enclose each other completely in a concentric manner; roundish-ovate, brownish white or yellowish grey in color externally.

</td><td>

Bulb of *L. hyacinthoides.*

1. It is a *scaly* bulb, made of very smooth and fleshy scales, which are so imbricated that they might be mistaken for coats if not carefully examined; roundish-ovate generally, sometimes slightly compressed on sides; and whitish brown externally.

</td></tr>
<tr><td>

2. Generally about the size of a small orange, and some times as big as a pomegranate.

</td><td>

2. Generally about the size of a large nutmeg, and very seldom attains the size of a lime.

</td></tr>
<tr><td>

3. It is generally a simple bulb.

</td><td>

3. Though it is not a multiple bulb like *Garlic*, yet 2 or 3 smaller bulbs often unite together at the base, and are inclosed in a thin membranous coat.

</td></tr>
<tr><td>

4. Taste slightly bitter.

</td><td>

4. Taste very bitter and slightly acrid.

</td></tr>
<tr><td>

5. However small the bulb is, the rudiment or base of the leaves, which is generally found in it, is 1 or 1½ inches in breadth.

</td><td>

5. However large the bulb is, the base of the leaves (or the dry leaves themselves, which are generally found attached to it), is not more than 1 or 2 lines in breadth.

</td></tr>
</table>

6. It is very seldom to find this bulb to have the remains of the *scape*. When it does so, the latter is about an inch in breadth, and 4 or 5 lines in thickness.

7. When dug out, these bulbs are generally found in clusters, each of which contains many of various size. The mother-bulb, which is the largest, is in the centre and surrounded by many smaller ones. In this condition, some of the smaller bulbs are much compressed on 2 or 3 sides from the pressure of others.

6. In addition to the leaves, this bulb occasionally contains the dry *scape* in its centre, which is about the thickness of a broom-stick.

7. I have always found these bulbs growing singly. They are probably propogated by seeds.

L. hyacinthoides is a better substitute for the *Officinal Squill* than *U. Indica*, and it is particularly so if selected soon after it has flowered. If cut into slices and dried, it is yellowish white or pale grey, slightly translucent, scentless, and very bitter. When recently dried, it bears some resemblance to the *Vermiform Tragacanth* of the European shops.

U. Indica possesses little or no action when it is old and large, as is generally found in the bazaar. To ensure its good action, it should either be very young and not larger than a lime in size, or its innermost coats alone should be selected. The outer coats are quite useless.

630. UVÆ, *Syn.* Uvæ passæ. *(Raisins.)*

Zabíb زبيب ; Mavéz مويز ; Monaqqá منقّي . *(Arab.)*
Bédánah بيد ا نه ; Angúre-*khushk* خشکـ انگور ا . *(Pers.)*
Kishmish كشمش ; Monaqqá منقّي ; Bédánah بيدأنه ; Sákhé-
angúr سوكهـ انگور . *(Hind.)* Monaqqá منقّي ; Bédánah
ايدا نه : . *(Duk.)* Ularnda-dirákshap-pazham உலர்ந்த

செபபழம். *(Tam.)* Endu-draksha-pandu ఎందుద్రాక్షపండు; Dipa-draksha-pandu దీపద్రాక్షపండు; Sanna-draksha-pandu సన్నద్రాక్షపండు. *(Tel.)* Muntirinnap-pazham മുന്തിരിങ്ങപ്പഴം; Unanniya-muntirinnap-pazham ഉണങ്ങിയമുന്തിരിങ്ങപ്പഴം. *(Malyal.)* Dipa-drakshi ದೀಪದ್ರಾಕ್ಷಿ. *(Can.)* Kismis; Monakkha; Saska-drakhya. *(Beng.)* Kismis; Kismis-drak. *(Guz.)* Vellich-cha-mudra-palam; Vellich-cha-mudra-ka. *(Cing.)* Ṣabí-ṣí, Ṣabyá-ṣí *or* Ṭabí-ti. *(Bur.).*

See the remarks under *Pyrus Cydonia.*

V.

631. VALERIANÆ RADIX. *(Valerian Root.)*

Sunbuluṭṭib سنبل الطيب; Sunbulul-aaṣáfír سنبل العصافير *(Arab.)* Sunbuluṭṭíb سنبل ا لطيب. *(Pers.)* Viláyati-jaṭámásí ولا يتي با ل جهڑ; Viláyati-búlchar ولا يتي جٹا ماسي *(Hind.)* Viláyati-*j*haṭámáṅsí ولا يتي جهٹاماننسي. *(Duk.).*

In Arabic and Persian, *Sunbul* سنبل is the name of *Valerian Root* and also of the root of *Nardostachys Jatamansi;* but in Dukhni, it is often applied to *White Arsenic (Arsenicum Album).* As this confusion might lead to some serious errors, I have omitted the name *(Sunbul)* from the text under all these drugs.

632. VALERIANA HARDWICKII, *Wall.*

633. VATERIA INDICA, *Linn. (Resin of—Piny or White Dammer.)*

Suféd-ḍámar سفيد ڌامر *(Hind.)* Vellai-kunṛikam வெள்ளைகுன்றிகம்; Vellai-ḍámar வெள்ளைடாமர். *(Tam.)* Dúpa-dámaru దూపదామరు; Tella-dámaru తెల్లదామరు. *(Tel.)*

Payana പയന; Vella-kunturukkam വെള്ളകന്തുരുക്കം
(*Malyal.*). Hal; Hal-dumula. (*Cing*).

634. VATICA TUMBUGAIA, *W. et A.* (*Resin of.*)

Kálá-ḍamar كالا دمر. (*Hind. and Duk.*) Karuppu-
ḍamar கருப்புடாமர். (*Tam.*) Nalla-dámaru నల్లదామరు. (*Tel.*)
Kara-kundurukkam കരകന്തുരുക്കം. (*Malyal.*).

635. VERNONIA ANTHELMINTICA, *Willd.* (*Seeds of.*)

Aṭarílál آطريلال; Itrílál اتريلا. (*Arab. and Pers.*)
Sómráj سومراج; Bukchí بكچي. (*Hind.*) Káli-zírí
كروي زيري; Káli-jírí كالي جيري; Karví-ziri كالي زيري
(*Duk.*) Káṭṭu ṣhíragam காட்டுசீரகம். (*Tam.*) Aḍavi-
jilakara అడవిజిలకఱ; Visha-kanṭa-kálu విషకంటకాలు. (*Tel.*)
Káṭṭu-jirakam കാട്ടുജീരകം. (*Malyal.*) Kádu-jirage ಕಾಡು
ಜೀರಗ. (*Can.*) Somráj. (*Beng.*) Aṭaví-jírakaha. (*Sans.*)
Ráṇácha-jíré. (*Mah.*) Káli-jírí; Kaḍvo-jíri. (*Guz.*) Sanni-
náegam; Sanni-náͦsang. (*Cing.*).

See the remarks under *Nigella Indica* with respect to the
Dukhni name *Káli-zírí*, &c.

636. VILLARSIA INDICA, *Vent.*

Kamúdní كمودني; Kamúdí كمودي. (*Hind.*) Baṛá-
antargangá بڑا انترگنگا. (*Duk.*) Periya-ákáṣha-támarai
பெரியஆகாசதாமரை. (*Tam.*) Pedda-ákáṣha-támara పెద్ద
ఆకాశతామర; Pedda-antara-támara పెద్దఅంతరతామర. (*Tel.*)
Nírámpal നീരാമ്പൽ; Naiͭtalánpal നൈയ്തലാമ്പൽ.
(*Malyal.*) Antara-gange ಅಂತರಗಂಗೆ. (*Can.*) Baṛa-pán-
chúlí. (*Beng.*).

637. VINUM. *(Fermented juice of grapes—Wine or Port Wine).*

Khamr خمر ; Sharáb شراب . *(Arab.)* Mai مي ; Bádah باده ; Mul مل . *(Pers.)* Angúri-sharáb انگوري شراب. *(Hind. and Duk.)* Diráksha-shárayam சராக்ஷசாருயம். *(Tam.)* Dráksha-sáráyi ராక்ஷஸாராயి ; Dráksha-rasam ராக்ஷரஸம். *(Tel.)* Muntiriṇṇap-pazham-cháráyam ഉന്തിരി ങ്ങപ്പഴംചാരായം. *(Malyal.)* Drákh-nu dáru. *(Guz.)* Múdira-ká-araku ; Múdiraka-pána. *(Cing.).*

638. VIOLA ODORATA,————.

Banafshaj بنفشج Banafsaj بنفسج . *(Arab.)* Banafshah بنفشه . *(Pers. Hind. and Duk.)* Váyileṭṭu வாயிலெட்டு. *(Tam.)* Bonosá. *(Beng.)* Baga-baṇósá. *(Mah.)* Banaphsá. *(Guz.).*

639. VIOLA SUFFRUTICOSA, *Linn.*

Ratan-purs رتن پرس . *(Hind.)* Ratan-purus رتن پرس . *(Duk.)* Órilait-támarai ஓரிலைத்தாமரை. *(Tam.)* Kéoki-biṇ. *(Bur.).*

640. VISCUM MONOICUM, *Roxb.*

Kuchlé-ká-malang کچلےکاملنگ . *(Hind.)* Kuchlé-kí-soukan کچلے کی سوکن . *(Duk.)* Pullurivi புல்லுரிவி ; Pullúri புல்லூரி. *(Tam.)* Pullurivi పుల్లురివి. *(Tel.).*

The above Tamil and Telugu names are applied in Madras to any small plant which grows on another plant, without much discretion, and they are also misapplied occasionally to *Cassyta filiformis* and another plant. They ought to be, however, restricted to *V. monoicum.*

641. VITEX NEGUNDO, *Linn.*

Aslaq ا ثلق ; Fanjangasht فنجنگشت ; Zúkhamsatil-ouráq ذ و خمسة الا و ر ا ق ; Zúkhamsate-asábeạ ذوخمسةا صابع . (*Arab.*) Panj-angusht پنج انگشت ; Banj-angasht' بنجنگشت ; Sisbán سيسبان . (*Pers.*) Sanbhálú سنبهالو ; Nirgandi نرگنڈي . (*Hind.*) Shanbáli شنبا لي ; Shambáli شمبا لي ; Shamálú شمالو . (*Duk.*) Vellai-noch-chi வெள்ளைநொச்சி ; Noch-chi நொச்சி. (*Tam.*) Tella-vávili తెల్లవావిలి ; Vávili వావిలి. (*Tel.*) Vella-noch-chi വെള്ളനൊച്ചി ; Vel-noch-chi വെൽനൊച്ചി ; Noch-chi നൊച്ചി. (*Malyal.*) Lakki-gidá ಲಕ್ಕಿಗಿಡ. (*Can.*) Nishindá ; Sámálú. (*Beng.*) Shvéta-surasa-vrikshaha. (*Sans.*) Nikka ; Sudu-nikka. (*Cing.*) Kiyou-bhán-biṇ *or* Kiyubán-biṇ. (*Bur.*).

See the remarks under the next plant.

642. VITEX TRIFOLIA, *Linn.*

Aslaqe-ábi ا ثلق آ بي . (*Arab.*) Panj-angushte-ábi پنج انگشت آبي ; Banj-angashte-ábi بنجنگشت آبي . (*Pers.*) Páni-ki-sanbhálú پاني کي سنبهالو سفيدسنبهالو ; Sufed-sanbhálú . (*Hind.*) Páni-ki-shanbáli پاني کي شنبالى ; Ujli-shanbáli ا جلي شنبا لى . (*Duk.*) Nír-noch-chi நீ:நொச்சி ; Shiru-noch-chi சிருநொச்சி. (*Tam.*) Niru-vávili నీరువావిలి ; Shiru-vávili శిరువావిలి. (*Tel.*) Nír-noch-chi നീർനൊച്ചി. (*Mal-yal.*) Níra-lakki-gidá ನೀರಲಕ್ಕಿಗಿಡ. (*Can.*) Páni-samálú. (*Beng.*) Surasa-vrikshaha ; Jala-nirgundi. (*Sans.*) Vaturu-nikka. (*Cing.*) Kiyoubhán-biṇ ; Ye-kiyubán-biṇ. (*Bur.*).

The native synonymes of *V. negundo* and *V. trifolia* are confounded with each other, particularly with respect to the words *white* and *water*, which are applicable to the latter only. See the remarks under *Justicia Gendarussa.*

643. VITIS INDICA, *Linn.*

Jangli-angúr جنگلي انگور . *(Duk.)* Shembára-valli
వొంబరవళ్లి. *(Tel.)* Chempára-valli ചെമ്പാരവള്ളി. *(Malyal.)* Ámoluká. *(Beng.).*

644. VITIS QUADRANGULARIS. *Wall.*

Hár-jórá ہا رجورا ; Had-jórá ھڈ جورا ; Nallar نلر .
(Hind.) Nallér نلير . *(Duk.)* Pirandai பிரண்டை. *(Tam.)*
Nalleru నల్లేరు. *(Tel.)* Verantá വെരണ്ട ; Piranta പി
രണ്ട. *(Malyal.)* Mangaruli ಮಂಗರೂಱ. *(Can.)* Hórjórá ;
Hárbhángá. *(Beng.)* Vajra-valli. *(Sans.)* Chodhári. *(Guz.)*
Shazávn-lese. *(Bur.).*

645. VITIS VINIFERA, *Linn.* (*Fruits of—Grapes.*)

Ainab عنب *or* Aanab عنب . *(Arab.)* Angúr انگور .
(Pers.) Angúr انگور ; Dák داک ; Dákh داکه . *(Hind.)*
Angúr انگور ; Dák ڈاک . *(Duk.)* Diráksha-pazham திராக்ஷ
பழம் ; Kodi-mundirip-pazham கொடிமுந்திரிப்பழம். *(Tam.)*
Dráksha-pandu ద్రాక్షపండు; Góstini-pandu గోస్తినిపండు. *(Tel.)*
Muntirinnap-pazham മുന്തിരിങ്ങപ്പഴം ; Pach-cha-muntirin-
nap-pazham പച്ചമുന്തിരിങ്ങപ്പഴം. *(Malyal.)* Drákshi-
hannu ದ್ರಾಕ್ಷಿಹಣ್ಣು. *(Can.)* Drakhyá ; Ángur. *(Beng.)*
Dráksha-phalam. *(Sans.)* Dráksha. *(Mah.)* Drákh. *(Guz.)*
Mudra-palam ; Mudraká. *(Cing.)* Sabí-sí, Sabyá-sí *or* Tabí-
ti. *(Bur.).*

The Hindustani and Dukhni names *Dák* and *Dák* are properly the general names of *Grapes*; but are commonly applied
in many places of India to only one variety of them, which is
black, and very large and long. The correct name for the
latter is *Habshí-angúr* حبشي انگور .

For the names of *Port wine*, *Wine vinegar*, and *Raisins*, see under *Vinum*, *Acetum*, and *Uvæ*.

646. VIVERRA ZIBETHA, *Linn.* (*Zibeth, or Zibeth Civet Cat.*)

Mushk-billí مشک بلی . (*Hind.*)   Mushak-billi or Mushaq-billi مشق بلي . (*Duk.*) مشکـبلي

647. VIVERRA ZIBETHA, *Linn.* (*Inspissated and dried Secretion of.*)

Billi-ká-mushk بلی کاـمشک . (*Hind.*).

W.

648. WITHANIA (PUNEERIA) COAGULANS, *Dunal.*

649. WITHANIA (PHYSALIS) SOMNIFERA, *Dunal.*

} *Seeds of.*

Habbul-káknaje-hindí حب الكا كنج هندي . (*Arab.*) Tukhme-káknáje-hindí تخم کاکنج هندي . (*Pers.*) Punir-ké-bij پنیر کی بینج . (*Hind.*)   Hindí-káknaj-ké-bínj هندي كاكنج کی بینج ; Nát-kí-asgand-ké-binj نات کی اسگند کے بینج . (*Duk.*) Amukkurá-virai அமுக்குறாவிதை. (*Tam.*) Pennéru-gadda-vittulu పెన్నేరుగడ్డవిత్తులు. (*Tel.*) Ashvaganda-bichí. (*Beng.*).

Káknaj کا کنج and *Asgand* اسگند are the names of another drug not indigenous to India, and therefore cannot be correctly applicable to the above seeds without the addition of the word *Indian* or *Country*.

650. WRIGHTIA TINCTORIA, *R. Br. (Seeds of.)*

Lasánul-aaṣáfir لسان العصا فير ; Laṣánul-aaṣáfirul-ḥaló لسان العصا فير الحلو . *(Arab.)* Indarjou الندرجو ; Indar-jouve-shírín اندرجوشيرين ; Tukhme-ahar تخم اهر ; Tukhme-ahare-shírín تخم اهرشيرين ; Zabáne-kunja*shk* زبان كنجبشك ; Zabáne-kunja*shke*-shírín زبان كنجبشك شيرين . *(Pers.)* Indarjou الندرجو ; Miṭhú indarjou ميتها الندرجو . *(Hind. and Duk.)* Veṭpá-lariṣhi வெட்பாலரிஷி ; Veṭpála-virai வெட்பாலவிளை. *(Tam.)* Koḍiṣha-vittulu కొడిశవిత్తులు ; Kalinga-vittulu కళింగవిత్తులు. *(Tel.)* Koṭakappála-vitta കൊടകപ്പാലവിത്ത. *(Malyal.)* Indarjou. *(Beng.)* Indrajou. *(Mah.)* Indarjou. *(Guz.)* Vepál-arsi ; Vepál-pál. *(Cing.)*

There are two kinds of *Indar-jou* اندر جو in the bazaar, *sweet* and *bitter*. According to some native works and many native practitioners and druggists, they are the produce of one and the same plant,. viz., *W. tinctoria;* but this is contrary to the fact. *W. tinctoria* is found in several gardens of Madras, and it always produces only one kind of seeds which are the *sweet Indar-jou.* The *bitter Indar-jou* is the produce of *Holarrhena antidysenterica* and *H. pubescens,* whose vernacular names will be found under the head of those plants*.

---

* The plant *Wrightia tinctoria,* which was until lately considered as *W. antidysenterica,* and which, as I have just stated above, is found in several gardens at Madras, quite corresponds with the distinctions pointed out by Dr. Wight in his able remarks in the Pharmacopœia of India, pages 456 and 457. In addition to these, there is another, which although not strictly a botanical distinction, it is a very practical one, viz., the taste of the seeds. The seeds of *W. tinctoria,* if not distinctly sweet, are quite free from bitterness ; while those of *Holarrhena antidysenterica* and *H. pubescens* are very bitter.

The seeds of *W. tinctoria,* which constitutes the sweet variety of *Indar-jou* in the bazaar, are not distinctly sweet, as they are supposed to be or as their names imply ; but being quite free from bitterness, they are named *Sweet Indar-jou* only to distinguish them from the bitter variety (*Bitter Indar-jou*), which is actually very bitter.

X.

651.   XANTHOCHYMUS PICTORIUS, *Roxb.*

Tamál-*chedi* தமால்செடி ; *Chíkati-*maram சீகழிமரம். *(Tam.)* Tamála-*chettu* తమాలచెట్టు ; *Chíkati-*mánu చీకటిమాను. *(Tel.).* Goraka *or* Gorakka. *(Cing.).*

652.   XYLOCARPUS GRANATUM, *Kon.*

Pórus*h.* *(Beng.)* Kadól. *(Cing.).*

The Burmese name given to this plant in Mason's Natural Productions of Burmah is more applicable to *Lodoicea Sechellarum* or *the sea-cocoanut plant.*

The Bengali name in the text is from the Hortus Suburbanus Calcuttensis, which is of rather doubtful acceptation, and as it is given in that work it signifies *a man.*

653.   XYRIS INDICA, *Linn.*

Koc*h*-*chilittip*-pullu கொச்சிலித்திப்புல்லு. *(Tam.)* Koch-*chilach*-*chipulla* കൊച്ചിലച്ചിപുല്ല. *(Malyal.)* Dábi-dúbi. *(Beng.).*

The literal meaning of the above Bengali name, which is from the Hortus Suburbanus Calcuttensis, is *champoing,* and it is not therefore, generally recognised as the name of any plant.

Z.

654. ZEA MAYS, *Linn. (Seeds of—Maize or Indian Corn.)*

Khandarús خندروس ; Khálávan خالاون ; Zurratul-makkah ذرة المكه ; Hintahe-rúmi حنطه رومي . *(Arab.)* Gandume-makkah گندم مكه ; Khóshahe-makki خوشه مكي . *(Pers.)* Makkah-javár مكه جوار ; Makkah-*bhuttah* مكه بهته . *(Hind.)* Makkah-jári مكه جارى . *(Duk.)* Makká-shólam மக்காசோளம். *(Tam.)* Makká-zonnalu మక్కాజొన్నలు. *(Tel.)* Chólam ചോളം. *(Malyal.)* Bhútá ; Makká-javár ; Makká-*bhútá*. *(Beng.)* Piyaanbu. *(Bur.)*.

655. ZINCI CARBONAS. *(Impure Carbonate of Zinc, or Calamine.)*

656. ZINCI SULPHAS. *(Sulphate of Zinc or White Vitriol.)*

Suféd-tútah سفيد توته ; Suféd-*thútháh* سفيد تهوتها . *(Hind.)* Suféd-tuttá سفيد تتا . *(Duk.)* Vellai-tuttam வெள்ளைத்துத்தம் ; Pál-tuttam பால்துத்தம். *(Tam.)* Pálu-tuttam పాలుత్తుం. *(Tel.)* Tuttam തുത്തം. *(Malyal.)* Bile-tutyá ಬಿಳೆತುತ್ಯ. *(Can.)* Sudu-tuttam. *(Cing.)*.

657. ZINCUM. *(Zinc.)*

Dastá دستا ; Jastá جستا or Jast جست . *(Hind.)* Jas جس . *(Duk.)* Tutta-nágam துத்தநாகம். *(Tam.)* Tuttunágam ತುತುನಾಗం. *(Tel.)* Nágam നാഗം. *(Malyal.)* Sattu ಸತ್ತು. *(Can.)* Nágam. *(Sans.)* Tutti-nága. *(Mah.)* Tutti-nága. *(Guz.)* Dastá. *(Beng.)*.

658. ZINGIBER OFFICINALIS, *Roxb. (Dried root of—Ginger.)*

Zanjabil زنجبيل ; Zanjabíle-yábis زنجبيل يا بس *(Arab.)* Zanjabíle-khushk زنجبيل خشك *(Pers.)* Sónṭh ; Sindhi سند هي *(Hind.)* Sónṭ سو نٹ سو ندّه ; *(Duk.)* Shukku சுக்கு. *(Tam.)* Sonṭi సొంఠి. *(Tel.)* Chukka ചുക്ക. *(Malyal.)* Vaṇa-sunṭhi ವಣಸುಂಠಿ. *(Can.)* Sónṭ. *(Beng.)* Vishva-bhéshajam. *(Sans.)* Súnṭ. *(Guz.)* Veḷicha-inguru or Inguru. *(Cing.)* Gínsi-khiáv. *(Bur.)*.

659. ZINGIBER OFFICINALIS, *Roxb. (Fresh root of—Green Ginger.)*

Zanjabíle-raṯab زنجبيل رطب *(Arab.)* Zanjabíle-tar زنجبيل تر *(Pers.)* Adrak ادرك *(Hind. and Duk.)* Iṇji இஞ்சி. *(Tam.)* Allam అల్లం. *(Tel.)* Inchi ഇഞ്ചി. *(Malyal.)* Hasísunṭhi ಹಸಿಸುಂಠಿ. *(Can.)* Ádrok. *(Beng.)* Árdrakam. *(Sans.)* Ala. *(Mah.)* Ádu. *(Guz.)* Amu-inguru. *(Cing.)* Giṇ sín. *(Bur.)*.

660. ZIZYPHUS JUJUBA, *Linn. (Fruit of.)*

Sidr سدر ; Nabiq نبق ; Aunnábe-hindí عنابـهندي *(Arab.)* Kunár كنار *(Pers.)* Bér بير *(Hind. and Duk.)* Elandap-pazham எலந்தப்பழம். *(Tam.)* Régu-paṇḍu రేగుపండు ; Ganga-régu-paṇḍu గంగరేగుపండు ; Karkandhuvu కర్కంధువు. *(Tel.)* Elantap-pazham ഏലന്തപ്പഴം. *(Malyal.)* Yalachi-haṇṇu ಯಲಚಿಹಣ್ಣು. *(Can.)* Kúl ; Bér ; Bór. *(Beng.)*

Badari-*phalam. (Sans.)* Bóra *(Mah.)* Bór. *(Guz.)* Ilanda ;
Másáṇká. *(Cing.)*   Zi-ṣi. *(Bur.)*.

The Arabic names of the above fruit, *Sidr* or *Sadur*, and
Nabiq, are misapplied in some books to *Pomegranate* and to
the fruits of *Cordia latifolia* and *C. myxa*. In a few others,
again, *Aunnáb* is considered as the name of this fruit *(Z. jujuba);*
but it is the name of another fruit, which does not grow in India.
It is often found in the bazaar, and as the fruit of *Z. jujuba*
is a good substitute for it, the latter, is correctly. named in some
works as *Aunnábe-hindi*.

The Malyalim synonyme *Perintoṭali* പെരിന്തൊാടലി or
' Perintodali' is found in the Hortus Malabaricus, in native
character in 2 places, (Vol. iv, Tab. 41 ; and Vol. v, Tab. 41).
It is not, however, generally recognised as the correct name of
either of the plants to which it is applied, viz., *Toddalia aculeata*
and *Zizyphus jujuba*. These plants are well known by the
Malyalim names inserted in this Catalogue under their respective
heads. If the name *(Perintoṭali)* is at all applicable to any of
these plants, it may be so to *T. aculeata*, but not to *Z. jujuba*.

ADDENDA.

A.

661. ACALYPHA INDICA, _Linn._

Kúpi كوپي ; Kuppi كپي . (_Duk._) Kuppai-méṇi குப்பைமேனி. (_Tam._) Kuppi-cheṭṭu కుప్పిచెట్టు ; Murukoṇḍa-cheṭṭu మురుకొండచెట్టు ; Puppaṇṭi పుప్పంటి ; Muruvpiṇḍi మురు పిండి ; Harita-manjari హారితమంజరి. (_Tel._) Kuppaman-cheṭi കുപ്പമൺചെടി ; Kuppa-maṇi കുപ്പമണി. (_Malyal._).

See the remarks under _Nardostachys Jatamansi_ and _Pimpinella anisum._

662. ACONITUM NAPELLUS, _Linn._
663. ACONITUM PALMATUM, _Don._ ⎱ _Root of._
664. ACONITUM LURIDUM, _H. et T._ ⎰

See the names and remarks under _Aconitum ferox._

In page 26, while describing some of the roots known generally as those of _A. ferox_, I expressed a doubt as to the whole of them being the produce of that species alone. Accordingly, I believe now, from the 3 plants given here in the text being included in the Pharmacopœia of India, that they are more likely the species producing some of those roots than _A. ferox_. But, until the roots of each of these plants are dried and described separately, no positive opinion can be given on the subject.

In many medical and other works ' Bikh' is given as one of the Hindustani names of the roots under discussion. Whether it is a corruption of ' Bish' (_Bish_ بیش) and ' Bis' (_Bis_ بس)

or not, it sounds like *Bikh* بيخ , which is a general name for a
root in Persian, and is often adopted in Hindustani, &c. It is
not, therefore, safe to apply it to the poisonous roots of *Aconite.*
The surest and safest native names in most parts of India for
these roots are *Bish* بيش , *Bis* بس , *Singyá-bis* سنگيا بس ,
Míthá-zahar ميتها زهر , *Buchhnág* بجهناگ , *Vasha-návi* ஐச
நாவி, and *Vasa-nábhi* வசநாபி.

665. AGATI GRANDIFLORA, *Desv.*

Agti اگتي ; Agtí-ká-*jhár* اگتي كا جهار . (*Duk.*)
Agatti அகத்தி. (*Tam.*) Avisi అవిసి. (*Tel.*) Agatti அகை
ணி. (*Malyal.*) Agashi అగశి. (*Can.*) Bako. (*Beng.*)
Agasti. (*Mah.*) Agatti. (*Guz.*) Kataru-murunga. (*Cing.*).

See the remarks under *Linum usitatissimum.*

666. AILANTHUS EXCELSA, *D. C.*

See the names and remarks under *A. Malabarica,* and also
the remarks under *Casuarina Muricata.*

667. ALŒ VULGARIS, *Linn. (Common Alœ plant.)*

See the names and remarks under *A. Indica.*

668. ALPINIA CHINENSIS, *Roscoe. (Root of—*
Lesser Galangal.)

Kĥúlanján خولنجان ; Kĥúl'anjáne-ạaqáribí
خولنجان عقاربي . ; Kĥúlanjáne-sagĥir خولنجان صغير
(*Arab.*) Kĥusrave-dárú خسرودارو ; Kĥusrave-dárúe-
kĥurd خسروے خرد . (*Pers.*) Chhótá-kulanján
چهوٹا كلنجن ; Chhótá-kulanjan چهوٹا كلنجن ; Chhótá-
kalijan چهو ٹا كليجن . (*Hind.*) Chhótá-kĥulanján·
چهوٹا خولنجان . (*Duk.*) Irattai இரட்டை ; Shitta-rattai
சித்தரட்டை. (*Tam.*) Dumpa-ráshṭrakam దుంపరాష్ట్రకం ;
Sanna-dumparáshṭrakam సన్నదుంపరాష్ట్రకం. (*Tel.*) Chitta-

latti ചിററലററി. *(Malyal.)* Sanṇarásmi ಸ೦ರಾಶ್ಮಿ. *(Can.)*
Rastama. *(Sans.)* Sitta-rattai. *(Cing.)*.

This root, which is commonly found in all the large bazaars
of India, is imported from China, and is quite identical with the
Lesser Galangal of European shops.

This is a much smaller root than the *Greater Galangal*
(Alpinia galanga), but possesses a much stronger smell and
taste, and is therefore a more active medicine than the latter.

It is generally about the thickness of a finger, from $1\frac{1}{2}$ to
3 inches in length, thicker at one end than at the other, reddish
brown externally and brownish-white internally, marked with
white rings, and has a peculiar aromatic smell and a strong
peppery and pungent taste. It is often knotty and occasionally
forked.

This is the real Ṣh*itta-rattai* சித்தரத்தை or 'Sittarittie' of
native druggists' shops, and not the root of *Hedychium spicatum*,
which I shall describe under that plant.

In the bazaars of Hyderabad and some other places, the
root of *Alpinia calcarata* is sold as Ḳhúlanjáne-ḡaqáribí, but this
name is correctly applicable only to the *Lesser Galangal* and to
the root I shall speak of in the next No. The root of *A. calcarata*
is a much smaller root, and does not possess any peppery or
pungent taste.

See the remarks in the next No. and also under *Alpinia*
galanga.

669. ALPINIA KHULANJAN, *(Root of—A variety*
of Lesser Galangal).

This plant is found growing in several gardens at Madras,
and its rhizome when dried resembles the *Lesser Galangal*
(A. Chinensis) so much, that it may be considered a variety of
it. The root is not sold in the bazaar, but when sent there, it
was recognised by the same native names as those of the *Lesser*
Galangal.

A few years ago, when I first found the plant, I thought
it to be *A. Chinensis;* but on examining it several times when in

flower, I found that it is a new species òf *Alpinia*, which has not been described by any body, as far as my knowledge extends. I have therefore named it *Alpinia khulanjan* after its native appellation Ḳhúlanjún خولنجان , and shall describe it here before speaking further of its root.

Bot. Des.——*Rhizome* perennial, creeping, jointed, forked, and annulated or marked with rings: *stem* 3–4 feet high, simple and unbranched, chiefly consists of the sheathing petioles of the leaves: *leaves* simple, almost sessile or shortly-stalked, oblong, rounded at the end and abruptly and shortly acuminate, smooth, margin slightly white and callous, 10–13 inches long, 3–4 inches broad: *petiole* sheathing: *inflorescence* terminal, spathaceous, raceme: *peduncle* bears 15–18 pedicels: *pedicels* alternate, single or double-flowered: *flowers* very small, white with some pink streaks and dots: *calyx* superior, tubular, 3-toothed : *Corolla* tubular below and divided above; the upper portion or limb is irregular with 6 segments in 2 whorls; the outer whorl 3-parted and equal, the inner whorl also 3-parted but very unequal ; the middle segment *(labellum or lip)* of the inner whorl is not only much larger than the 2 others, but is also the largest portion of the flower, being about ¾ inch long and ½ broad ; it *(labellum)* is slightly curved, divided into sides or surfaces by an intermediate thicker portion of a pale white color (yellowish-white inside and greenish-white outside), sometimes (when quite open) divided at the apex, and its sides are thin, marked with 5 or 6 streaks and some dots of a deep pink color ; the 2 other segments of the inner whorl are abortive, about 1½ lines in length, triangular, of a deep pink color internally : *Stamens* 3, 1 fertile and 2 abortive, the fertile stamen is situated opposite the labellum, the abortive stamens are very minute and only seen when the lower (tubular) portion of the carolla is carefully dissected ; the latter are about ½ a line in length, and possess no anthers : *anther* of the fertile stamen is oblong, 2–celled, opens longitudinally, its lobes embrace the upper part of the style : *style* filamentous : *stigma* small and round : *pollen* minute, white, soft: *berries* very small, about 1½ lines in length; oval or oblong, and pale yellow when quite ripe. Every part of the plant has a peculiar, sharp, and agreeable aromatic smell. , It generally begins to flower in April or May.

If the root of this plant is cut into pieces and dried, it presents the following characters :—

Slightly tuberous, about the thickness of the little finger, somewhat thicker at one end than at the other, from $1\frac{1}{2}$ to 3 inches long, often knotty and forked, reddish-brown externally and greyish internally, annulated or marked with white rings, slightly wrinkled, smell warm and aromatic, and taste strongly pungent and peppery.

This root is somewhat smaller and lighter in color than the *Lesser Galangal*, but slightly stronger in smell and taste.

The above plant is not *A. nutans*, because the latter is a much larger plant, and has a very large and showy flower with a yellow lip; and its root is also much larger *(like the Greater Galangal)*, and almost devoid of the pungent or peppery taste.

The only plant which approximates *A. Khulanjan* is *A. calcarata*, which is also found in some gardens of Madras growing together with the latter. It differs from it, however, in the following characters:—

First, the flower of *A. calcarata* is about 6 or 8 times larger than that of *A. khulanjan*.

Secondly, the leaves of *A. calcarata* are narrower, longer, and lanceolate.

Thirdly, the rhizome of *A. calcarata*, when dried, has almost the same appearance, but possesses no pungent, peppery or aromatic taste whatever.

Fourthly, the smell of the leaves and other parts of *A. calcarata*, when bruised, is something like that of *Cardamom*, while the smell of *A. khulanjan* is peculiar and different from it.

With regard to the medicinal properties of the root of *A. khulanjan*, it is not only stimulant, carminative, stomachic and expectorant like *Ginger*, but also a very good *stimulant-tonic*. In addition to all the diseases in which *Ginger* is indicated, it is very useful in some nervous disorders, as Neuralgia, Functional Impotence, Nervous Debility, &c. It has also proved useful in several cases of Incontinence of Urine. Its preparations and doses are the same as those of *Ginger*, to which it is also preferable in another respect, viz., that it is neither attacked by insects, nor destroyed by any length of time.

See the remarks under the preceding plant, and also under *A. galanga* and *Hedychium spicatum*.

670. ALTHEA ROSEA, *Cav. (Flower of)*.

Khiṭmi خطمي; Vardul-khiṭmi ورد الخطمي . (*Arab.*) Gule-khiṭmi گل خطمي; Gule-kh-airó گل خيرو . (*Pers.*) Gulkh-airó گل خيرو . (*Hind.*)　　Gulkh-airo-ká-phúl گل خيرو کا پهول . (*Duk.*)　Gulkhairó. (*Mah.*).

There are 3 or 4 varieties of this plant, which are recognised and named according to their color, as *red, white, purple, &c.*

671. AMOMUM AROMATICUM, *Roxb.*

Mórang-iláyechi مورنگ الا يحبي *or* Murang-iláyechi مرنگ الا يحبي . (*Hind.*).

672. AMOMUM XANTHIOIDES, *Wall. (Seeds of)*.

Through the kindness of Mr. Daniel Hanbury, I have received from London a sample of the seeds of *A. xanthioides*, and they are the same whose names are given in No. 47, under '*Amomum. Sp. of.*' I have described them in page 44, and this description corresponds with the seeds now received, except that the latter being comparatively very new, and apparently collected from immature capsules, are *pale-grey* in color instead of *pale-brown*, as is generally the case with the seeds (*Iláyechi-dáné* الا يحبي دا ني) of the Indian bazaars.

673. AMYLUM. *(Starch)*.

Nashástaj نشا ستج . (*Arab.*)　Nashástah نشا سله (*Pers. and Hind.*)　Nishastah نشسته . (*Duk.*).

674 ANISOMELES OVATA, *R. Br.*

675. **APIS MELLIFICA,** *Linn.*

676. **APIS SOCIALIS,** *Latr.*

677. **APIS DORSATA,** *Latr.* } *Honey Bee.*

678. **APIS NIGRIPENNIS,** *Latr.*

679. **APIS BICOLOR,** *Klug.*

Nahl نحل ; Zanbúre-aasl زنبور عسل . (*Arab.*) Magase-aasl مگس عسل ; Magase-shahad مگس شهد . (*Pers.*) Shahad-kí-makkhí شهد كي مكهى . (*Hind. and Duk.*) Téní தேன். (*Tam.*) Téne-tíga తేనెటీగ. (*Tel.*) Téni തേനി. (*Malyal.*) Jénu-noṇa ಜೇನುನೊಣ. (*Can.*) Módh-makkhí. (*Beng.*) Madú-cha-máṣhi. (*Mah.*) Madhá-ni-macha. (*Guz.*).

680. **APLOTAXIS AURICULATA,** *D. C. Syn.* AUCKLANDIA COSTOS, *Falc. (Root of.)*

Qusṭ قسط . (*Arab.*) Kósht كوشت or Kóst كوست . (*Pers.*) Pachak پچک ; Kút كوت . (*Duk.*) Góshṭam கோஷ்டம். (*Tam.*) Góshṭamu గోష్టము. (*Tel.*) Kóshtam. (*Sans.*).

The two varieties of this root sold in the bazaar, are recognised according to their taste as *sweet* (Shírín شيرين) and *bitter* (Taḷkh تلخ).

681. **ARGENTI NITRAS.** (*Impure Nitrate of Silver.*)

Kárí-khár كازي كهار . (*Hind. and Duk.*) Kádik-káram காடிக்காரம். (*Tam.*) Kádi-káramu కాడికారము. (*Tel.*) Káṭi-káram കാടികാരം. (*Malyal.*) Kádi-káram ಕಾಡಿಕಾರಂ. (*Can.*)

682. ARSENICUM BISULPHURETUM, *(Impure Bisulphuret of Arsenic, or Realger.)*

Zarníkhe-aḥmar احمر زرنيخ . *(Arab.)* Zarníkhe-sarkh زرنيخ سرخ . *(Pers.)* Mansal منسل ; Lál-hartál لال هرتال . *(Hind. and Duk.)* Manóṣilai மனோசிலை. *(Tam.)* Manúṣala మనూశల. *(Tel.)* Mansóla മനോല. *(Malyal.)* Mansalam. *(Sans.).*

683. ASTRAGALUS VERUS, *Oliver.*

Kotilla. *(Beng.).*

B.

684. BALSAMODENDRON MUKUL, *Hook.*

685. BALSAMODENDRON PUBE-SCENS, *Stocks.*

} *Resin of—Bdellium.*

See the names under *B. agallocha* (p. 64).

686. BDELLA NILOTICA, *Sav. (Indian Leech)*

See the names under *Hirudo.*

687. BIGNONIA XYLOCARPA, *Roxb.*

' Kúrsing' (?)

688. BLUMEA BALSAMIFERA, *D. C.*

Leverella or Leverella-gahá. *(Cing.).*

689. BOSWELLIA FLORIBUNDA, *Endl.*

See the names and remarks under *B. thurifera.*

690. BRAGANTIA WALLICHII, *R. Br.*

Alpam ആൽപം. *(Malyal.).*

691. BŒRHAAVIA DIFFUSA, *Linn.*

Thikri-ká-*jhár* تھکری کی جھار . *(Duk.)* Múkku-raṭṭai முக்குராட்டை. *(Tam.)* Aṭika-mámiḍi అటికమామిడి. *(Tel.)* Gadha-púrna.-*(Beng.)* Jan-tóps. *(Cing.).*

692. BRUCEA (NIMA) QUASSIOIDES, *Ham.*

Bahárangí بھارنگي ; *Bharangí* بھرنگي . *(Hind.).*

693. BUTEA PARVIFLORA, *Roxb.*

C.

694. CONVOLVULUS HIRSUTUS, *Roxb.*

E.

695. ELETTARIA MAJOR, *Smith. (Capsules of—Ceylon Cardamoms.)*

F.

696. FUMARIA OFFICINALIS, *Linn.*

697. FUMARIA PARVIFLORA, *Linn.*

Baqlatul-mulk بقلة الملك . *(Arab.)* Sháhtarah شاهتره . *(Pers.)* Pit-pápará پت پا پڑا . *(Hind.)* Shátrá شاترا . *(Duk.)* Turá தூரா. *(Tam.)* Cháta-ráshi చాతరాషి. *(Tel.)*

H.

698.   HEDYCHIUM SPICATUM, *Smith*. *(Root of.)*

Káfúr-kachrí كپورکچری ; Kapúr-kachrí كافورکچری . *(Hind.)*   Kapúr-kachrí كپورکچری ; Viláyatí-kachúr ولايتی کچپور . *(Duk.)*   Shímai-kich-chilik-kizhaṇgu சீமைகிச் சிலிக்கிழங்கு. *(Tam.)*   Síma-kich-chili-gaḍḍalu సిమకిచ్చిలిగడ్డలు. *(Tel.)*   Kapúr-kachri. *(Beng.)*.

This root, when entire, is reddish-brown and marked with white rings, and therefore resembles the ‘ Sit-ruttee’ or ‘ Sittarittie’ *(Lesser Galangal)* and the root of *Alpinia khulanjan* (No. 669), particularly the latter; but it is quite different from both of them.   It differs from them in being very white internally, amylaceous in structure, fragrant, and slightly warm or aromatic in taste, but not peppery or pungent.   Its smell, taste, internal color, and medicinal properties, are like those of the *Long Zedoary (Curcuma Zerumbet* of Roxburgh); hence its native names *Viláyatí-kachúr,* Shímai-kich-chilik-kizhaṇgu, and *Símakich-chili-gaḍḍalu,* which mean *Europe or Foreign Long Zedoary.*

Like *Long Zedoary,* this root is generally found in the bazaar in circular slices, 1 or 1½ lines in thickness, and about 2 Anna or ¼ Rupee piece in circumference, very white with a reddish-brown edge, and fragrant.   It is used for the same purposes as the *Long Zedoary,* but decidedly preferable to it.

In some works, one of the Hindustani names of this root, *Káfúr-kachrí* is used synonymously with ‘ Sittarittie’ and ‘ Sutruttee,’ which is incorrect, because the latter are the Tamil names of *Lesser Galangal,* which is a different root as I have just explained.

See the remarks under *A. galanga, A. Chinensis,* and *A. khulanjan.*

699. HYSSOPUS. *(Hyssop.)*

Zúfáé-yábis زونائے یابس . *(Arab.).*

J.

700. JAQUEMONTIA VIOLACEA, *W. Elliot.*

L.

701. LIQUOR SPIRITUS. *Indian Spirituous Liquor, Arrack, or Country Liquor.)*

 The names of this article are already given under *Arrack*, and I mention it again here chiefly to give the names of its varieties, which have been omitted under the latter head. It is distilled from many substances, the most common of which are the bark of *Acacia leucophlœa*, and a few other species of the same genus; the flowers of *Bassia longifolia; Toddy* of *Borassus flabelliformis, Phœnix sylvestris Cocos nucifera*, and *Caryota urens; Jaggery*; and *Rice*. The names of these varieties are as follows:—

 a. Liquor of Acacia leucophlœa.——*Kíkar-kí-sharáb* کیکر کي شراب . *(Hind.)* ; *Babúl-ké-sharáb* ببول کي شراب ; *Kíkar-kí-dárú* کیکر کي دارو ; *Paṭṭé-kí-sharáb* پتّے کي شراب ; *Kíkar-kí-sharáb* کیکر کي شراب . *(Duk.)* *Paṭṭai-ṣháṛáyam* பட்டைசாறயம். *(Tam.)* *Paṭṭa-sáráyi* పట్టసారాయి. *(Tel.)* *Paṭṭa-cháráyam* പട്ടചാരായം. *(Malyal.)* *Paṭṭe-sáráyi* ಪಟ್ಟೆಸಾರಾ ಯು. *(Can.)* *Babúl-suráp.* *(Beng.)* *Bávaḷ-dáru.* *(Guz.).*

 b. Liquor of Bassia longifolia--*Mohé-kí-sharáb* موھے کي شراب ; *Móhé-kí-dáru* موھے کي دارو ; *Móhé-kí-sharáb* موھے کي شراب *(Hind. and Duk.)* *Iluppai-ṣháṛáyam* இலுப்பைசாறயம். *(Tam.)*

Ippa-sárayi ఇప్పసారాయి. (Tel.) Irippa-chárayam ഇരിപ്പചാരായം. (Malyal.) Ippe-sárúyi ಇಪ್ಪೆಸಾರಾಯಿ. (Can.) Mohuvá-suráp. (Beng.) Madhúka-madyam. (Sans.) Móhácha-dáru. (Mah.) Mova-nu-dáru. (Guz.).

c. Liquor of Borassus flabelliformis——Tári-ki-sharáb تاڑي کی شراب ; تاڑي دارو. (Hind.) Tár-ki-dárú Túri-ki-dárú تاڑي کي دارو. (Duk.) Panan-chárayam பனஞ்சாராயம். (Tam.) Túri-sárayi తాటిసారాయి. (Tel.) Paná-cháráyam പനാചാരായം. (Malyal.) Pané-sárúyi ತಾಟಿಸಾರಾಯಿ. (Can.) Tál-suráp. (Beng.) Tálu-madyam. (Sans.) Taticha-dáru. (Mah.) Tád-nu-dáru. (Guz.) Tal-arak. (Cing.).

d. Liquor of Cocos nucifera————Nariel-ki-sharáb ناريل کي شراب ; Naréli-ki-sharáb ناريلي کي شراب. (Hind.) Nárél-ki-dárú ناريل کي دارو. (Duk.) Tennan-chárayam தென்னஞ்சாராயம். (Tam.) Tenkáya-sárayi తెంకాయసారాయి. (Tel.) Ténna-chárayam തെങ്ങചാരായം. (Malyal.) Tenginá-sárayi ತೆಂಗಿನಾಸಾರಾಯಿ. (Can.) Nárikél-suráp. (Beng.) Nári-kéla-madyam. (Sans.) Naralicha-dáru. (Mah.) Núryal-nu-dáru. (Guz.) Pól-arak. (Cing.).

e. Liquor of Phœnix sylvestris.——Séndi-ki-sharáb سيندي کي شراب. (Hind.) Séndi-ki-dárú سيندي کي دارو. (Duk.) Ich-chan-chárayam ஈச்சஞ்சாராயம். (Tam.) Íta-sárayi ఈతసారాయి. (Tel.) Ínte-cháráyam ഈന്തെചാരായം. (Malyal.) Indi-arak. (Cing.).

f. Liquor of Caryota urens.—Mari-ki-sharáb ماڑي کي شراب. (Hind.) Múri-ki-dárú ماڑي کي دارو. (Duk.) Kúndal-panai-shárayam குந்தல்பனைசாராயம். (Tam.).

g. Liquor of Jaggery.—Gur-ki-sharáb گُڑ کي شراب. (Hind.) Gúr-ki-dárú گُڑ کي دارو ; Gúr-ki-sharáb گُوڑ کي شراب. (Duk.) Vella-shárayam வெல்லசாராயம். (Tam.) Bellam-sárayi బెల్లంసారాయి. (Tel.) Vellam-chárayam വെല്ലംചാരായം. (Malyal.) Bella-sárayi ಬೆಲ್ಲಸಾರಾಯಿ. (Can.) Akuru-arak. (Cing.).

h. Liquor of Rice.—Chánval-ki-sharáb چانول کي شراب. (Hind.) Chánval-ki-dárú چانول کي دارو. (Duk.) Arishisháráyam அரிசௌறயம். *(Tam.)* *Biyyamu-sáráyi* వియ్యముసా రాయి. *(Tel.)* *Ari-chúráyam* ൟറിച്ചൂരായം. *(Malyal.)* *Akki-sáráyi* ಆ ಕ್ಕಿಸಾರಾಯಿ. *(Can.)*.

P.

702. PHARBITIS NIL RUBER. *(Red variety of P. Nil—Seeds of.)*

Suféd-zirki-ké-binj سفيد زركي كے بيذج . *(Duk.)* **Vellai-jiriki-virai** வெள்ளைஜிரிகிவிதை. *(Tam.)* **Tella-jiriki-vittulu** తెల్ల జిరికివిత్తులు. *(Tel.)*.

The chief difference between this plant and *P. Nil* of Choisy is the color of the seed, which is black in the latter and grey or reddish-brown in the former.

On account of the redness, the seeds of the above plant ought to be distinguished from *Kálá-dánah* كالا دانه or *Káli-zirki-ké-binj* كالي زركي كے بيذج *(the seeds of P. Nil)*, by the affiix red, as follows:—

Lál-dánah لال دانه . *(Hind.)* *Lal-zirki-ké-binj* لال زركي كے بيذج *(Duk.)* *Shirappu-jiriki-virai* சிவப்புஜிரிகிவிதை. *(Tam.)*, and *Erra-jiriki-vittulu* ఎఱ్ఱజిరికివిత్తులు. *(Tel.)*.

But, according to the usage, the seeds are known in the bazaars of Southern India with the word *white* as marked in the text, although neither the seeds themselves, nor any other part of the plant producing them, is white. See the remarks under *Clitorea ternatea* and *Pharbitis Nil.*

703. PHARBITIS. *Sp. of ? (Seeds of.)*

Shab-pasandú شب پسند . *(Hind.)* **Shuppasandu.** *(Beng.)*.

704. PICRORRHIZA KURROA, *Roy. (Root of.)*

Kharbaqe-hindi خربق هندي . *(Arab. and Pers.)* **Kutki** كٹكي . *(Hind.)* **Káli-kutki** كالي كٹكى . *(Duk.)*

Kaṭuku-rógaṇi கடுகுரோகணி. *(Tam.)* Kaṭuku-róni கటుக
ரோని; Kaṭuka-rógani கటుகரోகணి. *(Tel.)* Kutki. *(Beng.)* Kaṭu-
róhani. *(Sans.)* Kalú-rana. *(Cing.)*.

The root sold in the bazaars of Calcutta, Hyderabad, and
Bombay, under the name of *Kuṭki* كٹكی is identical with the
Káli-kuṭki كالی كٹكی and *Kaṭuku-rógaṇi* கடுகுரோகணி or
' *Kada-groganie*' of Southern India. If the quantity is large,
it varies much in size and appearance in each specimen, but the
essential characters are invariably the same.

Although this drug is commonly known as a root, it consists
partly of root and partly of stem; therefore, if it is *entire*, the
upper portion *(stem)* differs from the lower *(root)* in external
characters. The upper portion is about 2 to 3 inches long;
very rough from thin scales; brown or reddish-brown in color
if the scales are not worn out, but paler if they are so; in the
latter condition it bears circular or semi-circular marks of the
scales, which occasionally make it look slightly annulated;
varies in thickness from 1 to 3 goose quills; beset with
the remains of leaves; and often curved and sometimes bent
upon itself. The lower portion is much thinner, varying in
thickness from a quill of a fowl to that of a goose; paler in
color, being generally brownish-grey or brownish-white; nearly
of the same length as the upper portion; more or less compressed; wrinkled longitudinally; and beset with elevated
marks of rootlets. There is no difference between the color and
taste of the internal substance of both portions, which are black
and extremely bitter, respectively. The root is generally cylin-
derical, but from having the upper portion much thicker than
the lower, it looks tapering sometimes. It is very light and
brittle, and easily powdered.

The root, however, is seldom entire, but generally found
in the bazaar broken into smaller pieces, which are from 1½ to
3 or 4 inches long. They vary in their characters according as
they are the pieces of the upper or lower portion of the root,
which I have just described.

It is imported to Madras from Calcutta, and the latter place,
I believe, is also the source of its supply to Hyderabad, Bombay

and many other places in India. It is' apparently the produce
of Northern India, and the plant yielding it is also supposed to
be found in some mountains near Chittoor in Central Carnatic,
but I have not as yet received any specimen from this place.
I have picked out some dry plants on 2 or 3 occasions from the
bundles of *Kaṭuku-rógaṇi*, but never found any flower or fruit
in them. The following is a description of these plants :—

Stem from 2 to 4 inches long ; about the thickness of a
large goose quill ; curved or bent ; rough from many thin circular
or semi-circular scales ; reddish-brown externally and black
internally ; very bitter in taste ; occasionally divided into
2 stems ; generally terminates in 2 or 3 small branches, which
are seldom longer than an inch ; soft and swollen when soaked,
which indicates its. fleshy condition when fresh : *leaves* when
moistened and opened, are obovate with a very long, narrow
and tapering base, which looks in the dry state like a petiole ;
sessile ; serrate ; angulinerved ; and glabrous.

This description agrees with the characters of the stem
and leaves of *P. Kurroa*, and I therefore, believe that it is the
plant which produces the *Kutki* of the bazaar, under whose
head it is already placed in the Pharmacopœia of India, p. 160.

With regards to its medicinal properties, it has completely
failed in my hands as a purgative. It does not deserve even the
title of laxative in 1 or 2 drachm doses. But it is a very valuable
tonic, in which respect it is equal if not preferable to *Gentian* and
Calumba, not to speak of *Chiretta* and other weak medicines of
that class. It is also a very good antiperiodic. Its dose as a
tonic is 10 to 20 grains, and as an antiperiodic from 20 to 40,
three times a day.

In some books, the Arabic and Persian names Ḳharbaqe-
asvad خر بق ا سود and Ḳharbaqe-*siyáh* خر بق سيا ٪, are applied
to the above root, but they properly belong to the root of *Helle-
borus niger*, the *black Hellebore* of European shops. The
root of *P. kurroa* is very different from *black Hellebore*, and is
the produce of India, as already explained. Although the
Hindustani or Dukhni name *Káli-kuṭki* کا لي کٹکي corresponds

in its meaning with the above Arabic, Persian, and English names, it is not applied to this root as a translation of any of them, but chiefly on account of the black color of its internal substance.

R.

705. RHUS CORIARIA. *(Dry seeds of—Sumach or Sumar).*

Samáq سماق ; Tamtam تمتم or Timtim تمتم . *(Arab.)* Samáq سماق . *(Pers.).*

The thin pericarp of the above seeds, which is one of the most useful astringent medicines in India, is sold in the bazaar under the Arabic name *Gardahe-samáq* گرد ه سماق .

706. ROSMARINUS *(Rosemary).*

Aklilul-jabal اكليل الجبل . *(Arab.).*

S.

707. SOLANUM NIGRUM, *Bl.* not *Linn.*

Aanabus-saalab عنب الثعلب ; Aanabus-saalabe-asvad عنب الثعلب أسود . *(Arab.)* Rúbáh-turbuk روباه تربك ; Rúbáh-turbuke-síyáh روباه تربك سياه ; Angúre-rúbah انگور روباه ; Angúre-rúbáhe-síyáh انگور روباه سياه ; Sag-angúr سگ انگور ; Sag-angúre-siyáh سگ انگور سياه . *(Pers.)* Makó مكو ; Kálá-makó كالا مكو ; Udá-makó اودا مكو . *(Hind.)* Kámúni كاموني ; Udí-kámúni اودي كاموني . *(Duk.)* Káli-kámúni كالي كاموني ; Maṇattak-

káḷi மணத்தக்காளி; Karuppu-maṇattakkáḷi கருப்புமணத்த
க்காளி. *(Tam.)* Kánchi-cheṭṭu కాంచిచెట్టు ; Nalla-kánchi-
cheṭṭu నల్ల కాంచిచెట్టు ; Kámanchi-chĕṭṭu కామంచిచెట్టు ; Nalla-
kámanchi-chĕṭṭu నల్ల కామంచిచెట్టు. *(Tel.)* Maṇattakáḷi മണ
ത്തകാളി ; Karup'pu-maṇattakáḷi കറുപ്പമണത്തകാളി ; Maṇattán-kaṇṇi മണത്താങ്കണ്ണി ; Karuppu-maṇattán-kaṇṇi
കറുപ്പമണത്താങ്കണ്ണി. *(Malyal.)* Kánchi ಕಾಂಜಿ; Karé-
kánchi ಕರೆಕಾಂಜಿ ; Gaṇiké ಗಣಿಕೆ ; Karé-gaṇiké ಕರೆಗ
ಣಿಕೆ. *(Can.)* Mako ; Kál-mako. *(Beng.)* Kóvidáraha ;
Krish̄ṇa-kóvidáraha. *(Sans.)* Kánguṇa ; Kála-kánguṇa.
(Mah.) Pillúdo, Káḷo-pillúdo. *(Guz.)* Simani-gahá ; Kalu-
símani-gahá. *(Cing.).*

This plant is confounded in many books with *S. nigrum*
of Linnæus, but fortunately the latter is not, at least, generally
found in India.   If not for this, the above confusion would
have been a source of great danger, because the juice of the
S. nigrum of Blume is not only given internally by ounces
(six or more) at one time by Hakeems and other native practitioners, but the plant itself is often made use of as a pot-herb
in many parts of India.   I have used myself a Decoction and
Extract of the leaves of this plant, as well as those of the next
(S. rubrum,) in very large doses, in the treatment of chronic
enlargement of liver, with or without Dropsy, and with very
encouraging results.   In fact, the medicine promises to become
very useful in some hepatic affections.   The Decoction and
Extract are prepared from the juice of the fresh leaves.   In the
former case, after the leaves are bruised and the juice pressed
out, it is warmed in an earthen vessel for 10 or 15 minutes, or
until it loses its green color and becomes reddish brown.   When
it is cool, it is strained and given every morning in 6 or 8 ounce
doses.   It acts as a hydrogogue cathartic and diuretic.   The
same juice, instead of being warmed, if evaporated on a sand
or water bath to the consistence of a soft mass, forms an extract.
Used in 1 drachm doses, twice or thrice a day, this Extract

acts as a diuretic and laxative, and exercise a great influence over the enlargement and other chronic diseases of the liver.

I shall now describe the plant here to remove all doubts about its nature.

Bot. Des.——*Annual*, if cultivated with care perennial; erect, from 1½ to 3 feet high; branches occasionally and slightly angular and somewhat tubercular at the angles: *leaves* ovate, soft, slightly wavy, occasionally and partially dentate; petiolate; petiole short and slightly margined : *flowers* very small and white, drooping, lateral, pedunculate, pedicellate, and 3 or 4 form together a kind of umbel; *calyx* persistent, green, sepals 5 : *corolla* white, petals 5, stamens 5 : *berries* drooping, small, purple or black, many seeded, juicy, and slightly sourish in taste. It is always found in flower and fruit.

The above description also corresponds with *S. rubrum* of Miller, with the exception of the following minor characters :—

In *S. rubrum*, the berries are red and slightly sweet, the leaves generally and distinctly dentate, larger, thicker, paler in color, not wavy, and possess a slight disagreeable smell; branches more spreading and not distinctly angular or tuburcular.

Both these plants are cultivated in Southern India, but *S. Nigrum* is more common and cheaper, and therefore more frequently used. There is not much difference in the medicinal properties of these plants, and they are consequently used together on many occasions.

They are generally known by the same names in native languages, but in case of necessity, are distinguished by the color of their berries, as *black* and *red*, which correspond with the Latin words *nigrum* and *rubrum*.

See the remarks under the next plant (*S. rubrum.*)

708. SOLANUM RUBRUM, *Mill.*

Ạanabuṣ-ṣaạlab عنب الثعلب ; Ạanabuṣ-ṣaạlabe-aḥmar عنب الثعلب احمر . (*Arab.*) Rúbáh-turbuk روباه تربك ; Rúbáh-turbuke-surkh روباه تربك سرخ ; Angúre-rúbáh

; انگور روباه سرخ Angúre-rúbáhe-surkh انگوررو با ;
Sag-angúr سگ انگور سرخ ; Sag-angúre-surkh
(Pers.) Makó مکو ; Lál-makó لال مکو . (Hind.) Kámúni
کاموني ; Lál-kámúní لال کاموني . (Duk.) Maṇattakkáḷi
மணத்தக்காளி ; Shivappu-maṇattakkáḷi சிவப்புமணத்தக்காளி.
(Tam.) Kánchi-cheṭṭu కాంచిచెట్టు ; Erra-kánchi-cheṭṭu
ఎఱ్ఱకాంచిచెట్టు ; Kámanchi-cheṭṭu ; కామంచిచెట్టు ; Erra-
kámanchi-cheṭṭu ఎఱ్ఱకామంచిచెట్టు. (Tel.) Maṇattakáḷi മണ
ത്തകാളി ; Chovanna-manattakáḷi ചൊവന്നമണത്തകാളി ;
Maṇattán-kaṇṇi മണത്താൻകണ്ണി Chovanna-maṇattán-kaṇṇi
ചൊവന്നമണത്താൻകണ്ണി. (Malyal.) Kánchi ಕಾಂಚಿ ;
Kempu-kánchi ಕೆಂಪುಕಾಂಚಿ ; Gaṇiké ಗಣಿಕೆ ; Kempu-gaṇiké
ಕೆಂಪುಗಣಿಕೆ. (Can.) Mako ; Rakta-mako ; Lál-mako. (Beng.)
Kóvi-dáraha ; Rakto-kóvi-dáraha. (Sans.) Símani-gaha ;
Rata-símani-gahá. (Cing.) Kánguṇa ; Támbaḍa-kánguṇa.
(Mah.) Pillúdo ; Lál-pillúdo. (Guz.).

Aanabus-saglab عنب الثعلب, Rubáh-turbuk روباه تربك
and Sag-angúr سگ انگور, are the Arabic and Persian names
of S. rubrum and S. nigrum, but by some mistake, they are
applied to Atropa Belladonna (Deadly Nightshade) in some works,
including the Materia Indica. This is a very dangerous error,
and should be avoided with the greatest care.

In addition to the above, the Hindustani name of these
plants (S. rubrum and S. nigrum), viz., Makó مکو or Makóé
مکوي is misapplied in some books to Country Sarsaparilla
(Hemidesmus Indicus, p. 152) and Jamaica Sarsaparilla (Sarsa
Radix, p. 224).

See the remarks under the preceding plant (S. nigrum).

TABLE

OF THE

METHOD OF TRANSLITERATION

ADOPTED IN THE

CATALOGUE.

TABLE *of the method of transliteration adopted in the Catalogue for expressing the vernacular synonymes in English character.*

No.	Description of Letters.	Arabic, Persian, Hindustani, and Dukhni.	Tamil.	Telugu.	Malyalim.	Canarese.	Bengali.	Sanscrit.	Mahratti.	Guzratti.	Cingalese.	Burmese.	English letter or letters corresponding with each Vernacular character.	Examples of the sound of each character.	Remarks.
						VERNACULAR CHARACTERS.									
1	Vowels and Symbolic Vowels.	ı	அ	అ	അ	ಅ							a	(*Short*) sounding as *a* in *about*, as *u* in *upper*, as the second *a* in *Grammar*, and as the final *a* in *Calcutta*, pronounced quickly.	See Notes II, III, IV, V, VII, and VIII, at the end of the Table.

Vowels and Symbolic Vowels.

2		á	(*Long*) sounding as *a* in *all* and *call*, as *o* in *r̄od*, and as *aw* in *draw*.	See Notes II, IV, and IX.
3		i	(*Short*) sounding as *i* in *ink* and *bid*, and as *y* in *every*.	See Notes II, and IV.
4		í	(*Long*) sounding as *ea* in *east*, and as *ee* in *feed* and *free*.	See Note II.

No.	Vowels and Symbolic Vowels									Sound		
5		[illegible]	[illegible]	[illegible]	[illegible]	[illegible]	[illegible]			u	(*Short*) sounding as *wo* in *wolf*, as *u* in *full*, and *o* in *to*.	See Notes II, and IV.
6		[illegible]	[illegible]	[illegible]	[illegible]	[illegible]	[illegible]			ú	(*Long*) sounding as *oo* in *ooze*, *fool* and *too*.	See Notes II, and VI.
7		[illegible]	[illegible]	[illegible]	[illegible]	[illegible]	[illegible]			e	(*Short*) sounding as *a* by itself, as *e* in *elbow*, as the first *e* in *never*, and as *ay* in *say*, pronounced quickly.	See Notes II, and IV.

Vowels and Symbolic Vowels.

8	ó	(*Long*) sounding as *a* in *able*, as *ai* in *fair*, ānd as *ay* in *play*.	See Note II.
9	o	(*Short*) sounding as *o* in *opacity*, *approbate*, and *go*, the latter being pronounced quickly.	See Notes II, IV, and VII.
10	ó	(*Long*) sounding as *o* in *opium* and *home*, and as *ow* in *bow*.	See Note II.

No.	Vowels and Symbolic Vowels.									Roman	Sounding	Reference
11	آيْ أَيْ ـَيْ ي	ஐ ண உ	உ ண	ஐ ஐ	ஐ ൈ					*ai*	Sounding as *i* in *island* and *silent*, and as *y* in *by* and *fly*.	See Notes II, and IX.
12	آو أَو ـَو و	ஒள ஔ	ஊ ள	ஒள ஔ	ஒ ൗ					*ou*	Sounding as *ou* in *out*, *our*, *house*, *hour*, and *thou*.	See Note II.
13											When this small vowel (˘) is placed over any letter, the latter should be pronounced double or twice.	See Note IV.

14	Vowels and Symbolic Vowels.			When these small signs or vowels are placed over any letter, it is considered to be *quiescent*, that is, having no vowel to be sounded after it, and it necessarily unites with the preceding letter.	See Notes II, and IV.
15		am	Sounding as *a* (*short*) with *m*.	See Note VI.
16		áá	Sounding as double *á* (*long*.)	
17		an	Sounding as *a* (*short*) with *n*. When this sign (·) is placed over the final *alif* (١ or ١), which is always the case, the English representative of the letter preceding the *alif* should be added to *an* to express its sound; as (١ﺟ) *dan* and (ﻟ) *ban*.	See Note II.

	Vowels and Symbolic Vowels.							
18		ၜ					This sign serves to unite two *words* together.	See Notes II, and IV.
19		ဪ ၜ	ဪ	ဪ		*aha* *ha*	This sign (ः), the visarga, which is represented by *ha*, is always final and sounds like the final *h*.	See Note II.
20		ၰ ၢ	ၰ ၢ	ၰ ၢ		*ru*	(*Short*) sounding as *r* with *u* (*short*).	See Note II.
21		ၱ ၵ	ၱ ၵ	ၱ ၵ		*rú*	(*Long*) sounding as *r* with *ú* (*long*).	See Note II.
22						*ri*	(*Short*) sounding as *r* with *i* (*short*).	

No.	Vowels and Symbolic Vowels									
23									rí	(Long) sounding as r with i (long).
24				ఌ		౬			lu	(Short) sounding as l with u (short).
25				ౡ		౬			lú	(Long) sounding as l with ú (long).
26									li	(Short) sounding as l with i (short).
27									lí	(Long) sounding as l with í (long).

28	un	Sounding as *u* (*short*) with *n*. When this sign (ᵕ) is placed on a letter, the English representative of that letter should be added to *un* to express its sound; as (ॢ) *mun*.	See Note II.
29	in	Sounding as *i* (*short*) with *n*. When this sign (ᵕ) is marked below a letter, the English representative of that letter should be prefixed to *in* to express its sound; as (ॢ) *min*.	See Note II.
30	lri	Sounding as a *liquid* *l* with *r* and *i* (*short*).	
31	lrí	Sounding as a *liquid* *l* with *r* and *í* (*long*).	
32	oyi	Sounding as *o* (*short*) with *y* and *i* (*short*) together.	

Vowels and Symbolic Vowels.

	Consonants, Mute Consonants, and Symbolic Consonants.		Sounding	
33		k	Sounding as *k* in *kind*.	See Notes III, VI, and IX.
34		*kh*	Sounding as *k* with aspiration.	See Notes VI, and VIII.
35		g	Sounding as *g* in *good*.	See Note VI.

No.	Consonants, Mute Consonants, and Symbolic Consonants.						Rom.	Power.	Reference.
36	༪ ༪ ༪ ༪	ཀ	ཨ	ཨ			gh	Sounding as g (*hard*), with aspiration.	See Note VI.
37		ཨ	ཨ	ཨ	ཨ ཨ		ṅ	A strong nasal tone sounding somewhat like *ng* in *ring*.	See Notes III, and IX.
38	ཨ ཨ ཨ	ཨ	ཨ	ཨ	ཨ ཨ		ch	Sounding as *ch* in *chair*.	See Notes III, VI, and VIII.

Consonants, Mute Consonants, and Symbolic Consonants.

39	ç h	The sound of this letter is intermediate between that of *ch* and *s*.				
40	*chh*	Sounding as *ch* with aspiration.	See Note VII.			
41	j	Sounding as *j* in *joy*.	See Notes VI, and VII.			

	Consonants, Mute Consonants, and Symbolic Consonants.														
42	ز ز	జ								s	Sounding as z in zinc.	SeeNotes VI, VII, and VIII.
43	ఛ ఝ ఞ	ఝ	ఞ	ఝ						jh	Sounding as j with aspiration.	
44	ఌ ౡ	ౝ	ౠ	ఴ						ŋ	A slight nasal tone sounding softer than the n̤ (No. 37.)	SeeNotes III, and IX.

	Consonants, Mute Consonants, and Symbolic Consonants.								Sounding as t in *two*.	See Notes III, VI, and IX.
45				ɛ	s	ɜ			t	
46				ↄ	c	ↄ			*th*	Sounding as t in *two*, with aspiration.
47				ↄ	ε	ↄ			ḍ	Sounding as d in *do*. See Note VI.

48	Consonants, Mute Consonants, and Symbolic Consonants.	ڈھ ڈھ ڈھ		ఢ	ഢ	ಢ							*ḍh*	Sounding as *d* in *do*, with aspiration.	
49			ண ண்	ణ	ണ	ಣ							ṇ	Sounding as *n* (*hard*) pronounced by touching the palate with the tip of the tongue.	See Note III.
50		ث ثـ ـثـ ث ثـ ـثـ	த த்	థ ్	ഥ	ಥ ್							t	Sounding as *th* in *thin*.	See Notes III, VI, and VIII.

No.	Consonants, Mute Consonants, and Symbolic Consonants.							Value	Sound	Note
51	[glyph]	[glyph]	9	[glyph]				*th*	Sounding as *th* in *thin*, with aspiration.	
52	[glyph]	[glyph]	6	[glyph]				d	Sounding as *th* in *the*.	See Note VI.
53	[glyph]	[glyph]	3	[glyph]				*dh*	Sounding as *th* in *the*, with aspiration.	

	Consonants, Mute Consonants, and Symbolic Consonants.										
54	௰	ஃ	௳	௲	௩	௨				n	Sounding as *n* in *not*.	See Notes III and VI.
55	௴	௵	௶	௷	௪	௫				p	Sounding as *p* in *put*.	See Notes III and VI.
56	௸	௹	௺	௻	௼	௽				*ph*	Sounding as *p* with aspiration.	See Note VII.

No.	Consonants, Mute Consonants, and Symbolic Consonants.							Sounding	See Note
57	ج	ف	۴	و	బ	బ	b	Sounding as *b* in *book*.	See Note VI.
58	۴	۴	۴	۴	ఒ	భ	bh	Sounding as *b* with aspiration.	See Note VI.
59	۹	٩	و	భ	౨	మ	m	Sounding as *m* in *mind*.	See Notes III and VI.

60	Consonants, Mute Consonants, and Symbolic Consonants.	ي ـي ـيـ يـ	ய ய்	య ్య	യ ്യ	ಯ ್ಯ							y	Sounding as *y* in *you.*	See Notes III, V, and VI.
61		ر ـر	ர ர்	ర ్ర ృ	ര ്ര ൎ	ರ ್ರ ೃ							r	Sounding as *r* in *rain.*	See Notes III and VI.
62		ل ـل ـلـ لـ	ல ல்	ల ్ల	ല ്ല	ಲ ್ಲ							l	Sounding as *l* in *life.*	See Notes III, V, and VI.

No.	Consonants, Mute Consonants, and Symbolic Consonants.												Roman		See Notes
63													v	Sounding as *v* in *voice*	See Notes III, V, and VI.
64													sh	The sound of this letter is intermediate between that of *s* and *sh*.	See Note VI.
65													sh	Sounding as *sh* in *she*.	See Notes III, VI, VII, and IX.

66		౩	౩	౩	౩	ஸ ஸ்	౯	౩	౩			s	Sounding as *s* in *sun*.	See Notes III VI, VII, and VIII.
67						ஐ	౩	౩	౩			h	Sounding as *h* in *he*.	See Note VIII.
68						ஏ ள்	౩	౨	౯			ḷ	Sounding as *l* (*hard*) pronounced by touching the middle of the palate by the tip of the tongue.	See Note III.

Consonants, Mute Consonants, and Symbolic Consonants.

No.	Consonants, Mute Consonants, and Symbolic Consonants.							Sounding	
69		ஜ	ணஸ	ஜ			*ksh*	Sounding as *k* and *sh* pronounced simultaneously.	See Note IX.
70	ز ر	ధ ·ధ	౨	C			r	Sounding as *r* (*hard*) pronounced by touching the middle of the palate by the tip of the tongue.	See Note III.
71	ژ ڗ	ఫ ·ఫ		౯			*zh*	Sounding as *z* in *azure* and as *s* in *pleasure*.	See Note III.
72	ڌ ڍ ڈ						s	Sounding as *s* pronounced by pressing the tip of the tongue against the lower teeth.	See Note VIII.

Consonants, Mute Consonants, and Symbolic Consonants.

73	ح	ح ۶	ḥ	A peculiar sound, somewhat like that of *h* pronounced very forcibly by the throat.	See Note VIII.
7	ح ۶ ح	خ	*kh*	A peculiar sound somewhat like that of *kh* pronounced very forcibly by the throat. It is often heard in loud snoring during expiration.	See Note VIII.
75	ذ	ز	ẓ	Sounding as *z* pronounced by pressing the tip of the tongue against the lower teeth.	See Note VIII.

No.	Consonants, Mute Consonants, and Symbolic Consonants.				
76	ڡ			Sounding as *s* pronounced forcibly with a mixture of *w*.	See Note VIII.
77	ż			Sounding (*commonly*) as *z* pronounced forcibly; but its proper sound is that of *th* (*hard*) pronounced by pressing the tip of the tongue against the upper lip.	See Note VIII.
78	ظ			Sounding as *th* (*soft*) pronounced with a mixture of *w*, by pressing the tip of the tongue against the upper lip.	See Note VIII.

No.	Consonants, Mute Consonants, and Symbolic Consonants.															
79	ظ								z̤	Sounding as z pronounced with a mixture of *w*, by pressing the tip of the tongue against the upper lip.	See Note VIII.
80	ع								a̤	A very peculiar sound, somewhat like that of *a* pronounced very forcibly by the throat.	See Note VIII.
81	غ								*gḥ*	A peculiar guttural sound, somewhat like that made in gargling, or that produced by pronouncing *gh* very forcibly by the throat.	

Consonants, Mute Consonants, and Symbolic Consonants.	82	ف		f	Sounding as *f* in *fine*.	See Note VII.
	83	ق		q	A very peculiar sound somewhat like that produced when the water is suddenly poured out from a bottle or goglet.	See Note VIII.
	84	غ		*khy*	Sounding as *kh* with *y*, pronounced simultaneously.	See Note IX.

	Consonants, Mute Consonants, and Symbolic Consonants.			
85		ng	Sounding as *ng* in *ring*.	
86	ɔ ɔ	ṅ	Sounding as *n*, but very short, as if only half pronounced.	This letter corresponds with the *nú-ne-ghunnah* in Arabic and *chándí-búndú* in Bengali.
87	ț. ț. ț. ɛ.	nh	Sounding as *n* with aspiration.	

Consonants, Mute Consonants, and Symbolic Consonants.

88	*mh*	Sounding as *m* with aspiration.	
89	a	This letter corresponds with a mute consonant in some-languages; it is often silent, and sometimes has a sound which is intermediate between that of *a* and *o*.	See Note V.

Notes.—I. The foregoing Table is chiefly according to Sir William Jones' method, modified by Sir Charles Trevelyan and some other gentlemen, and published in 1834, at Serampore, in a work entitled 'The application of the Roman alphabet to all the Oriental languages, &c., &c.'. The few alterations and additions I have made, were quite necessary to make it more complete and clear, and suit *uniformly* the whole languages in the Catalogue.

II. The vowels are not placed in this Table according to the order in which they occur in native and other works, but arranged according to their frequency and usefulness in writing. The small letter or letters placed under each vowel are its symbols (*symbolic vowels*), and they are nothing but its representatives in a different and smaller form. This is the case in all the languages in the Catalogue, except the first four (Arabic, Persian, Hindustani, and Dukhni,) in which the small letters, viz., *zabar* (ˊ), *zér* (ˏ), *pésh* (ˏ), *tashdíd* (ˏ), *jazm* (o, ˯, or ˓) *madd* (~), *alife-maqsúrah* (ˈ or ﯼ), &c., are vowels themselves. The other letters inserted in these languages as vowels, viz., *alif* (ا), *yá* or *yé* (ی), *váv* (و), &c., are indirect vowels, not being able to produce any sound without the assistance of the small vowels. By the combination of these two kinds of vowels, the sounds of the long vowels are produced. The vowels which produce the sounds of *i* and *é* (*long*) are the same (ای, &c.) but the difference is that the *yá* (ی) in the former (*i*) is the *yáe-maarúf*, and that in the latter (*é*) *yáe-majhúl*. In the like manner, the sounds of *ú* and *ó* (*long*) are produced by the same vowels (او, &c.) and the difference here is that the *váv*

(ؚ) in the first (ú) is the *váve-maqrúf*, and that in the second (ó) *váve-majhúl*. The combinations of vowels which produce the sounds of *á (long)* are named *alife-mamdúdah* (آ, &c.) and *alife-maqṣúrah* (اٰ, &c.). When the small vowels (´ and ˋ) are doubled, thus (˝ and ˏ), they are named *Tanvín* in Arabic, because they take the sound of *n* (ن) after them when the letter to which they are attached is pronounced, as is already explained in the Table opposite to each of these signs.

III. The letters written under each consonant in the Tamil column, are the mute consonants. They differ from the common consonants only in not having the vowel *a (short)* attached to them. They are generally found in combination attached to the common consonants, when their sounds are required to be doubled. The small letters in the Telugu, Canarese, and Malyalim columns, are the Symbols of the consonants under which they are placed. In the first column, the Arabic, Persian, Hindustani, and Dukhni consonants will be found printed in four or five different forms opposite to each No. These forms correspond with the position of each letter in words, viz., *initial, medial,* and *final*.

IV. In all the languages in the Table, some letters are not written, but are understood and pronounced in combination. For instance, the first vowel *a (short)* is considered in Tamil, Telugu, Malyalim, Canarese, Bengali, Sanscrit, Mahratti, Guzratti, Cingalese, and Burmese, to be inherent in every consonant, and is therefore always understood when *medial* and *final*, and only written when *initial*. It is almost the same case with all the small or short vowels in

Arabic, Persian, Hindustani, and Dukhni, which are generally understood, though required for every letter to produce a sound. These remarks are also applicable to the sign (ـٔ*) which is named *vaṣl* (وصل), for it serves to unite together two Arabic words. *In all such cases, when a letter is understood in native characters, it is written in the English.*

V. Some letters, again, though written are not pronounced. While such letters are not rare in some languages, their occurrence is frequent in others. The Arabic may be included among the former, and the Burmese in the latter. The Arabic letters which generally become silent, are *alif* (ا), *lám* (ل), *yá* (ي) , *váv* or *váv-e-maadúlah* (و), &c., *In all these cases, the silent letters are omitted in English character.*

---

*The second of the two words united together by this sign, has always the Arabic article *alif* and *lám* (١ ل) prefixed to it. The *alif* in this case is always silent, and the *lám* is either silent or pronounced according to certain conditions. These conditions are, when the second word begins with ا ب ج ح خ ع غ ف ق ك م و ه or ى the *lám* is pronounced; and when that word commences with س ز ر ن د ث ت ل or ن it is dropped in pronunciation. In the latter case, the initial letter of the second word becomes double as if the silent *lám* were converted into it. *Ḥabbul-mishk* (حب المشك) and *Ḥabbul-bán* (حب البان) are the examples in which the *lám* is pronounced and the *alif* silent; and *Ḥabbus-salátín* (حب السلا طين) and *Ḥabbuz-zabíb* (حب الزبيب) are the instances in which both are dropped in pronunciation. It will be seen from the latter examples, that the initial letter of the second word in each of them has taken a *tashdíd* to become double.

VI.   In several languages, particularly, the Burmese and Tamil, some letters are possessed with more than one sound, or in other words, their usual sound is altered in one or more ways in combination, under certain circumstances. Most of these letters will be readily observed from the following arrangement.

TAMIL.

K (க) also sounds like *g*, as in கங்கை (Gaṉgai) ; கனம் (Ganam)'; கணபதி (Gaṇapati) ; மகன் (Magan) and கமுகு (Kamugu).

Ch (ச) also sounds like *ṣh*, as in சகோதரன் (Ṣhagódáran); சிந்தல்கொடி (Ṣhindalkoḍi); மாசம் (Máṣham ;) and பசி (Paṣhi).

Ch (ச) also sounds like *j*, as in சயம் (Jayam); கஜேந்திரன் (Gajéndiran) ; and பஞ்சி (Paṉji).

T (ட) also sounds like *ḍ*, as in டப்பி (Ḍabbi); குடம் (Kuḍam) ; and வண்டி (Vaṇḍi).

T (த) also sounds like *d*, as in தர்மம் (Darmam) ; படம் (Padam) ; and செய்கிறது (Ṣheygiradu).

P (ப) also sounds like *b*, as in படில் (Badil) ; பஸ்மம் (Basmam) ; அபிமானம் (Abimánam); and வசம்பு (Vaṣhambu).

BURMESE.

The sound of the letter represented by *k*, is altered into that of *g*.

Do................................by k, ...do.........ṭ.
Do................................by *kh*, ...do.........g.
Do. ....by *kh*, ...do......*gh*.
Do................................by s, ...do.........ṭ.
Do . ...by ṭ, ...do.........k.
Do........................ by p,............. do ....ṭ.
Do................ .... by p,............. do ....k.
Do. .... by p, ...do.........b.
Do..........................by r, ...do ....y.
Do. .... by r, ...do........*sh*.
Do. .... by l, ...do........*sh*.
Do .... by v, ...do.........ú.
Do. .... by t, ...do........*sh*.

BENGALI.

The sound of the letter represented by *j*, is altered into that of *y*.
.... Do. .... by *y*, ... do. ....*j*.
.... Do. .... by *y*, ... do. ....*z*.
.... Do. .... by *b*, ... do. ....*v*.

GUZRATTI.

The sound of the letter represented by *m*, is altered into that of *bh*.

TELUGU, MALYALIM, CANARESE AND SANSCRIT.

The sound of the vowel represented by *am*, is altered into that of *m* or *n*, according to the consonant it precedes.

In all these and other similar cases, the altered sound is represented by its corresponding letter or letters in English character, and not the original or usual one.

VII. In some languages, the alphabet are differently pronounced in different localities. The Bengali is the best example of this kind, in which the pronunciation used for some letters in the *North Bengal*, is different from that adopted in the *South*. The following letters are generally subject to this difference of pronunciation :—

NORTH BENGAL.	SOUTH BENGAL.
chh	s
j	z
ph	f
s	*sh*
sh	s
a	o

The pronunciation of the Northern parts being that which is generally found in books, is adopted in the Table.

VIII. There are several letters in Arabic, which are not generally pronounced correctly, and their sounds are confounded with each other in speaking ; but, they are all used correctly in writing, particularly by educated persons. They are as follows :—

Letters,	Correct pronunciation.	Incorrect pronunciation generally used in speaking.
ث	As exemplified in the Table, No. 72 (s).	
س	...............do..........., No. 66 (s).	Like *s* indiscriminately.
ص	...............do..........., No. 76 (s).	
ذ	...............do..........., No. 75 (z).	
ز	...............do..........., No. 42 (z).	Like *z* indiscriminately.
ض	...............do..........., No. 77 (z).	
ظ	...............do..........., No. 79 (z).	
ح	...............do..........., No. 73 (h).	Like *h* indiscriminately.
ه	...............do..........., No. 67 (h).	
خ	...............do..........., No. 74 (*kh*).	Like *kh* indiscriminately.
ق	...............do..........., No. 83 (q).	
ع	...............do..........., No. 80 (a).	Like *a* indiscriminately.
ا	...............do..........., No. 1 (a).	
ط	...............do..........., No. 78 (t).	Like *th* (*soft*) indiscriminately.
ت	...............do..........., No. 50 (t).	

In cases like the above, the letters used in writing for each correct sound, are expressed in English character, without any regard to the common sound in speaking.

IX. The diacritical marks used in the Table are only three, and of the simplest kind; viz., *accents*, *dots*, and *alteration of type*. The *accents* are employed for the *long* vowels to distinguish them from the *short*. The *dots* are placed either below or above the letters, and in a number varying from 1 to 3, and thus a letter in English is made to represent several in native languages. By *alteration of type* is meant, that when two or more English letters are required to represent a single native character in any word, they should be distinguished by *Italics* if other letters in the same word are printed in the Roman or English, and *vice-versa*. The letters in the altered type are to show that they stand together for one native character, and require to be pronounced simultaneously. Without some distinction like this, it is very difficult for the reader to know in combination which of the letters stand *collectively* and which *individually* for each native character. The first Sanscrit word occurring in the Catalogue, viz., vri*ksh*a *(a plant)* may be taken as an example. In this word, three letters *(ksh)* are standing together for one character, and it will be, at least, very difficult to know them as such, unless the reader is well acquainted with that language.

The compound letters *sh* and *ch*, however, did not require any distinction, being very familiarly known in English; but, for the sake of uniformity, they are also indicated in an altered type in common with others.

When two or more compound letters occur together in any word, and when they are indicated in an altered type according to the above rule, they will not be distinguished from each other and will likely be considered as one. In this case, a *hyphen* is placed between the compound letters to separate them for the sake of distinction. *

It would have been better if no native character was represented by more than one or two English letters. With this view many characters have been reduced to fewer letters than they actually require. Those that are still found in the Table represented by two or three letters, cannot be represented by one or two, or in any other way, without a great deviation from their natural or proper sounds, and this deviation renders the pronunciation of the words in which they occur, very unintelligible. The latter is very objectionable, particularly, when the names of medicines are concerned.

There are similar and sufficient reasons for every addition and alteration I have made in the method; but, as their explanation in so many languages will necessarily extend these notes to a very great length, I have not entered upon it.

---

* In order to distinguish the compound letters (two or more English letters representing a single native character) readily, it was first proposed to place a line under each of them, as is the case with *gh* and *kh* in Shakespear's Hindustani and English Dictionary; but, a considerable delay having taken place in preparing and casting a few of such letters, I gave up the plan and substituted the *alteration of type* as explained above.

As the Catalogue is now finished, I can say that I have found no disadvantage whatever from following the latter plan, while it had the advantage of being very easy and cheap, and was therefore readily adopted in all the types used in the work.

EXPLANATION of the INITIALS and NAMES ATTACH-
ED to the BOTANICAL NAMES and SYNONYMES.

Ach. or *Achar.*—E. Acharius, author of Lichenographia
Universalis.

Adans.—M. Adanson, author of Histoire naturella du sene-
gal, &c.

Ait. or *Aiton*—W., author of Hortus Kewensis, &c.

Balfour—Dr. J. H., author of the Class Book of Botany, &c.

Benth.—M. Bentham, author of Labiatorum genera et
species, and Schorophularineæ Indicæ, &c.

Berk.—Berkeley, a Botanist or Naturalist.

Bl. or *Blum.*—C. L. Blume, author of Flora Javanensis, &c.

Br. or *R. Br.*—R. Brown, author of many Botanical works.

Burm.—N. L. Burmann, author of a Flora Indica.

Cav.—A. J. Cavanilles, author of Icones et descriptiones
plantarum, &c.

Chois. or *Choisy*—A. D. Choisy, a Swiss Botanist who
elaborated several of the Natural Orders for De
Candolle's Prodromus.

Colebr.—H. T. Colebrooke, author of several Memoirs in the
Linnean Society's Transactions, &c.

Colladon—Author of Histoire des Cassiæ.

Corr.—J. Correa de Serra, author of some botanical papers.

Dalz.—N. A. Dalzel, one of the authors of Bombay Flora.

D. C.—A. P. DeCandolle, author of numerous botanical
works.

Dec.—DeCandolle, Fil. (Son of DeCandolle).

Delile—A. R., author of Floræ de Ægyptiaceæ Illustratis, &c.

Desv.—N. A. Desvanx, author of some botanical papers and editor of the ' Journal de Botanique.'

Don—D., author of the Prodromus Floræ Nepalensis, &c.

Duch.—A. P. Duchesne, author of Histoire Naturelle des Fraisiers, &c.

Dunal—M. F., author of Monographie de la famille des anonacées, &c.

Endl.—S. Endlicher, author of Genera plantarum secundum ordines naturales dispositæ, &c.

Fabr.—P. C. Fabricus, author of Enumeratio Methodica Plantarum Horti Medici Helmstadiensis, &c.

Falc. or *Falconer.*—Dr. H., author of some botanical papers.

Forsk.—P. Forskaol, author of Flora Ægyptico-Arabica, &c.

Forst.—Forster, author of a Flora, &c.

Gœrtn.—J. Gœrtner, author of ' De Fructebus et Seminibus'.

G. Don—Editor of a new Edition of Miller's Gardner's Dictionary.

Greville—Dr. Greville.

Gris.—G. Grisley, author of Viridarium lusitanicum, &c.

Ham.—Dr. F. Hamilton (formerly Buchanan), author of a ' Journey to Mysore,' and some botanical papers.

Haw.—A. H. Haworth, author of Synopsis Plantarum Succulentarum.

H. B. et K.—Humboldt, Bonpland, and Kunth, authors of Nova genera et species, &c.

Herbert—H. W. Herbert, author of ' Herbert's Amarillideæ' &c.

H. et T.—Drs. J. D. Hooker and T. Thompson, author of a Flora Indica, &c.

Heyn. or *Heyne*—B. Heyne, a Botanist or Naturalist.

Hook. or *Hooker*—Dr. W. J. Hooker, author of Botanical Miscellany, and of his (Hooker's) Journal of Botany.

Jack—Dr. W., author of some papers on Penang plants, &c.

Juss.—Bernard de Jussieu, author of Genera Plantarum, &c.

Koen., Kon. or *Kün.*—J. G. Koenig, a Danish Botanist.

Kth. or *Kunth*—A Prussian Botanist.

Labill.—J. J. Labillardiere, author of Icones plantarum Syriæ rariorum decades.

Lam.—J. B. Lamarck, editor of the botanical portion of the Encyclopedia Methodic.

Lehm.—J. G. C. Lehman, author of Plantæ é familia asperipoliarum nuciferæ, &c.

Lesch.—Leschenault de la Tour, a Director of the botanical garden at Pondicherry.

Lindl. or *Lindley*—Dr. J., author of the 'Vegetable Kingdom,' &c

Link—H. F., author of Philosophiæ botanicæ novæ prodromus, &c.

Linn.—Carl von Linnæus, the founder of Botanical Science.

Maton—Dr. W. E. Maton.

Meisn. or *Meissner*—Leon Fred. Meissner, author of some botanical papers.

Miers—J. Miers, author of a work.

Miq. or *Miquel*—F. A. W., a Botanist.

Mill.—P. Millers, author of the Gardener's Dictionary.

Moen.—C. Moench, author of a few botanical works.

Müll or *Mull.*—Otto Fred. Muller, author of some botanical works.

Nees—G. G. Nees von Esenbeck, author of several botanical works

Oliver—G. A., author of a botanical work.

Pavon—J., author of a botanical work.

Pell.—Pelletier, author of some botanical papers.

Pers.—C. II. Persoon, author of Synopsis plantarum seu enchridium botanicum, &c.

Planch—A Botanist.

Pohl—J. J. author of ' Brazilian plants', &c.

Retz.—A. J. Retzius, author of Fasciculus Observationum Botanicarum, &c.

Risso—A., author of Histoire naturelle des Oranger.

Rœm. or *Röm.* et *Schult.*—J. J. Rœmer, and J. A. Schultes, authors of Linnœi systema vegetabilium, &c.

Rosc. or *Roscœ*—W. Roscœ, author of ' Monandrian plants of the Order Scitamineæ.'

Roth—A. W., author of Novæ Plantarum, and several other works.

Rott.—Dr. Rottler, an Indian Botanist.

Roxb.—Dr. W. Roxburgh, author of Flora Indica, and Plants of the Coromandel Coast, &c.

Roy. or *Royle*—Dr. J. F. Royle, author of the Illustrations of the Botany of the Himalyan Mountains, and of a work on the fibrous plants of India.

Salisb.—R A. Salisbury, author of the Prodromus Londinensis, &c.

Sav. or *Savi*—C., author of several botanical works.

Schott—H., author of a few botanical works.

Schrad.—II. A. Schrader, author of many botanical works.

Sch. or *Schult.*—C. F. Schultz, author of Prodromus Floræ Stadgardiensis, &c.

Seb.—A. Seba, author of a book.

Ser.—N. C. Seringe, who has elaborated several difficult Tribes in De Candolle's Prodromus.

Sm. or *Smith*—Sir J. E. Smith, author of several botanical works.

Spr. or *Sprengel*—K. Sprengel, author of Systema Vegetabilium, and many other botanical works.

Stocks—author of some botanical papers in Hooker's Journal of Botany.

Stok.—J. Stokes, author of Botanical Materia Medica.

Swt.—R. Sweet, a Botanist.

Swz. or *Swartz*—O. Swartz, author of Prodromus Descriptionum Vegetabilium Indicæ Orientalis, &c.

Thunb.—C. P. Thunberg, author of Flora Japonica, and many other works.

Tourn.—J. P. Tournefornt, author of Elements de Botanique, &c.

Vahl—M., author of Symbolæ botanicæ, &c.

Vent or *Ventn.*—E. P. Ventenat, author of Principes de Botanique, &c.

Vill. or *Villars*—D., author of Histoire des Plantes du Dauphine, &c.

W. et *A.*—Dr. R. Wright and Mr. G. A. Walker Arnott, authors of the Prodromus Floræ Peninsulæ Indiæ Orientalis.

Wall.—Dr. N. Wallich, author of Plantæ Asiaticæ rariores, and Tentamen Floræ Nepalensis Illustratæ.

Wedd.—Weddell, author of Histoire naturelle des quinquinas.

W. Elliot—Sir, author of Flora Andhrica.

Wight—Dr. R., author of Icones Plantarum Indiæ Orientalis, Illustrations of Indian Botany, and Contributions to Indian Botany, &c.

Willd.—C. L. Wildenow, author of Species Plantarum, and several other works.

———————

NAMES OF THE BOOKS, &c., CONSULTED IN PREPARING THIS CATALOGUE.

Abdool Cawder's (Druggist) Lists of Cingalese names of th
bazaar medicines in Ceylon (MSS.).

Abel's (F. A.) System of Tables for Qualitative Mineral
Analysis.

Ainslie's (Sir Whitelaw) Materia Indica.

Alfázul-adviyah—a Catalogue of Arabic, Persian and Hindustani synonymes of Medicines in India, with brief
notes on their uses, &c.

Amaramu—a Sanscrit Vocabulary.

Baḥrul-javáher—an Arabic Medical Dictionary.

Bailey's Malyalim and English Dictionary.

Do.   English and Malyalim Dictionary.

Balfour's (Dr. E.) Cyclopædia of India, and of the Eastern
and Southern Asia, Commercial, Industrial, and
Scientific.

Balfour's (Dr. J. H.) Class Book of Botany.

Bowman's (J. E.) Practical Chemistry.

British Pharmacopœia.

Brown's (Mr. C. P.) Telugu and English Dictionary.

Do.   do.   English and Telugu Dictionary.

Do.   (R. N.) Hand Book of Madras plants, 2nd Ed.,
edited by Sub-Assistant Surgeon, J. J. Wood.

Burháne-qátea—a Persian Dictionary.

Campbell's Telugu and English Dictionary.

Carter's (Dr. Vandyke) List of Mahratti synonymes of
native medicines, (MS.)

*Ch*adura-agarádi—a Tamil Materia Medica.

Cleghorn's (Dr. H.) Hortus Madraspatensis.

Dalíle-sátea—a Hindustani and Persian Dictionary.

*Dh*anmantri-van*ou*-*sh*ada-ni*kh*anṭu—a Telugu Materia Medica.

*D*hananja-padárd*h*a-ni*kh*anṭu—a Telugu Materia Medica.

Don's (G.) new Edition of Miller's Gardener's Dictionary.

Drury's (Col. Heber) Useful Plants of India.

    Do.   do.   Hand Book of the Indian Flora.

D'Rozario's English, Bengali and Hindustani Dictionary.

Elliot's (Sir Walter) Flora Andhrica.

    Do.   do.   List of Tamil synonymes of some medicinal plants (MS.)

Forbes' latest Edition of Hindustani and English Dictionary.

Fown's (G.) Manual of Elementary Chemistry, Theoretical and Practical, 9th Ed., edited by Drs. Jones and Hofmann.

Garrot's Canarese and English Dictionary.

    Do.   English and Canarese Dictionary.

Gilchrist's Hindustani Philology.

*Gh*iyásul-log*h*at—an Arabic and Persian Dictionary.

Graham's Catalogue of Bombay plants.

Hanbury's (Mr. Daniel) Notes on Chinese Materia Medica.

Hooker and Thompson's (Drs. J. D. and T.) Flora Indica.

Hooper's (Dr. R.) Medical Dictionary.

I*kh*tiyáráte-badia—a Persion Materia Medica.

Jámaae-antáki—an Arabic Medical work.

Jámaae-bog*h*dádi—an Arabic Medical work.

Jámaae-béṭár—an Arabic Materia Medica.

Judson's Burmese Dictionary.

Key's (Dr. Thomas) Chemistry.

Ḳhámús—an Arabic Dictionary.

Ḳhulásatun-nafáyas—a Hindustani, Persian and Arabic
Dictionary.

Lindley's (Dr. J.) ' Vegetable Kingdom'.

List of Hind. Synonymes of the bazaar medicines at Bombay.

Do.   do.   do.   Calcutta.

Do.   do.   do.   Hyderabad.

Mackenzie's (Dr. William, c. b. &c.,) Náfeạul-amráẓ—a
Hindustani work on some native medicines.

Maḳhzanul-advíyah—a Materia Medica in Persian.

Malai-agrádi—a Medical Vocabulary in Tamil.

Mason's Natural Productions of Burmah.

Mírán Labbé's (Native Medical Practioner and Druggist)
Notes on the drugs of Colombo and Kandy (MS.).

Molesworth's Mahratti and English Dictionary.

Montgomerry's (Dr. H. B.) Materia Medica and Therapeutics.

Mubárak Ạalí's (Moonshee) List of Bengali and Hindustani
synonymes of the drugs at Islámábád (MS.).

Mufarredát dar ạilme-ṭib—a work on Botany, &c., in Persian.

Mufarredáte-móminá—a Catalogue of Simple Medicines in
Persian.

Mufarre-dáte-sikandrí—a Persian work on Simple Medicines.

Múligai-nigaṇḍu—a Tamil work on Medicinal plants.

Muntaḳhabul-advíyah—a Materia Medica of Hyderabad in
Persian.

Muntaḳhabul-logḥát—an Arabic and Persian Dictionary.

Náma-lingánu-shásanamu—a Sanscrit Vocabulary in Telugu.

O'Shaughnessy's (Sir B. W.) Bengal Dispensatory.

Do.   do.   Bengal Pharmacopœia.

Do.   do.   Manual of Chemistry.

Padartaguna-*chintámani*—a Tamil Materia Medica.

Pereira's (Dr. Jonathan) Elements of Materia Medica and Therapeutics.

Pharmacopœia of India.

Qánúne-búaali-siná—an Arabic Medical work by Avicenna, or ' Canons of Avicenna'.

Qarábádine-qádarí—a Pharmacopœia of Indian medicine in Persian.

Qarábádine-shifáí—a Persian work on Pharmacy.

Qarábádine-sikandarí—a Pharmacopœia in Persian.

Reeve's Canarese and English Dictionary.

Do. English and Canarese Dictionary.

Regnier's (Rev. M.) List of Burmese synonymes of some medicinal plants and drugs (MS.).

Rheed's Hortus Malabaricus.

Richardson's Persian, Arabic and English Dictionary.

Rottler's Tamil and English Dictionary.

Roxburgh's (Dr. W.) Flora Indica.

Do.   do.   Plants of the Coast of Coromandel.

Royle's (Dr. J. F.) Illustrations of the Botany of the Himalyan Mountains.

Royle and Headland's Materia Medica.

Shakespear's latest edition of Hindustani and English Dictionary.

Sura—an Arabic Dictionary.

Talife-sharifí—a Catalogue of Indian medicines in Persian.

Thwaites' (Mr. G. H. K.) List of Cingalese synonymes of the medicinal plants and drugs in Ceylon (MS.).

Tohfatul-mominín—an Indian Materia Medica in Persian.

Turner's (Dr. E.) Elements of Chemistry.

Voigt's Hortus Suburbanus Calcuttensis.

Waring's (Dr. E.) Lists of the Medicinal plants proposed to be included in the Pharmacopœia of India.

    Do.   Manual of Materia Medica and Therapeutics.

Wight's (Dr. R.) Icones Plantarum Indiæ Orientalis.

    Do.   Contributions to Indian Botany.

    Do.   Illustrations to Indian Botany, (Vol. I.)

Wight and Arnott's (Dr. R., and Mr. G. A.) Prodromus Floræ Peninsulæ Indiæ Orientalis.

William's English and Sanscrit Dictionary.

Wilson's Sanscrit and English Dictionary.

Winslow's Tamil and English Dictionary.

Zakhírahe-khárizmsháhí—a Persian medical work.

APPENDIX

APPENDIX.

INDIGENOUS CATHARTICS.
PHARBITIS NIL RUBER.

(Page 277.)

Although the seeds of this plant are known to some native practitioners and druggists in Southern India as a very good and better purgative medicine than the *Káli-zirki-ké-binj* or the seeds of the common variety of *P. Nil* (p. 196), yet they are seldom or never used in their practice, and are extremely rare in the bazaar. In fact, they are not to be found at all in the bazaar at present. A few years ago, I had obtained a sample of them with a great difficulty and from a great distance, and from these raised a few plants in my own compound. After collecting a sufficient quantity of the seeds, I have used them in many cases and found them decidedly superior to *Kálá-dánah* or *Káli-zirki-ké-binj*.

As this plant and its seeds are not noticed in any work, native or English, I shall describe them here :—

Bot. Des.—*Annual*, herbaceous, hairy and twining plant : *root* small and tapering with many thin rootlets : *stem* branched, about the thickness of a fowl's quill, twining from right to left, and slightly hairy: *leaves* triangular, petiolate ; not exactly downy, but covered with many thin, short, and weak hairs on both sides ; 3—lobed, lobes ovate and pointed, the two lateral lobes smaller than the middle, and the middle slightly dilated at the base: *flowers* axillary, pedunculate, pedicellate, bracteate: *peduncle* long, hairy, and 1—2 flowered: *pedicel* very short: *calyx* divided, sepals 5, lanceolate, slightly hairy, persistent, about twice longer than the capsule: *corolla* pale or purple blue, 2—3 inches long, monopetalous, companulate, hypogynous, plaited before expansion ; deciduous, expanding in the morning and remaining so only for a few hours, and then, as soon as the sun gets warmer, closes, and generally falls off before next morning: *Stamens* 5, erect, filiform, hypogynous; attached to the base of the corolla, with which they fall off: *anthers* oblong, bilocular, oscilating: *style* simple, included, filiform, persistent: *stigma* terminal, capitate, 2 lobed: *capsule* circular and broadly and slightly cordate, 1—3 celled, 1—3 valved, dehiscent: *cells* 1—2 seeded, triangular; each closed with a thin, smooth and curved valve: *seeds* irregular, angular, grey in color at the commencement and reddish-brown afterwards.

With the exception of color, there is no difference between these seeds and *Kálá-dánah*. They are about 2 lines long and 1 or 1¼ broad; their shape is that of the segment of an orange; the average weight of each is about half a grain; and their taste is mucilaginous with a peculiar and acrid sensation, quite like that of *Kálá-dánah*. In the centre of the posterior or broadest surface of the seeds, there is a slight longitudinal depression or groove. When very old, these seeds assume a brownish color, and there is some difficulty then to distinguish them from *Kálá-dánah*.

I have compared the above plant with the black or common variety of *P. Nil (Kálá-dánah plant)*, which was growing together, and found it to differ only in some minor points, as follows:—

P. Nil ruber.	*P. Nil.*
1. Seeds grey or reddish-brown.	1. Seeds black or dark-brown.
2. Stem generally pale-green, and often exceeds 25 or 30 feet in length.	2. Stem generally blue or greenish blue, and much shorter.
3. Leaves about the size of a palm, and of a pale-green color.*	3. Leaves, which are of the same form (triangular, not cordate), are generally smaller and of a deeper color.*
4. Peduncle generally bears but one flower, and some times two.	4. Peduncle generally bears two flowers, and some times three or more.

** In these, like in many other twining plants, whose stem is very thin and the leaves pretty distant from each other, the position of the latter (leaves), whether *opposite* or *alternate*, cannot be made out.

The above differences are very slight, and I therefore consider the plant under discussion as a mere variety of *P. Nil* of Choisy. To avoid the confusion that would necessarily arise if both plants and their seeds have the same names, I have named the present variety and its seeds as *Pharbitis Nil ruber* and *Pharbitis Seeds,* respectively.

I have used this medicine, as well as *Kálá-dánah* or *Káli-zirkí-ké-bínj*, in many cases, in the same dose, and under the same condition with regard to age, &c., and found the former *(Pharbitis Seeds)* to be decidedly preferable to the latter; or in other words, it is more speedy, certain, regular, and stronger in its action than the *Kálá-dánah*. It is also preferable to *Jalap* in some respects, viz., it is an efficient purgative by itself, while the latter is not so when used alone; and that it possesses no nauseous smell or taste.

Preparations.—Simple Powder of Pharbitis Seeds *(Pulvis Pharbitis Simplex).* This powder should be prepared in the ordinary way, passed through a fine sieve or cloth, and kept in a stopper-bottle.

Dose.—From 40 to 50 grains.

Compound Powder of Pharbitis Seeds *(Pulvis Pharbitis Compositus).* Take of Pharbitis Seeds and Rock Salt or Cream of Tartar, in powder, each seven ounces; Ginger or Lesser Galangal, in powder, one ounce. Rub them well together, and pass the powder through a fine sieve or cloth.

Dose.—From a drachm to drachm and a half. This powder is more efficient than ' Pulvis Kaladanæ compositus' and equal to the corresponding preparation of *Jalap*.

I have not yet used *Pharbitis Seeds* in any other form, but have no doubt that it can be used in all the forms that *Kálá-dánah* is used, viz., Extract, Tincture, and Resin; which are described in the Pharmacopœia of India, pages 155 and 156. I believe also that the action of these seeds depends upon a resinous principle similar to that found in *Kálá-dánah*, *(Pharbitisin).*

CONVOLVULUS HIRSUTUS.

(Page 273.)

This plant is neither known to possess any medicinal property, nor any part of it is sold in the bazaar.; but finding, accidentally, its seeds to bear a resemblance to, and have a taste somewhat like that of, *Kálá-dánah,* I thought they were a purgative, and found them to be really so on some trials, which I first began upon myself. I have used them since in numerous cases, and am now satisfied that they are a safe, certain, and active cathartic, and therefore one of the best cathartics in India.

This plant is the *Convolvulus hirsutus* of Roxburgh, and is described by him in his Flora Indica, Vol. I, page 479. It is also figured by Dr. Wight in his Icones Plantarium Indiæ Orientalis, Vol. III, page 834 ; but there is some confusion about its name in this work. ‘ Batatus pentaphylla’ is the only name found with the *Fig.* in page 834, but it is referred to, in the Index of the same Volume (III), by two other names, viz., ‘ Convolvulus pentaphyllus’ and ‘ C. Hirtus.’   Whatever may be the cause of this confusion, there is no doubt that the plant figured in page 834 of the above volume, is the one under examination, and that the word ‘ Batatus’ or *Batatas* is not applicable to it, for it possesses no tuberous root whatever, which will be seen immediately from its description.

I have raised this plant in my own compound to collect the seeds, and had it under my constant observation for the last few years. I shall therefore describe it minutely, and then speak of its seeds.

Bot. Des.—*Annual ;* if cultivated with care lives more than 8 or 9 months : *root* small and tapering with many thin fibres or rootlets: *stem* round, twining from right to left, often branched, herbaceous ; generally about the thickness of a goose-quill, but often as thick as a finger if cultivated with care ; length unlimited, one plant being sufficient sometimes to cover the whole of a small tree ; very hairy, each hair rising from a small reddish brown gland or papilla ; and these papillæ are very apparent and render the stem rough for a few months, and then disappear gradually : *leaves* petiolate, slightly hairy on both sides, digitate or quinate (not palmate) ; leaflets entire, diverge separately from the top of the petiole ; broadly lanceolate, with a point which is generally long and slightly acute ; unequal in size, the first lateral pair being smaller than the middle leaflet, and the second pair smaller than the first ; and there is occasionally a very small leaf or leafy appendage between the second pair just opposite to the middle leaflet : *petiole* generally longer than the leaf, and thicker than the stem for some time at the commencement ; hairy : *flowers* axillary, pedunculate, pedicellate, bracteate : *bracts* unequal, one being very small and almost abortive, and the other occasionally grows to the size of a small leaf : *peduncle* axillary, hispid, bracteate ; dichotomous 2 or 3 times, *i. e.* it divides first into 2 pedicels, and then each of the latter divides again into 2 smaller ones, and so on 2 or 3 times ; many-flowered, and jointed at the bracts just before it is divided into pedicels : *pedicel* 1—flowered, bracteolate, hairy ; thin and round at the base, but gradually becomes flat and thicker near the calyx ; and dichotomous once or twice in the same manner as the peduncle : *calyx* extremely downy or tomentose, persistent, ovate, divided ; sepals 5, unequal in size and development, remarkably imbricated and appear to be divided into 2 whorls ; the two innermost sepals, which appear to form the internal whorl, are imperfectly developed, and are membranous, smooth, transparent, elastic, and twisted so as to form a kind of cone around the style when the corolla is fallen : *corolla* white, 1—2 inches long, mono-petalous, campanulate, hypogynous, plaited before expansion, deciduous ; expands in the morning and remains so till about the noon, and then gradually closes and falls off in the night or the next morning ; generally expands only once : *stamens* 5, erect, filiform, hypogynous ; attached to the base of the corolla, with which they fall off ; irregular in size, 1 being generally the longest, 2 shorter, and the remaining 2 shortest : *anthers* oblong, bilocular, oscilating, white : *style* simple, included, filiform, persistent ; *stigma* terminal, capitate, 2—lobed, white : *disk* glandular and cup-shaped : *capsule* broadly cordate ; 2—4 celled generally, and sometimes 1—celled, in which case the second cell appears absent from absorption : *cells* 1—seeded, triangular, each closed with a thin, smooth and curved valve : *seeds* small, irregular and of a reddish-brown color. The plant is in flower and fruit during the whole period it lives, except the hottest part of the year.

The seeds of this plant, which may be called *Convolvulus Seeds*, are irregular in their outline, slightly angular, smooth, and generally reddish-brown and sometimes reddish-grey in color. They have two surfaces, one of which is convex, and the other divided into two smaller, flat, and slanting surfaces by an intermediate ridge opposite to the hilum, which gives them the appearance of a quarter segment of any globular body. Their length and breadth is about 1 or $1\frac{1}{2}$, and $1\frac{1}{2}$ or 2 lines, respectively ; and their taste is mucilaginous followed by a peculiar and slight acrid sensation, similar to that of *Kálá-dánah*, but much less in degree. The average weight of each seed is almost 1 grain ; or in other words, if the seed is large it weighs 1 grain, and if small $\frac{3}{4}$ of a grain.

When these seeds are powdered, mixed with water and swallowed, they taste like a flour ; and the acridity which is sometimes felt in the throat, is very slight, lasts only a few seconds, and often not felt at all. So this medicine my be considered to possess no disagreeable taste, while it is quite free from smell. In this respect it is preferable to *Pharbitis Seeds*, *Kálá-dánah* and *Jalap*, though somewhat milder in its action if used in the same dose.

Preparations.—Simple Powder of Convolvulus Seeds *(Pulvis Convolvuli Simplex)*. Powder the seeds in the ordinary way, pass through a five sieve or cloth, and keep in a stopper-bottle.

Dose.—From a drachm to drachm and a half.

Compound Powder of Convolvulus Seeds *(Pulvis Convolvuli Compositus)*. Take of Convolvulus Seeds and Rock Salt or Cream of Tartar, in powder, each seven ounces ; Ginger or Lesser Galangal, in powder, one ounce. Rub them well together, and pass the powder through a fine sieve or cloth.

Dose.—From drachm and a half to two drachms.

I have not yet used this medicine in any other form, but believe that it can be used in the forms of Extract, Tincture, and Resin.

CAMBOGIA.

(Page 83.)

Gamboge is a much stronger cathartic than *Jalap*; but like the latter, it is not very useful or satisfactory when used alone. In combination with other medicines, it is one of the best purgatives we are acquainted with.

During the last several years, whenever *Jalap* was out, I have used this medicine in Triplicane Dispensary, with *Cream of Tartar*, and never felt the absence of the first named drug. I have also used it lately with Rock Salt, and with a greater satisfaction.

Preparation.—Compound Powder of Gamboge *(Pulvis Cambogiæ Compositus)*. Take of Gamboge, in powder, three drachms; Rock Salt or Cream of Tartar, in powder, three ounces and one drachm; Ginger or Lesser Galangal, in powder, two drachms. Rub them well together, and pass the powder through a fine sieve or cloth.

Dose.—From fifty grains to a drachm, according to the condition of the patients with regard to strength, habit, &c. It is a hydragogue and drastic cathartic. It can be used in youths and children in smaller doses according to their age ; but contra-indicated in pregnant women. It is much more efficient and satisfactory than the corresponding preparation of *Jalp* and *Kúlá-dánah*.

One drachm of this Powder contains, six grains of *Gamboge;* fifty grains of *Rock Salt* or *Cream of Tartar ;* and four grains of *Ginger* or *Lesser Galangal:* or in other words, there is one grain of *Gamboge* in every ten grains of it.

IPOMŒA TURPETHUM.

(Pages 161 and 162).

There are two varieties of the root known as *Turbud*, *Tikṛá* or Shiṛadai-vér in the bazaar. They are generally sold under the same names, and sometimes distinguished by the words *Viláyati* or Shímai (Europe or Foreign), and *Náṭ* or *Náṭṭu* (Country or Indian). Both these varieties are indigenous to India, but the above words are used merely to distinguish them from each other.

The real drug which is the root or the bark of the root of *I. turpethum*, is one of the best purgatives in India, and is superior to *Jalap* in some respects which I shall explain presently. The other variety *(Náṭ-ká-turbud)* is also the root of a convolvulous plant, but what particular species the latter is, I have not yet found out. It is considerably inferior as a purgative, and its action is very irregular and uncertain.

The resemblance between these roots is so great, that they cannot be easily distinguished from each other, unless a person is well acquainted with them. I shall first describe the real drug, and then point out some distinctions between this and the other.

The best sort of *Turbud* is not a root, but the bark of a root. In this condition it is seldom or never sold separately in the bazaar, but almost always found mixed with pieces of the root, and requires to be picked out. The pieces of this bark are from 2 to 3 or 4 inches long, curved or quilled, about the size of a finger and about a line in thickness, possess a slight agreeable smell if new, and taste feebly acrid.

With regard to the color, there are two kinds of the bark; one of which is grey or reddish-grey, and the other brown. These two kinds are recognised in some bazaars by the Hindustani names *Suféd-turbud* and *Kálá-turbud*.

If the woody part of the fresh root of *I. Turpethum* is removed by cutting into the bark longitudinally in one place, the latter (bark) assumes the above form when dry. The color of the bark depends upon the age of the root before it is cut and dried, the older the latter is the darker the former becomes, and *vice versa*.

The next form in which the real *Turbud* occurs is the pieces of a root. These pieces are cylindrical, 2 to 4 or 5 inches long; vary in thickness from the size of 2 or 3 goose quills to that of 3 or 4 fingers put together, but generally of the thickness of a finger; brown or dark-brown in colour, and smooth though wrinkled longitudinally in some places.

The native druggists in the bazaar try their best to make the *false Turbud* (*Nát-ká-turbud*) to resemble the best kind of the real drug *(bark of the root of I. Turpethum)* by cutting out the ligneous portion of the former; but they cannot accomplish this object. The bark in the *false Turbud* is too thin, and does not assume the same form when dry. Therefore, the best kind of the *genuine Turbud*, viz., the bark of the root of *I. Turpethum*, cannot be confounded with any other bark or root. It is only the pieces of the root of *I. Turpethum*, which constitutes the commonest kind of the *real Turbud*, that can be imitated by, and confounded with, the *false Turbud*. The following distinctions, however, will be sufficient to distinguish the one from the other:—

False *Turbud* or *Turbith-root*.	Real *Turbud* or *Turbith-root*.
1. It is a much larger root, varying in size from the thickness of a finger or thumb to that of an infant's fore-arm.	1. Much smaller, it being generally about the size of a finger or thumb.
2. Brown or pale-brown in colour.	2. Generally darker in colour.
3. Very rough and uneven on the surface.	3. Smooth, though wrinkled in some places.
4. The structure of this root is that of any common root, and it is comparatively very hard and heavy.	4. Both the cortical and ligneous portions of this root are composed of parallel and straight longitudinal fibres, and this contrasts much with the structure of the *false Turbud* or *Turbith-root*.

5. Never attacked by in-sects.

5. Often worm-eaten.

6. Possesses no parti-cular taste.

6. Its taste is slightly acrid.

I have lately used this medicine *(the real Turbud)* in many cases, and found it to be a very superior and valuable purgative. It is preferable to *Julap* in having no nauseous smell or taste, and in being a very efficient and satisfactory purgative when used by itself. It is true that it requires to be used in a larger dose than *Julap*, but this is no disadvantage as long as it is safe and free from nauseous taste and smell. The dose is larger only by 10 or 15 grains.

Preparations.—Simple Powder of Turbith-root *(Pulvis Ipomœœ Simplex)*. If it is the bark of Turbud, it should be powdered in the usual way, passed through a fine sieve or cloth, and kept in a stopper-bottle. But if it is the root, the cortical portion should be separated from it, and the latter alone selected for powdering, &c., as above. The bark is easily separated if the root is broken longitudinally.

Dose.—From fifty to seventy grains.

Compound Powder of Turbith-root *(Pulvis Ipomœœ Compositus)*. Take of the Simple Powder of Turbith-root and powdered Rock Salt or Cream of Tartar, each seven ounces; Ginger or Lesser Galangal, in powder, one ounce. Rub them well together, pass through a fine sieve or cloth, and keep in a stopper-bottle.

Dose.—From a drachm to four scruples, or more.

CLITOREA TERNATEA.

(Pages 108 and 109.)

The seeds of this plant, which are casually noticed as a purgative in some medical and other works, are very deservedly included and spoken of highly in the Pharmacopœia of India, page 80. The native druggists and practitioners consider them as a very good substitute for the seeds of *Pharbitis Nil ruber* (p. 277) and *P. Nil* (p. 196), and they are consequently often known in the bazaar by the same names as those of the two latter, which I have already mentioned in page 109 of this work. They are certainly a very good substitute for the above drugs, as well as *Jalap*, and are equal to *Convolvulus Seeds* in every respect, except the taste, which is disagreeable and much more acrid.

I gave a trial to this medicine on two different occasions, and on each occasion in pretty large number of cases. When I tried first a few years ago, the medicine almost failed to act as a good purgative, but on the second trial, very recently, it has proved itself much more efficient than anticipated. The cause of this difference is, that the seeds used on the first occasion were bought from the bazaar, and they were, as I found out afterwards, collected before they were quite matured and dried on the plant. They were flat, dark-brown, and oblong. On the second occasion, the seeds used were gathered from the pods which were quite dry before their removal from the plant. These seeds were nearly round or slightly compressed near the edges; oblong; dull green, greenish brown or brown in color, and minutely mottled. The ends of some seeds were round, and of some flat, as if it were cut off by a knife. Speaking comparatively, these seeds were much thicker and rounder, paler in color, and more disagreeable and acrid in taste, than those used on the first occasion.

These seeds are not sold in the bazaar of Madras by the common or proper druggists, but by those druggists who sell the fresh medicinal plants and consequently named *Kach-chá-pansárí* in Dukhni. Even these do not sell them always, and generally procure them only when they are ordered to do so. Under these circumstances, the seeds are often required to be collected from the plants when there is a need for a large quantity of them. The plants are cultivated in some places, and found wild in others; and are as follows:—

Bot. Des.—Perrenial; much branched and shrubby : *root* slightly fleshy, tapering, branched : *stems* several, twining from right to left, pubescent in young plants: *leaves* unequally pinnate, leaflets 2—3 pairs, oval, or slightly ovate: *flowers* large, blue or white; pedunculate, resupinate, bracteolate : *peduncles* short, about ¼ inch in length; axillary, solitary, 1—flowered: *bracteoles* roundish, about 2 lines in diameter, adherent to the base of the calyx : *calyx* about ¼ of the length of the corolla, 5—cleft, unequal, persistent, hypogynous : *corolla* papilionaceous; vexillum large, rounded with a cleft at the end, exterior, blue with a yellowish white color in the centre; alæ oval with a very thin and narrow stalk; keel slightly boot-shaped with two thin thread-like stalks : *stamens* varying in number from 5 to 10 or more, diadelphous, 1 being separate and the rest united by filaments; hypogynous : *anthers* very small, globular, white : *style* simple, longer than the stamens, slightly curved, dilated at the end : *legume* a few inches in length and a few lines in breadth, flat, straight, slightly pubescent, 2—valved; 1—celled, but divided into many partitions by cellular walls, each of which contains a seed; many seeded : *seeds* oblong, about 2 or 3 lines long, greenish brown or brown in color. The plant is always in flower.

There are two varieties of this plant, distinguished by the color of their flowers as *blue* and *white*. The blue, again, has another sub-variety, which is double-flowered. There is no apparent difference in the action of the seeds of these varieties, or if any at all, it is in favor of the white variety. But, from whatever variety they may be, the rounder and thicker the seeds are, the more energetic they prove in their action.

As these seeds are not known by any particular name, it is inconvenient to describe their preparations; and I have therefore named them *Clitorea Seeds*.

Preparations.—Simple Powder of Clitorea Seeds (*Pulvis Clitoreæ Simplex*). To be powdered in the ordinary way, passed through a fine sieve or cloth, and kept in a stopper-bottle.

Dose.—From a drachm to drachm and a half.. In this dose it produces 5 or 6 free motions, and its action is increased in proportion to the increase of its quantity up to two drachms, when the number of motions it generally produces is 8 or 9.

Compound Powder of Clitorea Seeds *(Pulvis Clitoreæ Compositus)*. Take of Clitorea Seeds and Rock Salt or Cream of Tartar, in powder, each seven ounces; Ginger or Lesser Galangal, in powder, one ounce. Rub them well together, pass through a fine sieve or cloth, and keep in a stopper-bottle.

Dose.—From drachm and a half to two drachms.

JACQUIMONTIA VIOLACEA.

(Page 275).

The seeds of this plant are a safe and mild aperient. It being a periennial and always in flower, which is of a beautiful blue color, it is used as an ornamental plant in many European bungalows, gardens, and other places at Madras. It is supposed to have been introduced first into the Horti-agricultural Society's and other gardens at Madras by Sir Walter Elliot, and he is, very likely, also the author of its botanical name.

The plant is very easily propagated by cutting, layers, or seeds; but in the first two cases, it does not generally produce seeds.

Bot. Des.—*Perennial*, spreading extensively, very ornamental: *stem* twining as well as creeping; about the thickness of the little finger near the root, but very thin in upper parts ; length unlimited, bluish-green, twining from right to left, and takes root if any part of it comes in contact with soil: *leaves* cordate or oblong-cordate, petiolate, smooth, soft, slightly wavy, entire: *flowers* axillary, pedunculate, pedicellate, bracteolate: *peduncle* twice or three times longer than the petiole, many flowered: *pedicels* very short, generally 2—3 ; each surrounded by several bracteoles, and form a kind of umbel, which is generally compound: *calyx* divided; sepals 5, 3 of which well developed and 2 almost abortive ; imbricated, broadly cordate, acuminate, longer than the capsule, pale green in color : *corolla* monopetalous, about an inch long, bright blue with a white eye, plaited before expansion : *stamens* 5, of equal size, attached to the base of the corolla : *anthers* oblong, white : *style* filiform, a little longer than the stamens, generally persistent : *stigma* small, 2—lobed, white : *ovary* very small, glandular, cup-shaped, of a pale-yellow color : *capsule* nearly round or broadly cordate, about the size of a coriander fruit, 1—2 celled, dehiscent: *cell* 1—2 seeded : seeds very small, angular, and of various color, generally brown or reddish brown.

The seeds are about $\frac{3}{4}$ of a line in length and breadth, angular, and bear a resemblance to *Kúlá-dánah* in their form. They are inodrous, and their taste is purely albuminous, without the least acridity or disagreeableness. This is the only advantage of this aperient over all other medicines of the same class. Their color is reddish-brown, brown, or yellowish white. The reddish brown and hard seeds should alone be selected for medicinal purposes. Their dose is from a drachm and a half to two drachms.

ACACIA CONCINNA.

(Page 21.)

The dry pod or legume of this plant is the commonest article used by native women in this country for washing their head, as soap is in Europe, &c. It is therefore found not only in every bazaar, but also in every family house.

The pod is either reddish-brown or brown in color ; varies much in length, generally from 3 to 6 inches ; about 1 inch broad ; many seeded ; 2—valved ; valves much contracted between the seeds ; much wrinkled ; and has a sourish and nauseous taste. The seeds are shining black, oval or oblong, and very hard.

This pod is a cathartic, nauseant, and also emetic to a slight extent. In its action as a cathartic, it is superior to *Senna*, but it is more nauseous and disagreeable in taste and smell. Like *Senna*, it is not an efficient purgative by itself, but a very good adjuvant to other purgatives, as *Sulphate of Magnesia, Rock Salt, &c.* In addition to the stronger action, its other advantages over *Senna* are, that its use is not attended with griping in the bowels, and that it is a very useful remedy in Jaundice not depending upon obstruction.

Preparations.—Simple Infusion of **Acacia** Concinna *(Infusum Acacia Concinnæ Simplex).* Take of the dry Pods of Acacia Concinna, without seeds, four ounces ; Boiling Water, 20 fluid ounces Bruise the pods, iufuse in a covered vessel for two hours, and strain.

Dose.—Four fluid ounces. This is a mild cathartic, and if four drachms of Sulphate of Magnesia added to it, acts as a strong purgative.

Compound Infusion of Acacia Concinna *(Infusum Acacia Concinnæ Compositum).* To be prepared in the same manner as the above preparation, with the addition of Coriander Fruits, bruised, four drachms ; and Ginger or Lesser Galangal, sliced, two drachms.

Dose.—The dose and manner of using this preparation as a cathartic is the same as those of the preceding. This Infusion is more suited to be used by itself in Jaundice, &c., in which case, it should be administered in three or four ounce doses two or three times in 24 hours.

PHARBITIS. *Sp. of ?*

(Page 277.)

I have obtained the seeds known in Calcutta as Sha*b-pasandú* or ' Shapussundo,' which are mentioned in the Pharmacopœia of India, page 157. I have sown a great many of them but only two plants were produced, and these too, died after 2 months without flowering. They had grown to the extent of 2 feet, and were as follows :—

Bot. Des.—Herbaceous : *root* small and tapering : *stem* twining, very hairy : *leaves* palmate with regard to the form, and septenate with reference to the number of leaflets ; hairy on both surfaces; leaflets entire, ovate or oval.

They were apparently Convolvulous plants, but from want of flowers I cannot say to what Genus of that Order they belong. They are, probably, either a species of *Convolvulus* or *Pharbitis.*

The dry seeds I have received from Calcutta, are of the form of a quarter segment of any globular body ; grey, dark-grey or reddish-brown in color ; woolly, being covered with small, thin, very soft, and cotton-like hairs; inodorous and almost tasteless. They bear a great resemblance to Convolvulus Seeds *(Convolvulus hirsutus)* in their form, and though somewhat larger than the latter, yet lighter in weight.

Although mild, this medicine is one of those cathartics which are preferable to many others for not having a bad smell or taste.

Preparations.—Simple Powder of Shab-pasandú Seeds *(Pulvis Shab-pasandú Simplex)*. To be well dried in the sun, powdered in the ordinary way, passed through a fine sieve or cloth, and kept in a stopper-bottle.

Dose.—From one drachm to drachm and a half.

Compound Powder of Shab-pasandú Seeds *(Pulvis Shab-pasandú Compositus)*. Take of Shab-pasandu Seeds and Rock Salt or Cream of Tartar, in powder, each seven ounces; Ginger or Lesser Galangal, in powder, one ounce. Rub them together, pass through a fine sieve or cloth, and keep in a stopper-bottle.

Dose.—From four scruples to two drachms.

ROCK SALT.

(Page 216.)

This Salt is well known now to be a mere variety of *Chloride of Sodium,* but why it is much more stronger as a cathartic than the latter I cannot explain. It is also stronger than *Cream of Tartar,* but like this drug, it is not a satisfactory cathartic by itself. Used in combination with other purgatives, it is more satisfactory than *Cream of Tartar*. I have already mentioned its entrance into the Compound Powders of *Gamboge; Pharbitis, Convolvulus, Clitorea,* and *Shab-pasandú Seeds;* and *Turbith Root;* and have also used it in the same manner with *Jalap* and *Kálá-dúnah* in lieu of *Cream of Tartar*.

Rock Salt occurs in large masses, varying in weight from 2 or 3 to 8 or 10 lbs. The masses are dull or brownish white externally, and white and crystalline internally. The salt has a pure saline taste. It is procurable in every large bazaar in India, and its price is about 4 or 5 annas per lb.

N. B.—In conclusion of my remarks on Cathartics, I wish to state that these medicines are generally required to be used in a larger dose to act satisfactorily among the natives of this country than Europeans. For example, the *Compound Powder of Kálá-dánah* prepared and used in fifty or sixty grain doses according to the Pharmacopœia of India, page 156, is, perhaps, sufficient to act as an efficient purgative in Europeans ; but it is not so in natives, in whom even drachm and a half of that Powder does not act quite satisfactorily.

According to my own experience, the best way of preparing the *Compound Powder of Kálá-dánah* is to combine it with *Rock Salt* or *Cream of Tartar*, in equal proportion, with a small quantity of *Ginger* or *Lesser Galangal;* or in other words, it should be prepared in the same manner as the corresponding preparation of all the purgatives I have described above, except *Gamboge*. Prepared in this proportion, it produces 6 or 7 motions satisfactorily in $1\frac{1}{2}$ drachm doses.

My remarks on all the above cathartics, particularly with reference to their action and dose, is solely based upon the experience among the natives of this country, who, as a rule, are not satisfied with any purgative, unless it acts briskly and produces some slime or bile.

INDIGENOUS EMETICS.

RANDIA DUMETORUM.

(Page 212.)

The dry nut of this plant is one of the most ancient emetics, and is not only found in India, but also in Arabia, Persia, and many other places of Asia. In latter places it is said to be sold under the Arabic name *Jouzul-qai*, which means *the emetic nut.* It is well known in the Indian bazaars by its Hindustani and Dukhni names *Mén-phal* and *Ménd-phal.* It is very cheap and procurable in many bazaars at about 2 annas a lb.

The nut is generally about the size of a small nutmeg, and often much larger; globular or oval; deep grey or reddish brown; and crowned with the rim of the calyx. It consists of a shell or pericarp, seeds, and mucus or pulp. The shell is hard and thick; 2—celled; contains numerous small seeds, which are very adherent to the mucus and to each other; wrinkled and divided externally into quarters by 4 distinct longitudinal lines, 2 of which are generally more marked and correspond with the division of the cells internally. The seeds are small and oblong; about 1½ lines in length; slightly flat; of a reddish brown color; very hard; and formed into a lump together with the mucus, which is hard and corresponds with the shape of the nut, and is divided symmetrically into 2 halves by a thin membranous layer, the septum of the cells. The mucus or pulp is generally grey or reddish brown and sometimes yellowish grey; very small in quantity; and possesses a very nauseous taste and smell; and is so adherent to the seeds, that it cannot be separated from them by any process in dry state. It is, however, very soluble in cold and hot waters, alcohol, and many other liquids.

The average weight of the nut is 1 drachm, and if the pulp is completely removed by dissolving in water, the shell and seeds generally weigh 45 grains, and thus show the weight of the pulp only to be 15 grains or $\frac{1}{4}$ of the nut.

This is one of the medicines I have paid much attention to during the last few years, and have now found out that it is, as an emetic, quite equal to *Ipecacuanha* if not superior to it.

It is certainly not a good emetic, nor quite free from irritation, if used, as is generally done, by powdering the whole nut. The thick shell and the numerous hard seeds of the nut are not emetic at all ; indeed, if any thing, they are slightly irritant ; but only the dry pulp or mucus, which is the least part of the nut, possesses the emetic and nauseant properties.

When the shell is broken, the lump of the mucus and seeds will be found hard and loose, and is easily removed from the former. But the mucus and seeds cannot be separated from each other, except by dissolving in water or powdering and passing through a cloth or sieve.

The lumps of 2 or 3 nuts is generally a dose of the medicine. They should be bruised, macerated for 10 or 15 minutes in 3 or 4 ounces of water, rubbed with fingers, and then strained through cloth. The mucus being very soluble in water, passes off with it, and the seeds with some resinous and other insoluble matters, remain on the cloth. The draught is now ready for use, and if given to a patient, it produces nausea and vomiting in about 10 minutes, and very free emesis is followed if assisted with warm water.

The best and most convenient way, however, of using this medicine is in powder, which I shall describe under the head of *Preparation.*

Sugar and *honey* do not seem to interfere with the action of this medicine, and they may therefore be added to it to cover the nauseous taste. This combination is very useful when it is administered to children as an emetic or expetorant, in smaller doses according to their age, &c.

When used as an emetic, the vomiting produced by this medicine contains a large quantity of frothy mucus. From this, and from its being a very nauseant vegetable emetic, I thought it will prove a good remedial agent in Dysentery, in the same way as *Ipecacuanha* is. On instituting a trial on some cases, this opinion was more than realized. Having now used it in many cases, I do not hesitate in considering the dry pulp of the *Emetic Nut* or *Randia Nut (Randia dumetorum)* equal to *Ipecacuanha* as a remedy in Dysentery.

The *modus operandi* of this medicine is the same as that of *Ipecacuanha*, viz., it relieves the Dysenteric Inflammation—

First, by reducing the force of general circulation, partly by depressing the system, and partly by determining the blood to the skin.

Secondly, by reverting or diminishing the peristaltic motion, and thereby giving rest to the inflamed bowel.

Thirdly, by increasing the secretion of mucus from the extensive surface of the bowels, and thus restoring to its normal condition the morbid capillary circulation of the affected part.

Every nauseant emetic or medicine will more or less possess the actions in the 1st and 2nd axioms, and, if it is not irritant at the same time, might subdue the dysenteric inflammation to some extent. But, unless it also possesses the action in the 3rd, it will not be so useful in Dysentery as to deserve a special notice. It is the latter action which makes the dry pulp of the nut of *Randia dumetorum*, *Ipecacuanha*, and also a few other emetics to be noticed in the following pages, peculiarly useful in that disease.

Like *Ipecacuanaha*, the pulp of *Emetic-nut* is not sufficient to effect or complete a cure in Dysentery by itself, but generally requires the assistance of other medicines, particularly the *Opium*. I almost always prescribe it with the latter from the commencement of treatment, and in ordinary cases they check the progress and mitigate the symptoms of the disease in 3 or 4 days, and then the cure is completed in 5 or 6 days more, either by the same medicines or by the use of *Dover's Powder* or some other preparations of *Opium*. In slighter cases, the disease itself is often checked in a few days, and requires little or no other medicine afterwards. In some severe and obstinate cases, however, when the disease lasts longer than a week or so, or assumes the chronic form, the use of other medicines is always necessary.

Even in Dysentery the most convenient way of using this medicine is to have it ready in powder. But in the absence of this preparation, it may be made into a draught as already described, and given 3 or 4 times in 24 hours. The pulp of 1 or 2 nuts is generally sufficient for a dose in Dysentery, and the draught is to be combined with 20 to 40 drops of *Tincture of Opium*, according to the frequency of motions.

Preparation.—Simple Powder of the Pulp of Emetic Nut (*Pulvis Pulpæ Randiæ Simplex*). After removing the shell, the lumps of seeds and pulp should be well bruised and passed through a sieve or thin cloth. By this means all the seeds will be separated. The coarse powder thus obtained should be powdered again and passed through a fine sieve or cloth. The powder is now fit for use, and should be kept in a stopper-bottle.

Dose.—Two scruples, as an Emetic; and from fifteen to thirty grains or more, in Dysentery, according to the severity of the disease.

Other preparations of this medicine are the same as those of *Ipecacuanha*, and as they are more nauseant, diaphoretic, and astringent than emetic, I shall not describe them here.

STRYCHNOS POTATORUM.

(*Page* 235.)

The berries or fruits of this plant are familiarly known in the Indian bazaars by the Hindustani and Dukhni names *Nirmalí* and *Chilbinj*. They are as common and cheap as the nut of *Randia dumetorum*, and their price is about the same, viz., 2 annas per lb.

These fruits are known as an emetic in Southern India, and often resorted to for that purpose by some native practitioners; but what they are very popular for in this, as well as many other places in India, is, their property of clearing the dirty or muddy water. This explains the meaning of their names *Nirmali, Clearing Nut, &c.*

The emetic property of these fruits is also noticed in some medical and other works, but in a very casual manner; and they do not appear to have been ever used in the English medical practice.

The cause of their not acquiring a repute as a valuable emetic is the improper way in which they are administered. The whole fruit is generally powdered and given in about half a tea spoonful doses, and there is no wonder if it does not act satisfactorily, because the seed which is by far the largest portion of the fruit, is not emetic. The *dry-mucus* or *pulp* and the thin *pericarp* or *testa* are the only parts endowed with the property of emetic, and if they be used separately, their action is highly satisfactory.

Of these two parts, again, the dry mucus is more efficient,. but it is so small in quantity and so adherent either to the seed or pericarp, that it cannot be separated from them. If it is adherent to the pericarp, so much the better, and they both can be used together very satisfactorily. But if it is adherent to the seed, it is not easily available for use.

The fruits of *Strychnos Potatorum* are a little smaller than a *Soap-nut*, round, smooth, shining, and of a greenish or yellowish brown color. They are 1—seeded, and the seed is slightly flat and circular, and yellowish grey or pale brown in color.

The seeds are found in the bazaar with or without the pericarp, but generally in the latter condition. If the fruit is entire, the pericarp can be easily removed from the seed with fingers, and the pericarp is also sold separately in some bazaars of Southern India.

When sold separately, it occurs in two conditions. In one condition it is found in thin, scaly, and shell-like pieces, which are shining externally, and of a greenish or yellowish brown color. This is nothing but the pericarp removed when the fruit is dry. In the second condition, it is formed together with the mucus into large balls or masses, each of which generally weighs a lb. If the pericarp is removed with mucus or pulp when the fruit is quite ripe, and made into balls and dried, it assumes the above form. In this condition, it contains a large quantity of dry mucus, and is much superior in its action than the other form. The dry mucus appears to be more efficacious in Dysentery than *Ipecacuanha*, but it is obtained with such a difficulty that the small quantity I received was sufficient only for a few cases, and was used in much smaller doses than desirable.

The dose of the Simple Powder of Pericarp, prepared in the usual way and kept in a stopper-bottle, is from 40 to 50 grains, as an emetic; and from 15 to 30, in Dysentery.

TYLOPHORA ASTHMATICA.

(Page 249.)

This is one of the commonest plant in Southern India, and found in almost every garden and field. It enjoys a great reputation as an antidote to snake-bites, &c., among the snake-catchers of this country, and is known to them as the plant resorted to by *Mongoose* when bitten by a snake. The natives are aware of its emetic property, but seldom employ it as such, and no part of the plant is sold in the bazaar. It is required to be collected for use.

Bot. Des.—*Perennia* *root* fibrous, fibrils numerous: *stems* several, twining from right to left; generally about the size of a fowl's quill, some times as thick as that of a goose; branched, slightly downy: *leaves* opposite, often decussate near the root, entire, 2 to $3\frac{1}{4}$ inches long and $1\frac{1}{2}$ to $2\frac{1}{4}$ broad, oblong-ovate, slightly bearded on the upper side at the base, occasionally and slightly cordate at the base, very shortly and abruptly acuminate, glabrous above and slightly downy below, petiolate: *petiole* short, downy, slightly channelled: *Flowers* small, about 3 or 4 lines in diameter, of the shape of a star; expanding morning and evening and in the night, but close during the day when the sun is hot; pedunculate, umbellate, involucrate: *peduncle* axillary, simple, generally alternate, longer than the petiole: *umbel* generally compound and irregular, surrounded at the base by involucres: *involucres* very small and persistent:

calyx hypogynous, persistent, poly-sepalous ; sepals 5, small, about a line or line and a half in length, green or pale green : *corolla* hypogynous, poly-petalous ; petals 5, triangular, about a line or line and a half in length, occasionally and slightly recurved ; pale yellow, except at their base internally, where they are of pink color or marked with pink dots : *stamens* and *pistil* unite together and form a common body *(gynandrous)*, which is about a line in diameter, and marked with 5 yellowish and elevated lines : *ovaries* 2 : *follicles* in pairs, opposite to each other and slightly adherent at the base (divaricate when young), tapering to a point, 2 to 4 inches long, about ½ an inch in thickness in the middle, glabrous, 1—valved, dehescent : *seeds* comose, being furnished with a tuft of hairs on the upper end or base which is towards the end of the follicle ; small, very thin, reddish brown, and slightly obovate. The plant flowers all round the year, particularly when cultivated.

There are two varieties of this plant, which differ from each other only in size and a few other minor characters. When placed under the same circumstances, one is always larger than the other. In the large variety, the petals are larger, more or less reflexed, and also slightly revolute some times; and the adult leaves are broader, thinner, deeper in color, and slightly recurved.

With regard to the root of this plant, it seems to have been confounded with another root in some books. For example, the following sentence occurs in the Materia Indica, Vol. II, page 83 :—

' The root of this plant, as it appears in the Indian bazars, is thick, twisted, of a pale color, and of a bitterish and somewhat nauseous taste.'

In the first place, the root of this plant is not sold in bazaars, at least, in the bazaars of Southern India. Secondly, it is not a thick root, but a *fibrous root* consisting of many round, thin, and brittle fibres or fibrils. These fibrils generally vary in their number from 5 to 15 or 20, and sometimes they are upwards of 50. They are from to 2 to 5 or 6 inches long, about ¼ or 1 line in thickness, and of a pale or dirty white color. These fibrils or roots issue from a woody part, which is the axis or centre between them and stems. They are seldom branched, but generally give attachment to very thin and hair-like fibres or rootlets.

The whole of the plant under discussion, including the stem and follicles, is emetic ; but the root and leaves are not only the best, but also easily powdered to be brought into use.

The root, again, is by far the best as a substitute for *Ipecacuanha* in Dysentery, and as an expectorant and diaphoretic.

About 4 years ago, when I had an occasion to make remarks upon some native medicines, my opinion of *Tyloph ra asthmatica* was as follows :—

‘ It is the best substitute we possess in this country for Ipecacuanha, both as an emetic and as a remedy for Dysentery in large doses. From 20 to 40 grains of its powder with the same quantity in minims of Tinctura Opii, 3 or 4 times a day in 24 hours, checks the disease as speedily and successfully as the Ipecacuanha. It is also a better medicine than the latter, to use as an emetic or expectorant in cases of Asthma.

‘ Next to Ammonia I have more faith in Tylophora Asthmatica as an antidote to snake-bites than any other medicine. The fresh juice should be administered frequently and in large doses till free vomiting is produced, and then be followed with strong and diffusible stimulants.’

From my subsequent and more extensive experience of native medicines, I have found that *Tylophora asthmatica* is not the best, but one of the 4 or 5 best emetics in India, and ranks after *Randia dumetorum* and *Strychnos Potatorum ;* and that although the whole parts of it are emetic, the root alone is a very good remedial agent in Dysentery. Its *modus operandi* in this disease is the same as already explained under *Randia dumetorum.*

Preparations.—Simple Powder of Tylophora Root (*Pulvis Tylophoræ Simplex).* To be prepared in the usual way, passed through a fine sieve or cloth, and kept in a stopper-bottle.

Dose.—From forty to fifty grains, as an emetic ; and 15 to 30 or more, in Dysentery.

Simple Powder of Tylophora Leaves *(Pulvis Tylophoræ Foliæ Simplex)*. The leaves are powdered with more difficulty than the roots. They should be first well dried in the sun or on a sand bath, powdered, and passed through a thin cloth. This coarse powder is to be pulverized again, passed through a fine sieve or cloth, and kept in a stopper-bottle.

Dose.—Same as the Simple Powder of the Root.

There are also other preparations of the root of *T. asthmatica,* as Compound Powder, &c., but as they possess more of other properties than emetic, they may not be described here.

CALOTROPIS GIGANTEA.

(Page 82.)

This is one of the commonest shrubs in India, and in S. India there is scarcely any waste, ruinous, or sandy ground which is not covered with it. Its medical properties are known to the natives of this country from the earliest period, and is particularly held in high estimation by the Hindu practitioners (V*ai*ddiyars) in the treatment of venereal and other skin diseases. So much so, that it is called by some of them ' the vegetable mercury.'

Although this plant is frequently used as a medicine, yet no part of it is sold in the bazaar. It being found in every place, it is resorted to whenever it is required.

Bot. Des.—*A large shrub,* much branched, abounding in a milky and acrid juice : *stem* and *branches* knotted at short intervals, slightly ash-colored : *leaves* opposite, decussate, entire, 3 to 6 inches long and 2 to 3 broad, cuneate-obovate or oblong-obovate, rounded and slightly pointed at the end, bearded on the upper side at the base, stem-clasping, subsessile, under surface is covered with a woolly down : *flowers* pedunculate, umbellate, involucrate ;

peduncle lateral or terminal, thick and long, simple, slightly clothed with a woolly down, nearly erect ; when lateral, it is alternate *i. e.* arising alternately between the opposite leaves : *umbels* generally simple, occasionally compound, surrounded at the base by involucres : *involucres* small and scaly : *calyx* hypogynous, deciduous, poly-sepalous, sepals 5, ash-colored, each sepal about a line and a half or 2 lines in length : *corolla* hypogynous, deciduous, poly-petalous ; petals 5, oblong, obtuse, reflexed, revolute, pale-blue or white : *stamens* indistinct, filiments combined and formed into a tube *(gynostegium)* which completely surrounds the pistils : *stamineous corona* 5—leaved ; leaflets keel-formed, recurved at the base, slightly incurved and dentate at the apex : *ovaries* 2 : *styles* 2, situated within the gynostegium : *stigma* common to both styles, dilated into a flat body which is about $1\frac{1}{4}$ lines in diameter, 5—angled, cartilaginous, and is situated just above the gynostegium : *follicles* in pairs, ventricose, smooth, dehescent, and one of the pairs generally abortive : *seeds* comose, very thin, slightly obovate, and have a tuft of hairs attached to their base or upper end which is towards the end of the follicle. The plant is seldom or never free from flower in any part of the year.

The two varieties of this plant met with in Madras, are distinguished by their color, which is pale-blue or bluish-purple in one, and cream-white in the other.

Almost every part of this plant is used in medicine, but the bark of the root and dry milky juice are by far the best. Of these two parts, again, the milk is the strongest, but it is very irregular and unsafe in its action ; therefore, the root-bark is the best and most useful for medicinal purposes.

According to my experience, the older the plant is, the more active is the bark in its effects ; and if it be powdered by simply drying it, as is generally done, it requires to be used in a much larger dose to act efficiently as an emetic. The thick, rough, and spongy epidermis, which the bark is covered with, and which is quite inert, should be scraped off with a knife before it is powdered. The powder prepared with this precaution, is white and bears a great resemblance to the flour of rice. It has a nauseous and slightly acrid smell, and a bitterish taste. It should be preserved in a stopper-bottle. The dose of this powder as an emetic, is from forty to fifty grains.

According to the suggestion of Sir W. B. O'Shaughnessy in the Bengal Dispensatory, I have used also this medicine in some cases of Dysentery, and found it in large doses to be a good substitute for *Ipecacuanha*. Its dose in this disease is the same as the Simple Powder of *Tylophora asthmatica*.

ALANGIUM DECAPETALUM

AND

ALANGIUM HEXAPETALUM.

(Pages 35 and 36.)

The root-bark of *A. decapetalum* is the chief ingredient in a few secret prescriptions which are in great vogue in the treatment of Leprosy, venereal and other skin diseases, at Arcot and Vellore. While using this bark myself in some cases of Lepra, I found it produce vomiting on many occasions, even in so small a dose as 5 grains, and this gave me a clue as to its being an emetic. On trials in larger quantities, which were as usual begun upon myself, it has proved itself an efficient and safe emetic. In smaller doses, it is a nauseant and febrifuge ; and in still smaller quantities one of the best alterative-tonic in India.

This bark is very bitter, and its repute in skin diseases is not without foundation. If it is continued for a sufficient period, its influence over them is greater than that of *Calotropis gigantea*.

The plant is pretty common in the jungles of Southern India, and also occasionally met with in the gardens. No part of it is sold in the bazaar.

Bot. Des.—*Tree*, size variable, generally small, spinescent when young; the young branches arising from the trunk of an old or adult tree are also spinescent : *leaves* alternate, oblong-lanceolate or narrow-oblong, 3— 5 inches long and 1—1½ broad.

glabrous, petiolate : *petiole* short, slightly pubescent, about ¼ inch in length : *Flowers* middle-sized, slightly fragrant, yellowish-white, generally axillary, pedunculate : *peduncle* short, simple : *calyx* epigynous, toothed, persistent, short : *corolla* poly-petalous ; petals 6—10, oblong, more or less reflexed : *stamens* twice the number of the petals; filaments hairy at the base ; anthers oblong : *style* generally longer than the stamens : *fruit* about the size of a small soapnut, globular, glabrous, druping, red in color, mounted with the calyx, 1—seeded, slightly and agreeably sweet to the taste : *seed* circular, slightly flat above and below, hard, and brown. Flowers about the beginning of the hot weather.

The native practitioners and druggists speak of 2 varieties of this plant, and call them *white* and *black*. The white is, the plant I have just described, but the black is not a variety, as considered by them, but a closely allied species, viz., *Alangium hexapetalum* of Lamarck. They call this plant as a black variety of *A. decapetalum*, because it bears some resemblance to it in its general appearance, its flowers are purple or purplish blue, and its bark is much darker in color.

The bark of this plant is considered as a much superior alterative and alexipharmic, and its use is said to be attended with occasional vomiting. I am induced from these circumstances to think that it is also an emetic ; but the plant not being found in Madras, and its specimens obtained with a great difficulty and cost, I have not as yet ascertained its properties by personal experience.

Preparation.—Simple Powder of Alangium Bark *(Pulvis Alangii Simplex)*. Dry the bark of the root without exposing it to the sun, powder in the ordinary way, pass through a fine sieve or cloth, and keep in a stopper-bottle.

Dose.—Fifty grains, as an emetic.

FICUS OPPOSITIFOLIA
FICUS DÆMONA
AND
FICUS POLYCARPA.

(Page 143.)

A few years ago, while examining the medicinal plants in some gardens and fields in Codumpock, a village about 6 or 7 miles from Madras, with a view to find out their native names in actual use, I eat a few fruits of *Ficus oppositifulia*, which bear a great resemblance to the common cultivated *fig (F. carica)* and are very sweet in taste. A few minutes afterwards, I felt sick in the stomach and vomited 2 or 3 times. This circumstance led to the discovery of the emetic and other properties of this plant, as well as of *F. polycarpa*, which are already noticed in the Pharmacopœia of India (p. 217) according to my remarks sent in a paper to the Committee of that work, together with some specimens of the plants.

I mention now these plants here merely to state that every thing I said about them before has been confirmed by subsequent experience, except the antiperiodic effect, which is very feeble; and that *F. dæmana* of Kœnig and one or two other closely allied species of Ficus are also possessed with emetic property.

It was my intention to describe all these plants, but from the long and continued dry weather in this place during the last 2 years, most of them are either dead, dying, withered, or not in fruit at present. I cannot, therefore, describe them with such minuteness as is necessary to show some clear and decided distinctions between them. They are, however, well described and figured by Drs. Roxburgh and Wight in their Flora Indica and Icones Plantarum Indiæ Orientalis, respectively, and the following is the description from the first named work, of *F. oppositifolia* and *F. dæmona*, which are by far the most common, and also more useful than the other plants :—

F. oppositifolia (Roxb.)

' A small tree, a native of the banks of rivulets, and other places vhere the soil is moist and rich, common about Calcutta.

' Trunk erect, seldom as thick as a man's body, branches opposite and sub-erect. Bark scabrous, ash-colored. Young shoots scabrous, and covered with much short white hairs, piped, and interrupted at the insertion of the leaves as in the Bamboo. Leaves opposite, short, round, petioled, oblong, slightly serrate, of a firm scabrous texture, shining above, downy below, and most beautifully reticulate, one of each pair is always considerably smaller than the other; they are from 5 to 9 inches long. Fruits on the young shoots axillary and peduncled, in the naked woody branches racemed, round, about the size of a large nutmeg, covered with much short white hairs, several equi-distant ridges running from the umbilicus to the base. Calyx of the fruit 3—leaved. Flowers, a few round the inside of the mouth of the navel. Filaments or peduncles single, with a proper three-parted perianth surrounding the middle. Female flowers numerous. Peduncles long. Perianth none. Style and stigma placed together on the side of the germ, funnel-formed.

F. dæmona (Kön.).

' Shrubby. Leaves generally opposite, cuneate, oblong or oblong-pointed, serrate, above scabrous, downy underneath, with a green gland in axills of the veins. Fruit in pairs on long radical racemes, above very hairy, of the size of a nutmeg.

' A native of the sandy lands near the sea on the coast of the Tanjore country. From thence Dr. Rottler sent plants to this garden (Calcutta garden) where they produce fruits all the year round. In its native barren soil it grows to be stout ramous shrub, or small tree.

' Young shoots densely clothed with thick, soft, appressed white hairs. Leaves in general opposite, petioled, oblong or oblong cuneate, acute, serrate, above smooth but hard, downy underneath, and elegantly reticulated with numerous, soft, hairy veins, and a deep-green smooth gland in their axills ; from 2 to 12 inches long, one of the pairs is always smaller than the other, and when single often oblique as in *Begonia*. Petioles round, clothed with appressed pubescence, in each side of their insertion is a green gland. Stipules within the leaves, caducous

Fruit for the most part in pairs, in radical withering racemes, and frequently of great length, with apices penetrating the earth. In the native soil the whole raceme and fruit often entirely under-ground ; also found single or in pairs on the trunk or branches, though less frequently than on the root. They are generally about the size of a large nutmeg, obovate, very hairy ; the mouth shut with numerous scales, the exterior ones glandular and more remote ; several obscure, equi-distant ridges run from the umbilicus towards the base. Calyx of the fruit of three minute scales. Male corrollets monandrous. In habit this plant is very much like *F. oppositifolia*, but the inflorescence is very different.'

As found in the vicinity of Madras, these plants differ in some minor points from the above descriptions, and they resemble so much in their general appearance, it is very difficult to distinguish them from each other, except by repeated and careful examination.

What is described as *fruit* by Dr. Roxburgh in the above plants, as well as in many other species of Ficus, is the *fruit-receptacle* of recent authors, which is fleshy, assumes a globular or fruit-like form, and therefore generally known as a fruit. It has a great many very small flowers and fruits attached to its inner surface within the cavity. The fruits or rather *achenes* of these plants are those small bodies, which are about the size and form of a poppy-seed, attached to the inner surface of the fruit-receptacle, and commonly known as seeds.

With regard to the bark of these plants, which is recommended for use, it is meant for the bark of the trunk and branches, and not the root-bark.

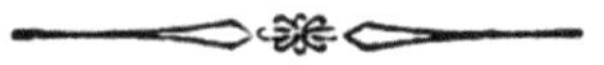

INDEX OF THE BOTANICAL NAMES USED AS SYNO-
NYMES, AND MENTIONED IN THE REMARKS,
ADDENDA AND APPENDIX.

INDEX OF ENGLISH SYNONYMES.

INDEX OF ARABIC SYNONYMES.

A, Á, Ạ.

B, Bh.

I.

L.

R.

S, Ṣ, Ṣ, Sh.

T, Ṭ.

INDEX OF PERSIAN SYNONYMES.

A, Á, Ạ.

B.

F.

K, *Kh.*

N.

P.

Q.

T, Ṭ.

Ch, Chh.

D, Ḍ, Dh, Ḍh.

K, *Kh*, *K̲h*.

M; M*h*.

N.

Ou.

P, Ph.

T, Ṭ, Th.

U, Ú.

INDEX OF DUKHNI SYNONYMES.

A, Á, Ạ.

B, *Bh.*

Ch, Chh.

H, Ḥ.

I.

J. Jh.

K, *Kh*, Ḵh.

L.

M, *Mh*.

P, Ph.

Q.

R.

S, Ṣ, Ṣ, Sh.

T, *Th*, *Ṭh*.

U, Ú.

INDEX OF TAMIL SYNONYMES.

A, Á.

<h2 style="text-align:center">B.</h2>

J.

K.

L.

M.

O, Ó.

P.

U, Ú.

INDEX OF TELUGU SYNONYMES.

A, Á, Am.

Ch.

D.

E, É.

J.

K, Kh.

R.

T.

U, Ú.

V.

INDEX OF MALYALIM SYNONYMES.

A, A.

P.

R.

ഉ

V.

INDEX OF CANARESE SYNONYMES.

A, A.

Ch.

D, ಧ.

N.

P, *Ph.*

V.

Y.

INDEX OF BENGALI SYNONYMES,

A, A̤, Á.

B, Bh.

Ch, Chh.

D, *Dh.*

H.

K, Kh.

L.

M.

S, Sh, Sh.

T. *Th*

INDEX OF SANSCRIT SYNONYMES.

A, Á.

B, Bh.

K, *Kh*, *Ksh*.

INDEX OF MAHRATTI SYNONYMES.

T, *Th.*

INDEX OF GUZRATTI SYNONVMES.

A, Á.

B, *Bh.*

II.

I.

J, Jh.

INDEX OF CINGALESE SYNONYMES.

A, Á.

II.

I.

J.

R.

S, Ṣh.

T, *Th.*

INDEX OF BURMESE SYNONYMES.

A, A, Á, Ạ.

B, *Bh*.

H.

K, *Kh.*

N, Ṇ.

O, Ó.

P, *Ph.*

S, Ṣ, Ṣ, Sh, Ṣh.

T, Ṭ, *Th.*

U, Ú.

LIST OF ERRATA.

———

Page 131, line   3, from below, for رگذ read رگز.
 ,, 134, ,,   16, for 'Burn,' read Burm.
 ,, 138, ,,   2, from below, for زهرگا و read زهرگا و.
 ,, 140, ,,   7, for 'terbinthinate' read terebinthinate.
 ,, 143, ,,   18, for 'Chiṛiya-pú atti' read Shiriya-pé-atti.
 ,, 153, ,,   11, for 'Indica' read Indicus.
 ,, 155, ,,   8, from below, for 'ODERATA' read ODORATA.
 ,, 157, ,,   9, from below, insert 'a' before the word 'more.'
 ,, 163, ,,   11, from below, for 'Solanacœ' read Solanaceæ.
 ,, 166, ,,   7, for 'fsequently' read 'frequently.'
 ,, 166, ,,   15, for 'Gai-nu-dúdh' read Gáí-nu-dúdh.
 ,, 171, ,,   13, for 'Phol' read Pohl.
 ,, 185, ,,   4, from below, for 'Jingam' read Jingan.
 ,, 188, ,,   14, for ಬ್ಯೂಠರ ಳ್ ಣ read ಬ್ಯೂಠರ ಳ್ ಣ.
 ,, 189, ,,   8, for 'Sesamam' read Sesamum.
 ,, 189, ,,   5, for 'Móḷu-yeranḍi-nu-tél' read Móṇu-yeranḍi-nu-tél.
 ,, 200, ,,   2, from below, insert (Arab.) after the words
    فلفل ا سو د.
 ,, 204, ,,   12, Consider the word 'POLANISIA' as obsolete.
 ,, 214, ,,   15, for Karaḷa-giḷá ಕರಗಿಡ read Haraḷa-giḍá ಹರ ಗಿಡ.
 ,, 217, ,,   21, for Rójáp-pú-tittíppu ரோஜாப்புத்திப்பு read Irójáp-pú-tittíppú இரோஜாப்புத்திப்பு.
 ,, 220, lines 11 and 12, for വെൺപഞ്ചസാര read വെൺപഞ്ചസാര.
 ,, 220, line   20, for Ráp-sharukkarai ராப்சருக்கரை read Iráp-sharukkarai இராப்சருக்கரை.
 ,, 221, ,,   5, for 'Pál-akuru' read Pol-akuru.
 ,, 222, ,,   3, for 'Willah' read Will.
 ,, 230, ,,   11, for 'Alæ' read Aloe.
 ,, 236, last line, for 'Dát gandak' read Dál-gandak.
 ,, 239, line   15, for 'Gazmájú' read Gazmázú.
 ,, 240, ,,   16, for 'Sagván' read Ságván.
 ,, 243, ,,   5, for ಟಗ ಲಫ್ಫು read ಟಗ ಲ್ ಹುಫ್ಸ.
 ,, 244, ,,   21, for 'Tél-koṭukka' read Téḷ-koṭukka.
 ,, 246, ,,   16, for 'Pál-rá' read Pol-rá.
 ,, 246, ,,   4, from below, for 'not yet began' read 'have not yet begun.'
 ,, 249, ,,   11, for 'Gahung' read Gahun.
 ,, 252, ,,   9, for 'propogated' read propagated.
 ,, 252, last line, for بایدنه read بیدنه.
 ,, 253, line   6, for 'Saská-drakhya' read Suká-drakhyá.
 ,, 256, last line, for 'Justhicia' read 'Justicia.'
 ,, 259, line   5, from below, in the foot-note, for 'constitutes' read constitute.

Page 272, line   2, for ' Realger' read **Realgar.**
  ,,   272, lines 5 and 6, for ' Manoṣilaï' and ' Manuṣala,' read
                       Manoṣhilaï and Manuṣhala, respectively.
  ,,   281, line   4, from below, for ' hydrogogue' read 'hydra-
                       gogue.'
  ,,   282, ,,   20, for ' tubercular' read ' tubercular.'
  ,,   315, ,,   8, insert ' of the' after the word ' whole.'
  ,,   315, ,,   3, from below, omit 'the' before the word 'like.'
  ,,   317, ,,   6, for ' written' read ' expressed,'
  ,,   340, ,,   4, for ' oscilating' read ' oscillating.'
  ,,   343, ,,   2, from below, for 'oscilating' read 'oscillating'
  ,,   345, ,,   6, from below, for '*Jalp* read' *Jalap.*
  ,,   351, ,,   10, for ' periennial' read ' perennial.'
  ,,   352, ,,   12, for ' inodrous.' read ' inodorous.'
  ,,   354, ,,   3, from below, omit ' more' before the word
                       ' stronger.'
  ,,   356,   5, from below, insert 'the' before the word 'dry.
  ,,   361   13, for ' plant' read ' plants.'
  ,,   362   17, for ' dehescent' read ' dehiscent.